The University of Kansas
Medical Center: *A Pictorial History*

The
University *of* Kansas
Medical Center
A Pictorial History

Lawrence H. Larsen and Nancy J. Hulston

Foreword by D. Kay Clawson, M.D., and Gene A. Budig

Published for the University of Kansas Medical Center

by the University Press of Kansas

Published by the University Press of Kansas (Lawrence, Kansas 66049), which was organized by the Kansas Board of Regents and is operated and funded by Emporia State University, Fort Hays State University, Kansas State University, Pittsburg State University, the University of Kansas, and Wichita State University

Library of Congress Cataloging-in-Publication Data

Larsen, Lawrence Harold, 1931–
    The University of Kansas Medical Center : a pictorial history / Lawrence H. Larsen and Nancy J. Hulston ; foreword by D. Kay Clawson and Gene A. Budig.
        p.   cm.
    Includes bibliographical references and index.
    ISBN 0-7006-0539-8 (hardcover)
    1. Hospitals—Kansas—History. I. Hulston, Nancy J. II. Title.
    [DNLM: 1. University of Kansas. Medical Center.—History.
2. University of Kansas. Medical Center. 3. Education, Medical—history—Kansas—
pictorial works. 4. History of Medicine—Kansas—pictorial works.   WZ 17 L421u]
RA981.K2L37 1992
362.1'1'0978139—dc20
DNLM/DLC
for Library of Congress   91-44669

Printed in the United States of America

10 9 8 7 6 5 4 3 2 1

The paper used in this publication meets the minimum requirements of the American National Standard for Permanence of Paper for Printed Library Materials Z39.48-1984.

Contents

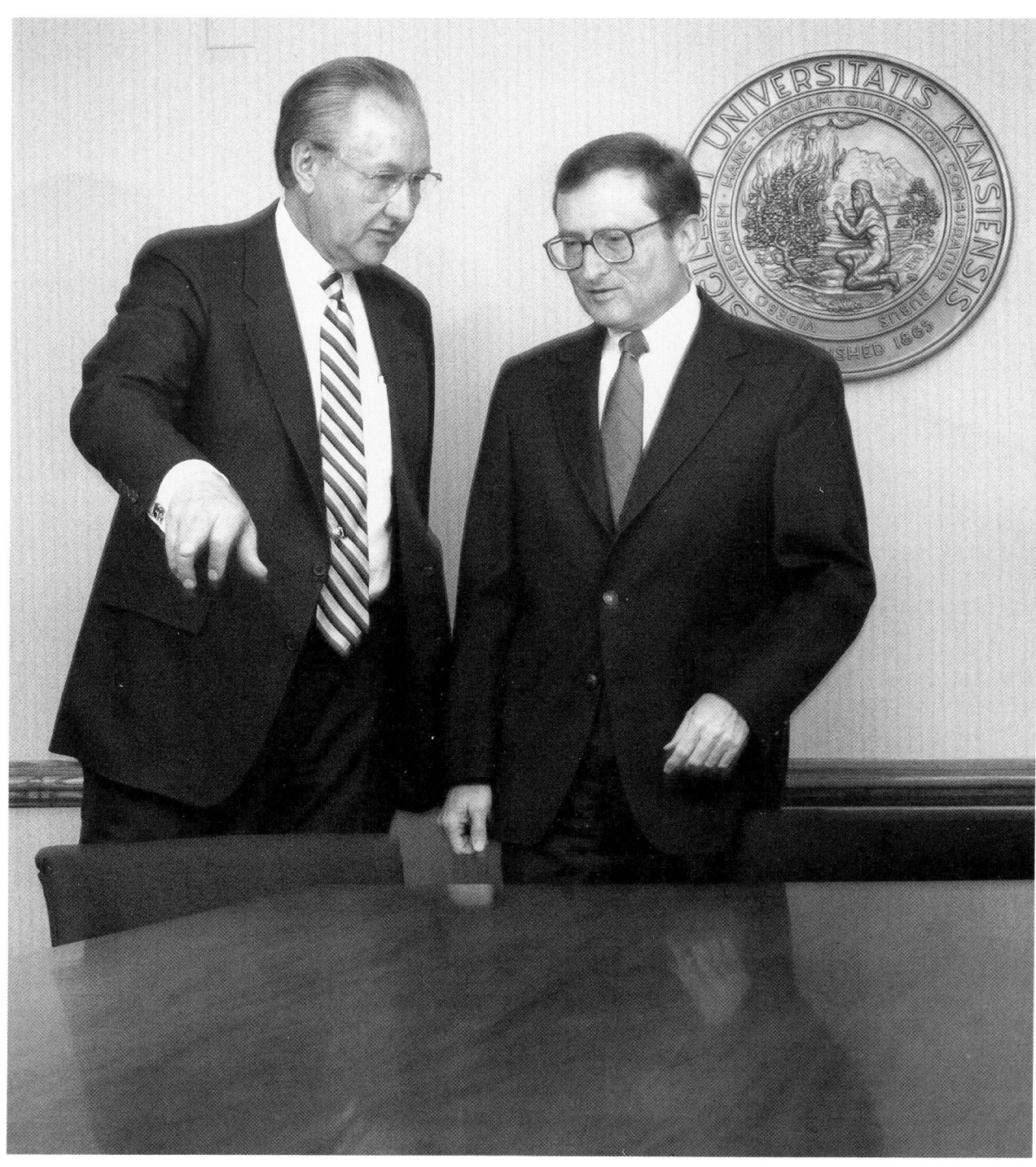

D. Kay Clawson, M.D., executive vice chancellor of the University of Kansas Medical Center, and Gene A. Budig, chancellor of the University of Kansas.

Foreword

The University of Kansas Medical Center's Clendening History of Medicine Library is known throughout the world as one of the finest and largest collections of rare medical books and manuscripts. The library holds some of the writings of outstanding faculty such as Peter Bohan, Logan Clendening, Ralph Major, Thomas Orr, Earl Padgett, and Richard Sutton; yet for the most part the colorful history of KU Medical Center has never been systematically preserved. Composite class pictures were stored in an inaccessible alcove in the Student Union building. Other photographs were maintained in the alumni office, audiovisual services, and university relations. Nowhere could one find a chronological history of the development of the medical school and its subsequent medical center. In contrast, the Lawrence campus of the University of Kansas had produced both a scholarly account of its history and an enjoyable pictorial history, *On the Hill*. Since the School of Medicine, established in 1905, is approaching its centennial, it seemed appropriate to begin collecting, preserving, and maintaining photographs and documents relevant to the history of the institution.

In March 1988, with no idea of what kind of records might be available, the executive vice chancellor hired Nancy J. Hulston as archivist. Her task was to establish an archival program in an effort to preserve the rich history of the University of Kansas Medical Center. Since one goal of the archives project was to produce a companion volume to *On the Hill*, Professor Lawrence H. Larsen, a professional historian, was commissioned to assist in the production of a photographic history of the medical center. While it was clear from the beginning that it could take years to accumulate the documents to write a comprehensive history of the institution, we hoped that a pictorial history would become a stimulus for alumni and friends to reminisce about the "good old days" and bring forth any

documents that could be the basis for a scholarly study of the KU Medical Center.

This photographic history demonstrates that there has never been enough money to provide for the most up-to-date facilities for the medical center. From its humble beginnings on the inauspiciously named "Goat Hill," the University of Kansas School of Medicine has been scrutinized and criticized, doubted and underfunded by a skeptical Kansas state legislature. There was difficulty agreeing on where the School of Medicine should be located and, at times, resentment that it abutted Kansas City, Missouri, where most of its medical faculty sustained themselves through the private practice of medicine. The photographs clearly show that by the early 1950s the medical school buildings still could not be considered modern by any standard and were inadequate to meet the needs of an aggressive and expanding young faculty and student population. Also clearly depicted in this book are the ubiquitous "temporary" buildings that eventually acquired an aura of permanence, as well as the large numbers of poor patients, particularly African Americans, who sought care in these out-of-date facilities.

At the close of World War II, the medical school remained a divided campus: The first two years of premedical curriculum and the basic science faculty were housed in Lawrence; the remainder of the curriculum was taught on the Kansas City campus, which consisted of a series of small buildings constructed in the 1920s and 1930s, with a handful of prewar barracks used for crowded clinics and laboratories. The Franklin Murphy/Clarke Wescoe era provided a new beginning for the medical school, with a flurry of building activity starting in the 1950s. Most of this activity related to the move of the basic science faculty from Lawrence to the Kansas City campus.

Depicted also are nursing school activities and the nurses' home that, although it was moved repeatedly, was an integral part of the medical center campus. While a nurses' training school had been under the School of Medicine since 1906, an independent School of Nursing was not established until 1974. Three years later, the School of Allied Health was organized. Neither program was housed in its own building, as was customary in other institutions; they were located throughout the institution where space allowed. A truly modern teaching hospital, the 850,000-square-foot Bell Memorial Hospital (now the University of Kansas Hospital), was not completed until the late 1970s; the 110,815-square-foot Orr-Major teaching facility opened in 1976; the 56,000-square-foot Dykes Library opened in 1983; the 40,438-square-foot research support facility and the 46,000-square-foot Kirmayer Fitness Center opened in the late 1980s and early 1990s, respectively. Despite the recent surge of building activity and now pleasant campus atmosphere, the issues of "catch up" continue as the KU Medical Center enters a new era of medicine. Although gradual improvements have occurred over the years, the facilities still remain behind many other modern medical centers.

It is often said that those who do not understand their history are condemned to repeat it. Surely this pictorial history will demonstrate to the alumni and the citizens of Kansas that there has been a century-long struggle to develop and maintain a high quality medical center to serve the state. By the time each new addition was completed, more space and new facilities were already needed to meet the ever-expanding demands of medical high technology and of the public's growing expectations for superior health care. Perhaps readers will appreciate that no matter how large or impressive the medical center appears today, it must continue to expand and change to keep up with future developments. We can only hope that as we enter the twenty-first century, the University of Kansas Medical Center can change from a mode of constant "catch up" to one of vision and leadership in medical science and medical care, therefore helping to create a better tomorrow for all Kansans.

Gene A. Budig
Chancellor

D. Kay Clawson, M.D.
Executive Vice Chancellor

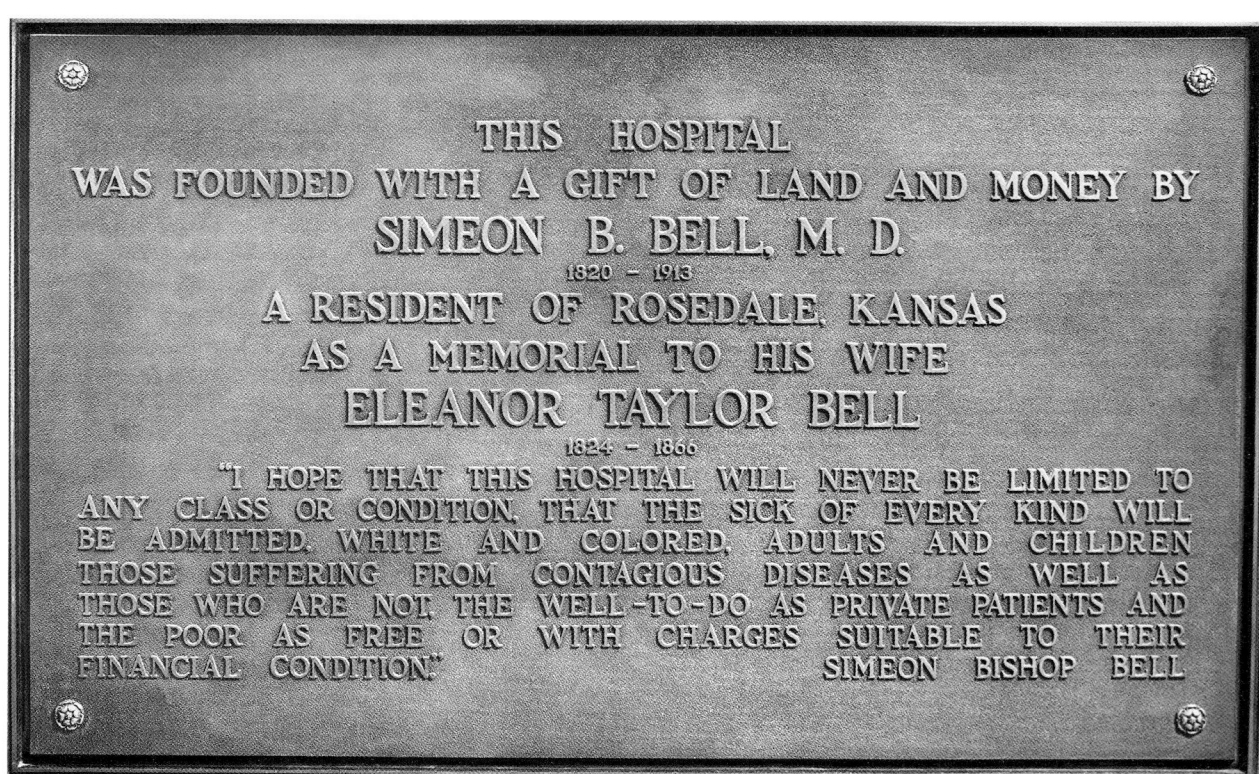

Original plaque of Eleanor Taylor Bell Memorial Hospital, now located in Hinch Hall.

Preface

The story of the University of Kansas Medical Center is one of growth and development. Its origins stem from a two-year medical preparatory program started in 1880 on the University of Kansas campus in Lawrence, Kansas, and from three proprietary medical schools on both sides of the state line in the Kansas City area that combined in 1905 to form the University of Kansas School of Medicine. For nearly twenty years, the institution operated out of four modest buildings at a rather uninviting location on "Goat Hill" in Rosedale. In 1924, the main campus moved to a new modern facility in Kansas City, Kansas, at 39th Street and Rainbow Boulevard, adjacent to the Missouri state line. During the Great Depression, a combination of New Deal programs and state funding resulted in the addition of a number of educational, clinical, and research buildings. Construction accelerated following World War II, especially during the 1960s and 1970s. Of special note was the largest building project ever undertaken by the state of Kansas—the new University of Kansas Hospital. By 1990 the Medical Center had over 2.3 million cubic feet of space at 39th and Rainbow, plus many thousands more in Wichita and at area health education centers throughout the state. Over a period of nearly one hundred years and from humble beginnings, the University of Kansas Medical Center has grown into a large and significant medical institution.

The thrust of this study is to use photographs to chronicle the rise of the University of Kansas Medical Center. We hope this book will provide guidance and a framework for a future comprehensive scholarly history of the institution. At the inception of the present project, we had no idea what existed in the way of photographs, as few had been collected and gathered into a central location. We knew that our goal was to produce a companion volume to *On the Hill: A Photographic History of the*

University of Kansas, which contains many arresting and memorable images of student life, athletic events, physical growth, campus landscapes, and educational activities. The Mount Oread campus, overlooking the rolling terrain of eastern Kansas, presented numerous photographic opportunities. The possibilities presented by a medical center in the heart of a vast urban area seemed at first glance less promising. Yet, as we soon discovered, a metropolitan medical facility, just like a residential college campus in a medium-size town, has a distinct life of its own, one that lends itself in the twentieth century to telling its basic story through photographic documentation.

Many aspects of the University of Kansas Medical Center proved fairly easy to illustrate. Our main problem was not, as we had initially feared, finding the photographs, but choosing from the thousands that became accessible to us. The Medical Center Archives (under the auspices of the Department of the History and Philosophy of Medicine), the Department of Audio-Visual Services, and University Relations proved great sources, as did the University of Kansas Archives in Lawrence and other area repositories. Many individuals associated in one way or another over the years with the Medical Center also assisted.

Although a medical center does not have the same type of student life as a traditional upper educational school—the students in medicine, nursing, and allied health are generally older, the course of study more rigorous, the hours longer, and the environment more serious—it does have student and faculty activities. Photographic evidence often relates to such things as fraternal organizations, social events, and recreational activities. Individual formal photographs are available for almost all medical and nursing graduates and many faculty members; we had little difficulty in documenting individuals. In some cases, we had available photographs of staff and faculty members taken at various stages during their careers. Additionally, we found many action photographs: medical doctors in white coats using complex equipment or conducting clinical examinations, nursing student demonstrations, children's rehabilitation activities, students listening attentively to lectures, patients undergoing various treatments, and nonmedical staff performing a variety of tasks. A significant run of photographs illustrated changes over the years in the operating rooms; others related to the construction of buildings from foundation to completion. The photographic evidence was so complete that, had we wanted to, we could have devoted an entire chapter to the development of the Medical Center power plant alone.

So, while our book stands as a companion volume to *On the Hill*, it has developed a life of its own, illustrating and detailing the historical evolution of a great medical center.

During the creation of this photographic history of the University of Kansas Medical Center, many people assisted in a variety of ways. Photographs relating to the history of the Medical Center that were housed in other area historical institutions came to light through the efforts of Gerald A. Motsinger, Jackson County Historical Society Archives; Lisa Schwarzenholz, Wyandotte County Historical Society and Museum Archives; and John Nugent and Barry Bunch, University of Kansas Archives. Both photographs and significant documentation emerged from the Kansas State Historical Society with the help of Eugene D. Decker and Robert Knecht. Dr. Philip H. Hostetter contributed many photographs taken at the Medical School while he was a student during the depression.

This project's completion is largely due to the invaluable cooperation of the Medical Center's Audio Visual Services Department. Our special appreciation goes to Burton W. Johnson, Stephen L. Spector, Dale Monaghen, Noel Klein, Elissa Monroe, John Kennison, Patricia Reed, Rick Robinson, and Larry Howell (Design and Illustration). Shari Hartbauer, photographer for the Medical Center's University Relations, loaned us a number of her photographs. Jack Reed, Director of Facilities Operations, graciously answered many of our questions on buildings, dates, and square footage.

The contributions, advice, and encouragement of many individuals were essential to the completion of this book. Doris Geitgey, R.N., Ed.D., Helen Sims, Max Allen, M.D., E. W. J. Pearce, M.D., James Denio, Ed.D., Frank Applegate, Tyler Motsinger, Barbara J. Cottrell, Pam Dupuy, and Patricia Walters all provided support in one way or another. Deborah Hickle, Oral History Program Coordinator for the Medical Center, gave much of her time to proofreading the manuscript. Robert P. Hudson, M.D., Susan Case, and Lou Gehlbach of the Department of the History and Philosophy of Medicine all provided indispensable advice, encouragement, and support. Julia Cook of the University of Missouri–Kansas City History Department assisted in typing the manuscript.

While images of all who were a part of the history of the University of Kansas Medical Center could not be included, we have attempted to show, through the photographs, a varied cross-section of those people who helped shape the history of this institution.

Lawrence H. Larsen   Nancy J. Hulston

The University of Kansas
Medical Center: *A Pictorial History*

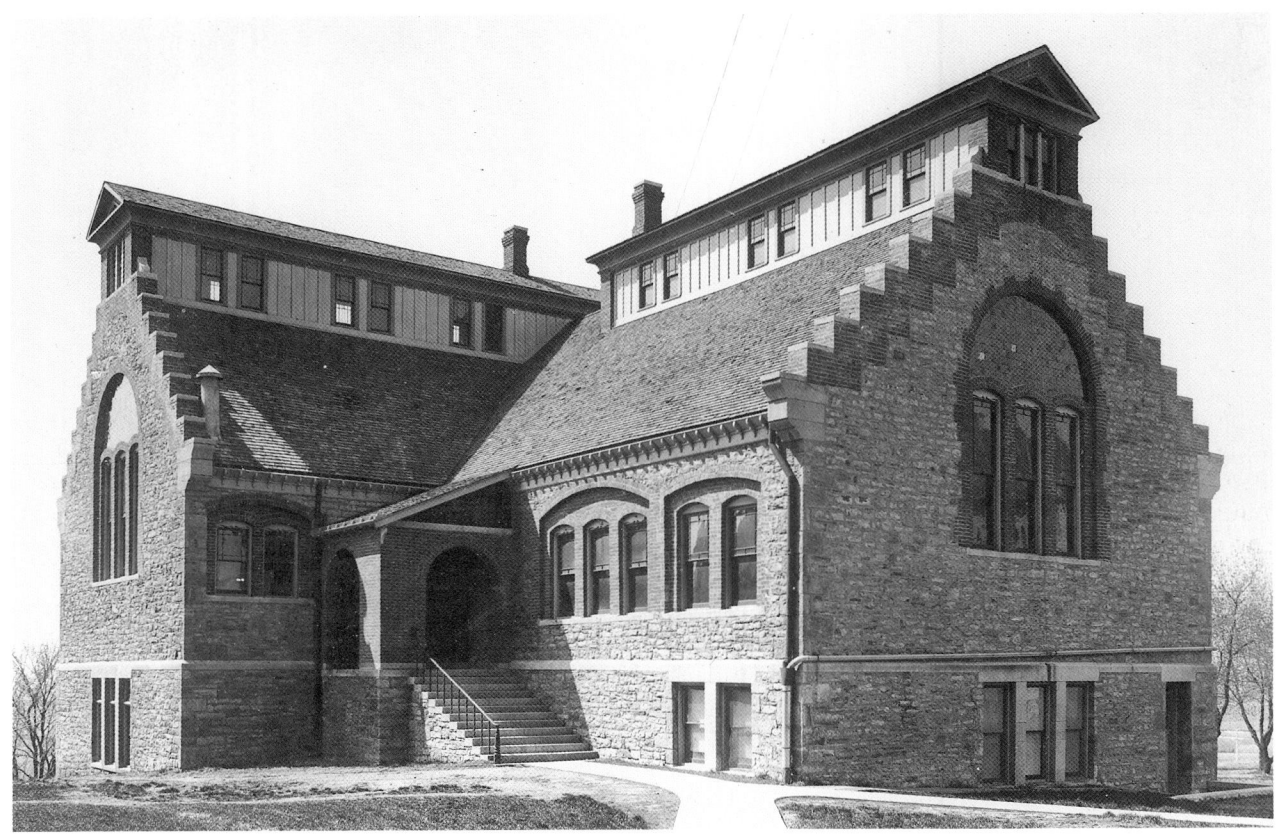

Chemistry Hall on the Lawrence campus, late 1890s.

1

Years of Marking Time

A University of Kansas medical school first became a reality in the early twentieth century. By then, the state of Kansas, with over a million inhabitants, was fifty years old. Legislation authorizing the establishment of the University of Kansas, which opened its doors in Lawrence in 1866, had envisioned a medical school. Initially this meant offering basic courses in chemistry, physiology, and biology—hardly a complete medical curriculum. During the 1880s, school officials started a one-year "preparatory medical course," adding special offerings in materia medica, human physiology, and comparative anatomy. Agreements with other institutions enabled some Kansas students to complete their initial preparation as physicians at either the Rush Medical College in Chicago or the Ohio Medical School in Cincinnati. After the University of Kansas preclinical program expanded to two years in the 1890s, it received formal approval from certain examining bodies, including the prestigious Association of American Medical Colleges. Even so, despite limited progress, Kansas remained increasingly outside what was then considered the mainstream of modern American public medical education.

A number of considerations explained the limited scope of state-supported medical instruction in Kansas. During the "Bleeding Kansas" days of the 1850s, hundreds of newcomers claimed to have impressive medical credentials. Some never attempted to practice medicine, instead becoming politicians and land speculators. Despite questions about quality, however, Kansas did not experience a statistical shortage of medical personnel during the nineteenth century. As a further complication, medical practitioners formed competing societies of regular, homeopathic, and eclectic physicians. Disagreements over the philosophy of medicine, coupled with controversies over alleged quacks, kept the Kansas medical community divided until a 1901 act of the state legislature provided for a Board of Examination and Registration designed to regulate the quality of practicing physicians in Kansas. Even more divisive was a growing schism over the location of a medical school, reflecting both old and new urban rivalries. Topeka, Wichita, Leavenworth, Kansas City, Rosedale, and Manhattan interests all claimed to deserve a medical school more than Lawrence. Meanwhile, University of Kansas officials had followed the course of slowly expanding the scientific curricula.

Wherever the eventual location or whatever the nature of a comprehensive institution of medical knowledge, the problem of financing was of prime importance. Kansas, an "area state"—meaning one with artificially drawn boundaries—had trouble developing an economic base. The colorful cowtowns brought only fleeting prosperity. The depression that followed the Panic of 1873, coupled with severe grasshopper plagues, impeded agricultural growth. The introduction of Turkey Red wheat led to an agricultural boom in the 1880s that ushered in a short period of prosperity and corresponding rapid settlement throughout the state. Unfortunately, the Panic of 1893 and several years of drought checked progress, causing acrimonious political turmoil. Prosperity returned, however, and the possibility of a national "Golden Age of Agriculture" improved the state's economic outlook. Given the new conditions, action regarding some sort of publicly supported medical facility seemed only a matter of time.

In 1894, Simeon Bishop Bell, a pioneer Kansas physician, farmer, and land speculator, offered to give land and money with a total estimated value of $75,000 to the state for a medical school in Rosedale, where he had large holdings. Rosedale, a suburb just south of Kansas City, Kansas, lay hard against the Kansas-Missouri state line. Parochial interests, especially in Topeka, had temporarily blocked the Bell proposal, but increasingly it became conventional wisdom that the high costs of modern medicine necessitated placing schools of medicine in large metropolitan districts. By 1900, some 305,000 people lived in the Kansas City metropolitan area compared to fewer than 35,000 in Topeka, the second largest city in Kansas. After Bell donated an additional $25,000, the legislature accepted it, providing for the formation in 1905 of the University of Kansas School of Medicine.

Political and educational considerations clouded the establishment of the institution, causing serious problems. The first two preclinical years of the program remained in Lawrence. The final two years, for the most part clinical, were in Rosedale. From a practical standpoint, this meant that Kansas, after trying for half a century to obtain a complete medical school, ended up with one school in two locations. Even more vexing was the composition of the faculty. Most of the instructors in the preclinical and first two years of medical school in Lawrence were scientists—one was a sometime polar explorer, Lewis Lindsay Dyche, who taught anatomy. In contrast, physicians constituted almost the entire instructional staff at the Rosedale campus.

Nearly all physicians affiliated with the new University of Kansas School of Medicine had previous proprietary medical school teaching experience. Proprietary schools of medicine, products of the entrepreneurial era of nineteenth-century American medicine, varied greatly in educational standards and clinical training. At best, groups of physicians, going beyond the preceptor system of "reading medicine," provided students with a broad range of practical experiences. At worst, the object was to crank out physicians for profit. A degree from one of the proprietary schools was better than nothing in an age before formal medical accreditation, but the system failed to guarantee quality medicine. Few of these institutions emphasized the importance of research. In the forty years following the Civil War, Kansas and western Missouri had at least twenty proprietary medical schools, many of which were classic diploma mills, attracting students eager to obtain a degree in the shortest possible time. A few provided substantive clinical training. Fortunately for American medicine, proprietary schools had seen their day by the dawning of the twentieth century; a consensus held that modern medical schools, even those with proprietary roots, should

be part of established universities. This happened in Kansas with unpopular consequences as a result of the formation of the new University of Kansas School of Medicine.

Unfortunately for the immediate future of the new institution, Chancellor Frank Strong of the University of Kansas adopted a controversial course. He worked out agreements combining three proprietary medical schools into the University of Kansas School of Medicine. Only one of the schools involved was in Kansas, the College of Physicians and Surgeons of Kansas City, Kansas. The two others, the Medico-Chirurgical College and the Kansas City Medical College, both reasonably respectable in terms of quality, were in Kansas City, Missouri. They had become receptive to a Kansas affiliation after attempts failed to have the University of Missouri establish a medical school in Kansas City, Missouri. Because of the realities of the merger process, most of the physicians on the first faculty of the University of Kansas School of Medicine lived and practiced in Missouri. In addition, the Missouri side of the state line furnished the bulk of the patients for the new Kansas school, many of whom were the so-called "packing house rabble." Indeed, the University of Kansas School of Medicine ran a dispensary on Independence Avenue in downtown Kansas City, Missouri. This outpatient clinic afforded medical students a wide variety of clinical experiences and had humanitarian overtones, but it fueled charges that the Kansas medical school primarily served Missourians.

The land donated by Simeon Bell furthered the impression that Kansas had embarked upon building a medical school for the poor of Kansas City, Missouri. To help finance construction projects, Bell had donated other lots, some of which were in Missouri. Placement of the University of Kansas School of Medicine on the eastern edge of the state raised serious political questions, especially in light of the widespread competition for the school. Moreover, the Rosedale campus was over four hundred miles from the western Kansas border. From across the state came charges that the school, despite receiving tax money, was not a true Kansas institution. A more inauspicious beginning could hardly be imagined.

The two-year clinical school opened for business in the fall of 1905 in the basement of a building in downtown Kansas City, Kansas, that had previously housed the College of Physicians and Surgeons.

The first dean, Dr. George Howard Hoxie, a young Lawrence physician who took the position primarily because he disapproved of proprietary schools, found himself on premises that had housed one such school only a few months earlier. A more complex consideration involved the faculty acquired from the three proprietary schools. There were approximately 100 faculty members, most inherited from the merger, for 96 medical students—to say the least, a low student-teacher ratio. Some of the proprietary school physicians had impeccable credentials, having studied at prestigious East Coast and European universities. They boasted successful private practices and were among the leaders of the Missouri medical profession. About their only flaw, from the Kansas perspective, was that they lived in

Missouri. These physicians, who performed their scholarly and clinical duties without salaries, formed the backbone of Hoxie's faculty. At the chancellor's suggestion, Hoxie weeded out less able instructors by temporarily making all courses elective. This method produced the desired results, but not before Hoxie became widely disliked within the Kansas City medical community. The situation created opportunities for Kansas enemies of the school.

Special interest groups in other cities continued to press their claims. Some argued that medicine was a trade rather than a profession and wanted a medical institution affiliated with the state agricultural college in Manhattan. More powerful political forces pressed for designating the Kansas Medical College, a proprietary school in Topeka that served

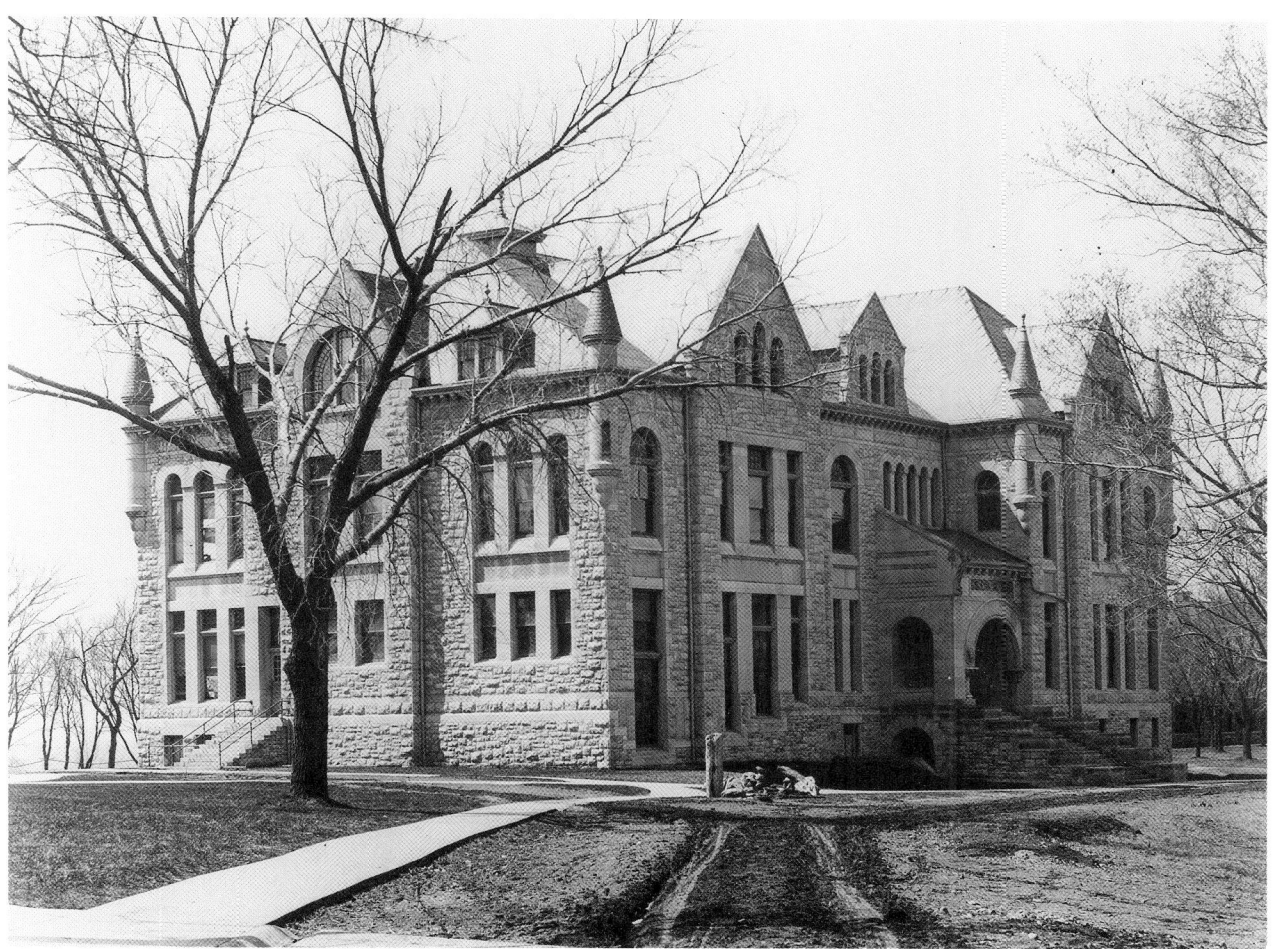

Snow Hall of Natural History, dedicated in 1886, Lawrence campus.

as the medical department of Washburn University, as the official school of medicine for Kansas.

Even though the Kansas City area school had a reasonably good faculty and a location in a regional metropolis with an abundance of clinical material, its future remained in doubt. Hoxie tried to consolidate most of the clinical functions at Bethany Hospital in Kansas City, Kansas. He negotiated an agreement with the hospital's administration, but the head nurse successfully killed it by refusing admission to patients transferred for teaching purposes by the University of Kansas School of Medicine. Her ruling stood because she had the backing of most of the physicians at Bethany Hospital, who represented a cross section of the medical community in Kansas City, Kansas, and by inference, in Kansas as a whole. This left Hoxie and the School of Medicine more isolated than ever.

In an atmosphere of uncertainty, planning proceeded for construction of a medical school on the land Bell donated in Rosedale. Because of a failed local bond issue and scant state funding, the project required scaling down. The $25,000 Eleanor Taylor Bell Memorial Hospital, which opened in 1906, fell short of being a full-scale medical teaching facility—the structure had fewer than thirty-five beds. The pavilion-style architecture had a utilitarian and undistinguished quality. The same was true of a three-story rectangular teaching and research laboratory erected close by in 1907 for $20,000. The two buildings were situated on a steep hillside called "Goat Hill," after a goat herd that lived at the bottom. The small and somewhat primitive medical school had a public budget of under $40,000 a year. In part to cut down expenses, Hoxie soon started a small training school for nurses. The first nursing

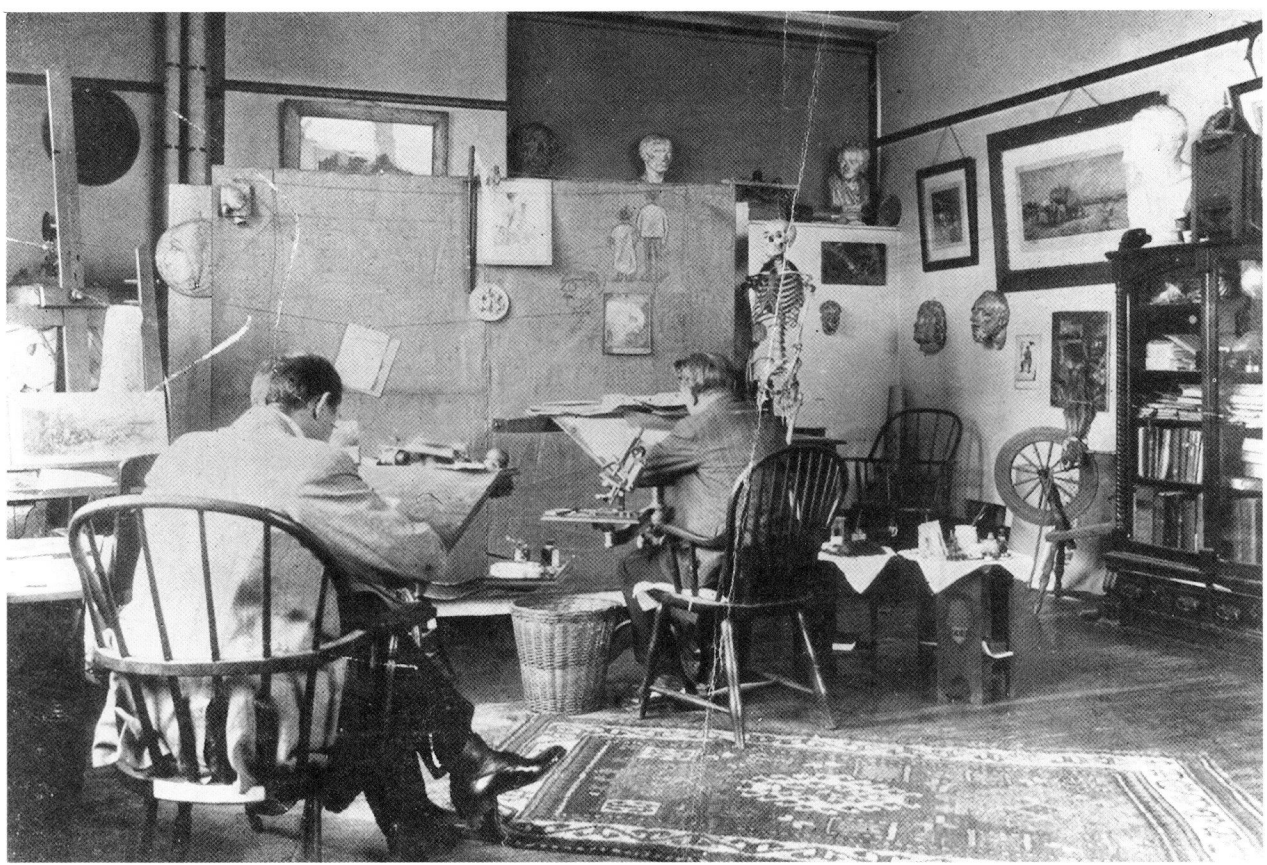

Medical illustrators, Medical Department, Lawrence campus, 1890s.

class of four students, all hand-picked by the nursing supervisor, graduated in 1909, only three years after the first medical class of fifty-six students. For all the troubles, Hoxie could point with some pride to the professional faculty he developed out of the remnants of the old proprietary medical schools, the building of a hospital and laboratory, and the sharply improved training of the first new physicians and nurses. The state legislature, dominated by members who wanted a different site, responded by cutting the already inadequate budget. Hoxie, who later called much of his tenure as dean of the school a "bad dream," resigned in 1911.

Photographs relating to the pioneering period of the University of Kansas School of Medicine document the institution's troubled beginnings and seemingly bleak future. Bell, his family, and his farm appear tranquil, but he survived Civil War bushwhackers, the death of his beloved first wife, Eleanor, and an unsuccessful second marriage during his long and prosperous life. The sorry state of the campuses of the proprietary schools, as shown in the photographs, graphically illustrates the need for educational reform. Student photographs, elaborately posed in a macabre tongue-in-cheek fashion, concentrate on anatomy classes, leaving a one-dimensional impression of turn-of-the-century medical training. Exterior and interior shots of the physical plant of the University of Kansas School of Medicine, especially of the Goat Hill campus, indicate the problems faced by pioneering medical educators in Kansas. With the first graduation ceremonies for medical students (including two women) in 1906, came new symbols: the granting of diplomas served to start traditions, providing evidence of annual renewal and hope of survival from small and unpromising beginnings.

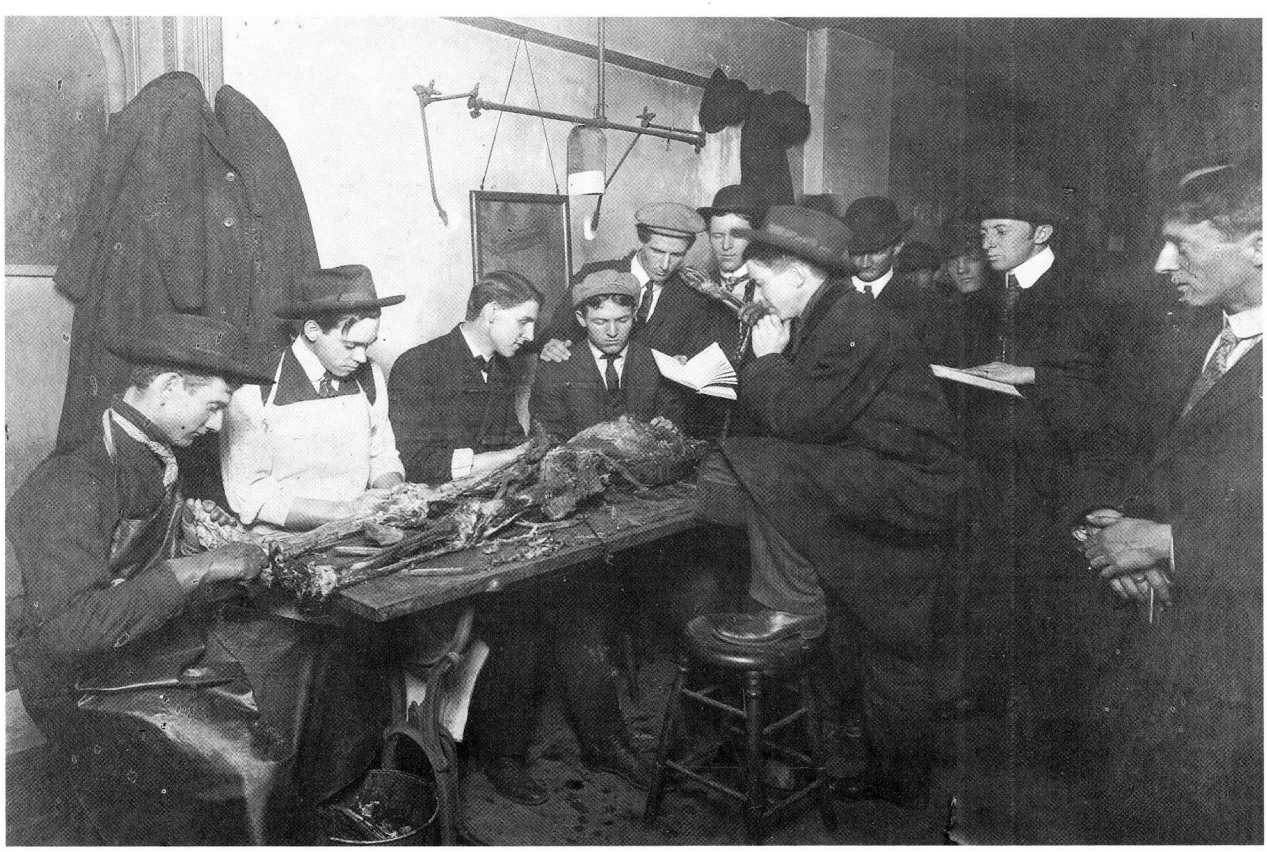

An 1890s anatomy class at Lawrence.

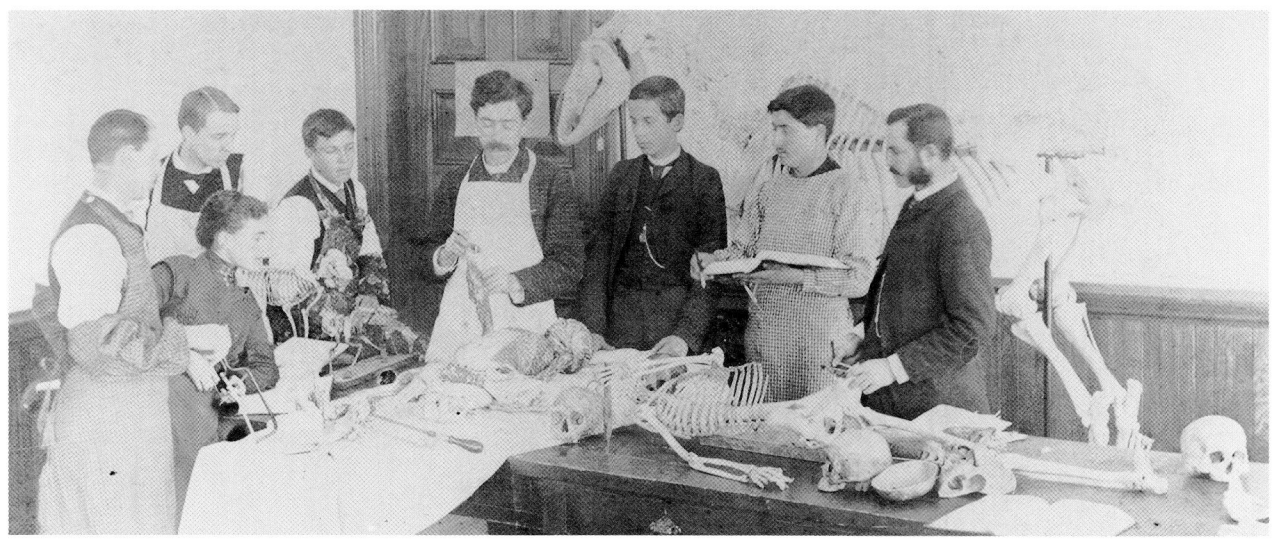

Professor Lewis Lindsay Dyche teaching anatomy at Lawrence, ca. 1900.

Not all of the state's doctors were happy about the cautious, hesitant policy of the University in advancing toward a full medical course. Some wanted a complete medical school from the first. Others were jealous of Lawrence as the site of the embryo school. Still others saw in medical education the prospect of making money. Across the nation there had sprung up in the 19th century a whole series of proprietary schools, usually physician-owned, which outrivaled each other in shortening curricula, reducing tuition, and setting easy requirements for degrees. The proprietary medical college fitted in perfectly with the rampant spirit of free enterprise and laissez-faire so characteristic of this age in America.
—Thomas Neville Bonner, *The Kansas Doctor: A Century of Pioneering*, 1959.

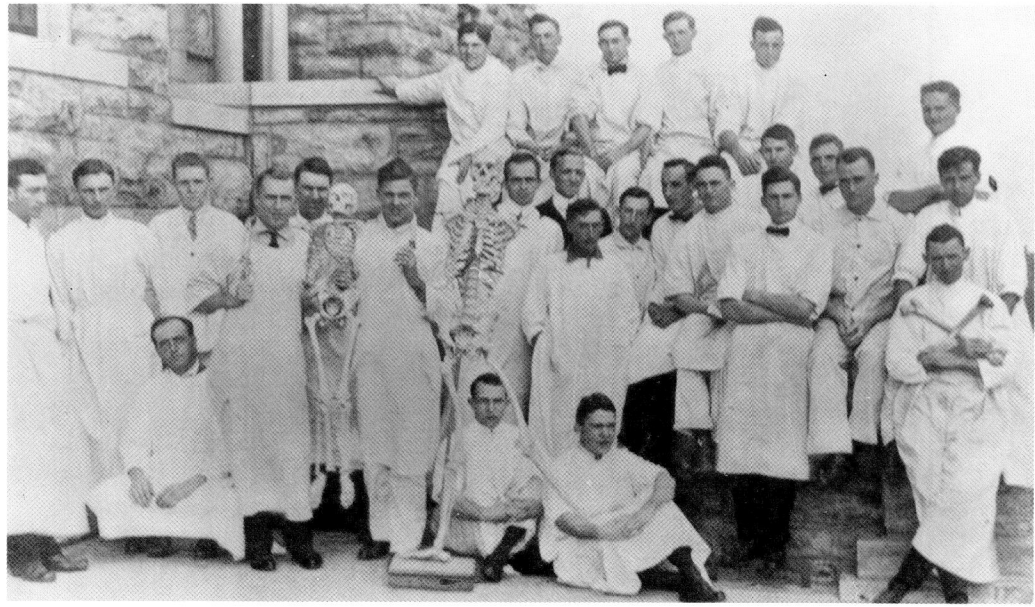

Medical students on the Lawrence campus, ca. 1900.

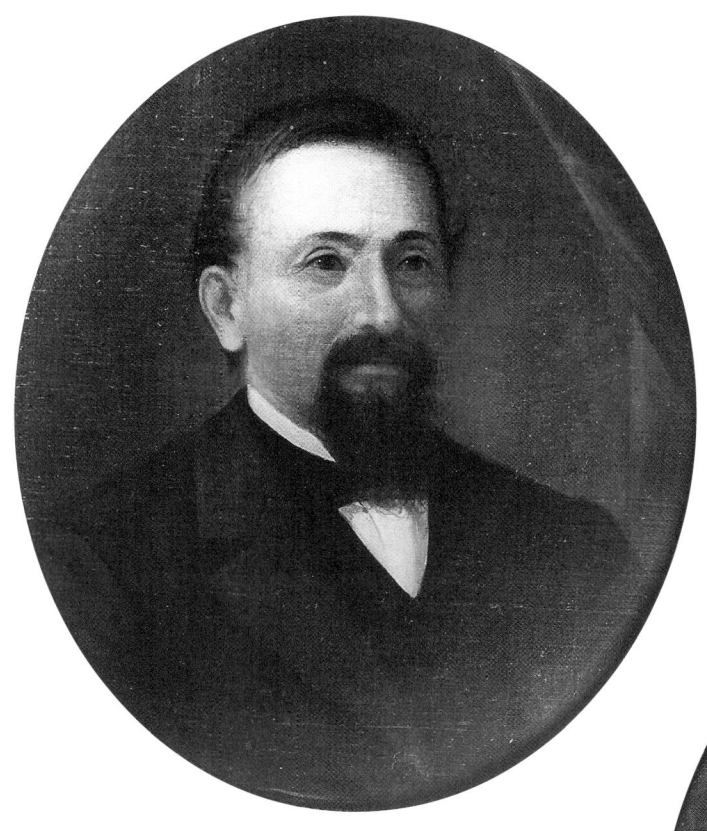

Simeon Bishop Bell, M.D., 1820–1913. Dr. Bell donated both land and money in 1894, thus making the four-year University of Kansas Medical School a possibility.

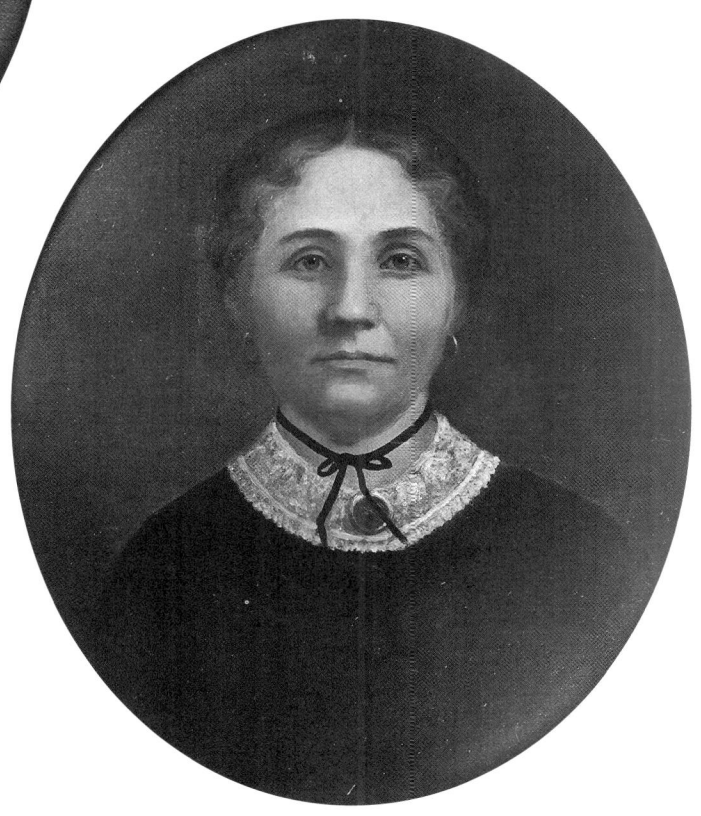

Eleanor Taylor Bell (1825–1866), the wife of Simeon Bell, M.D. Dr. Bell's donation to the University of Kansas was in her memory.

I wish to make some propositions for your own and others' interest—looking toward the establishment and building—first an Hospital—and secondly a Medical College . . . in Rosedale where Kansas City, Kansas, Rosedale, Kansas, Kansas City, Missouri and Westport, Missouri corner with each other. . . . I will donate a suitable site for Medical College buildings—all of which is respectfully submitted to the management of the Kansas State University.
—Simeon B. Bell, M.D., to Professor Sayre, August 24, 1894.

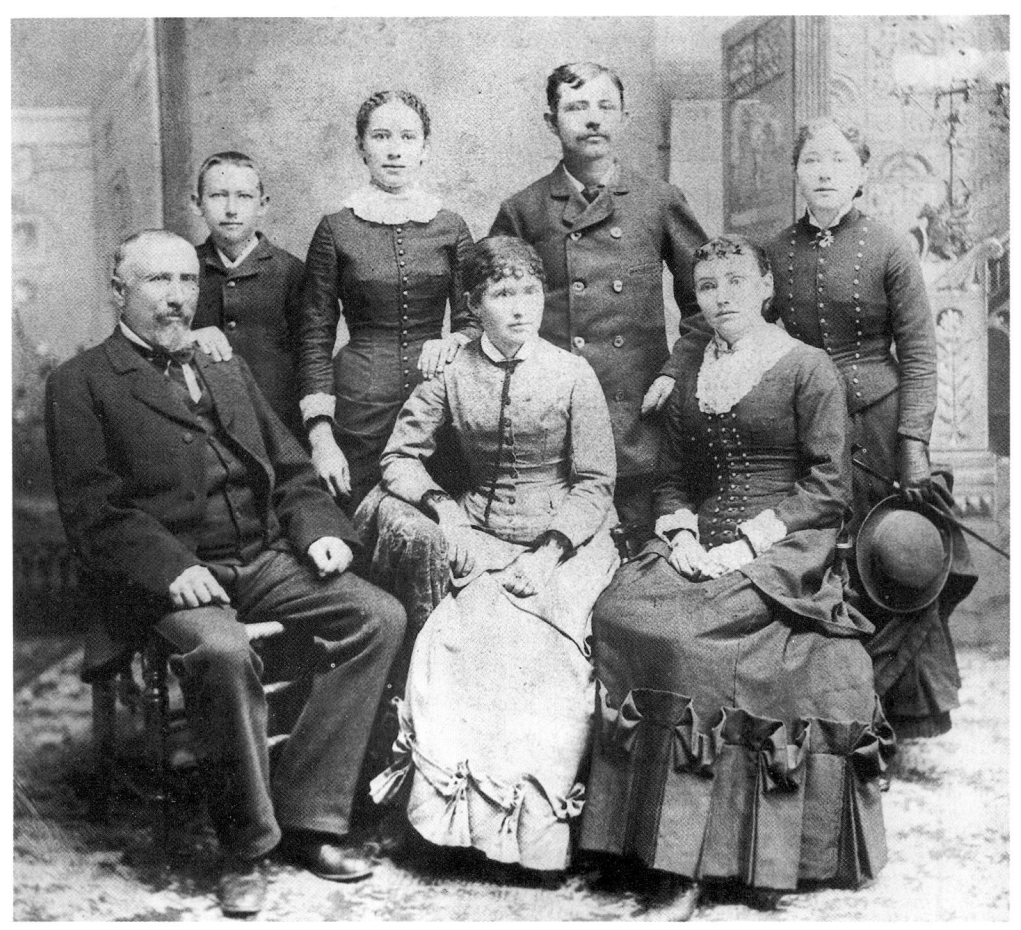

Dr. Bell with his children, ca. 1890.

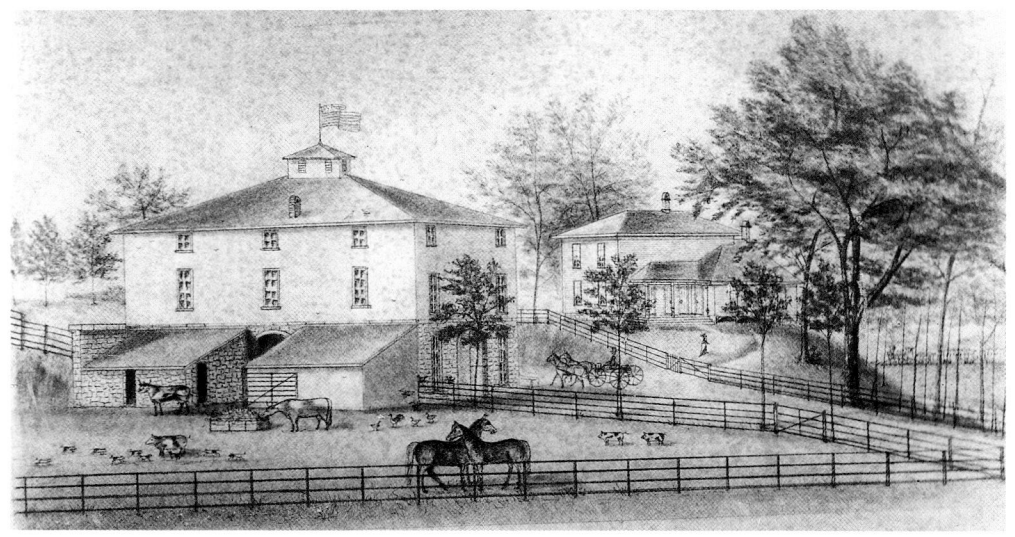

Dr. Simeon Bell's farm in 1882, located on what would become Southwest Boulevard in Wyandotte County, Kansas.

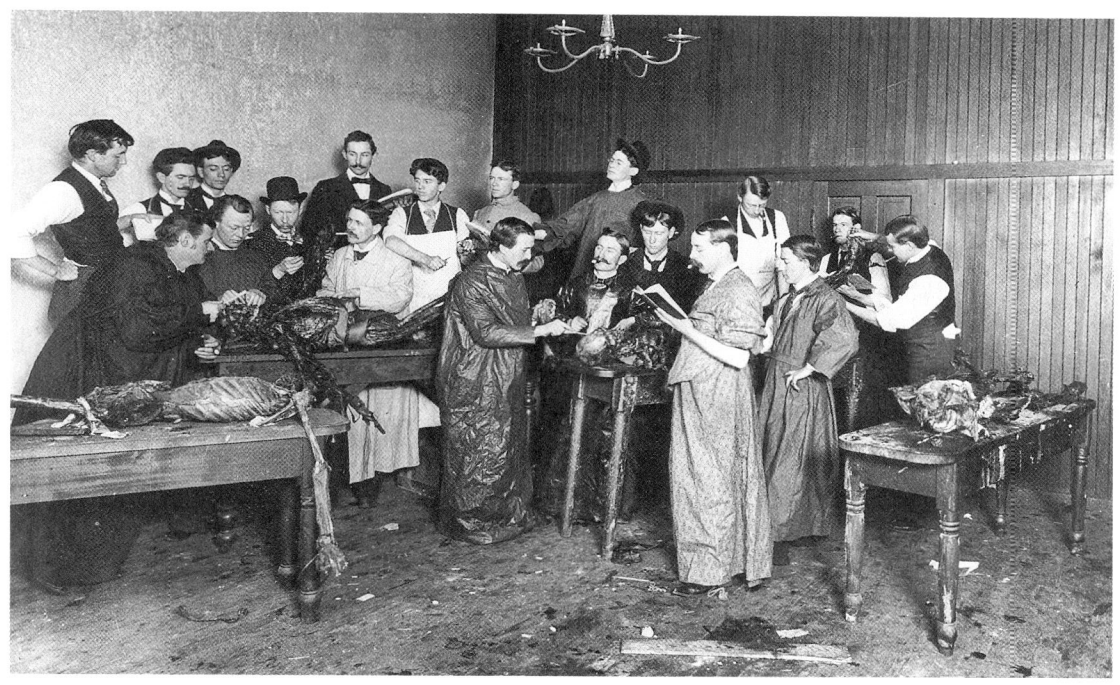

Kansas City Medical College anatomy class, 1896. Students often contrived photographs like this.

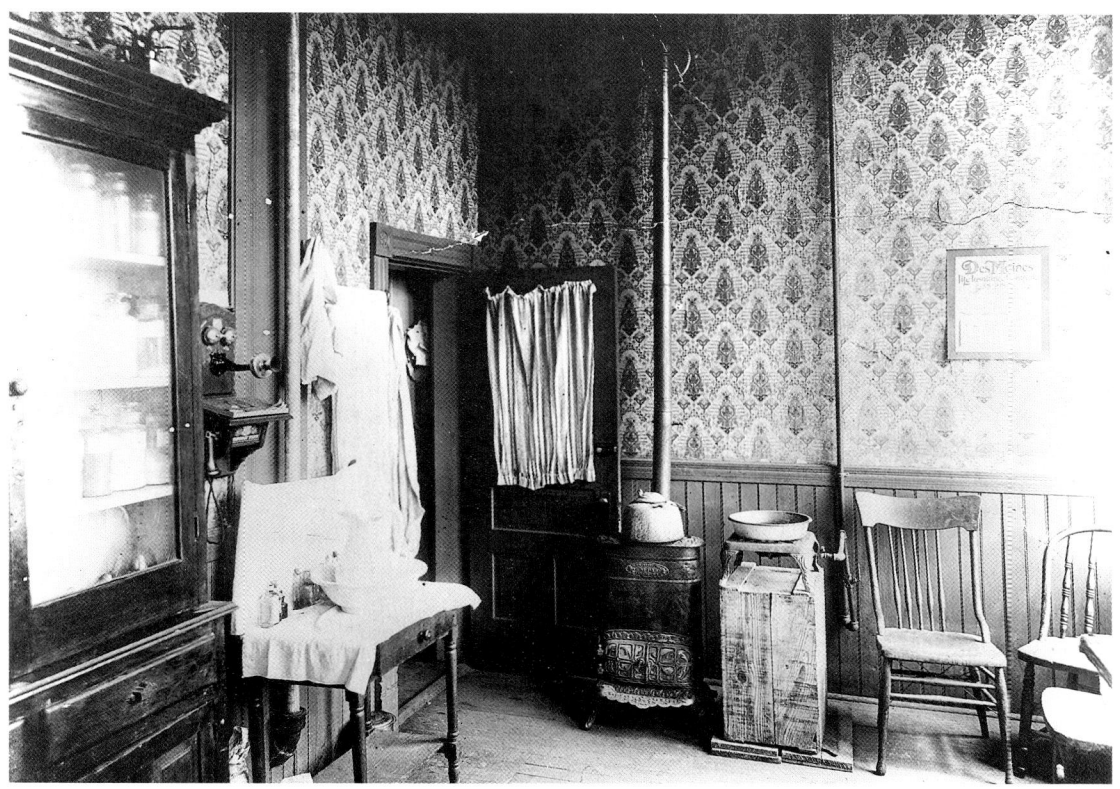

Kansas Medical College Dispensary, Topeka, Kansas, 1909.

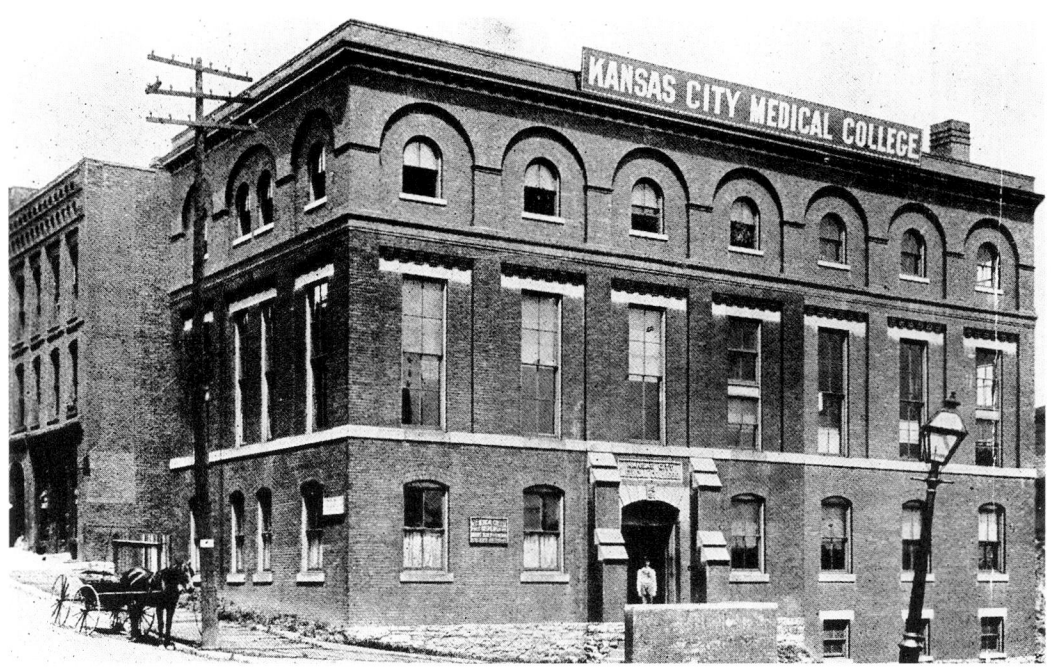

Kansas City Medical College, Kansas City, Missouri, near the time of the merger, 1905.

In 1869, when Kansas City was yet a comparatively small river town, a number of prominent businessmen and physicians united to establish the Kansas City Medical College. Its founding was an early manifestation of that public spirit for which the citizens of Kansas City have become famous and which has kept the school system and libraries and philanthropic institutions, as well as the public buildings and parks and boulevards of the city, fully abreast with its commercial growth.

The college set for itself a high ideal of thorough teaching and honest examinations long before any pressure was brought to bear by State Universities and State Boards to provide adequate standards and safeguards for medical education. It prides itself to-day on enforcing its entrance conditions and its requirements for graduation, irrespective of the policy of its competitors.
—Kansas City Medical College, Thirty-Sixth Annual Announcement, 1904–1905.

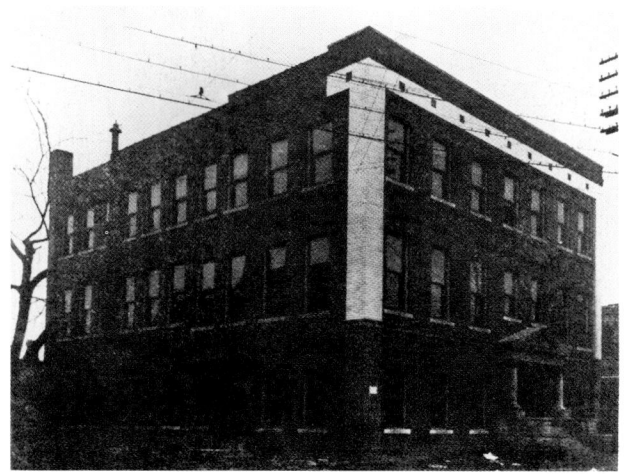

Medico-Chirurgical College, Kansas City, Missouri, ca. 1905.

The College building is located at 409–411 Cherry Street. It is admirably located and recognized as the best field for clinical material, easily accessible from all parts of the City, and about one block east from the County Court House. Street railways run nearby, which enables the students to speedily reach all parts of the City.

It is the intention of this institution to give instructions by lectures, clinics, practical courses in the dissecting room, laboratories, hospitals, recitations, and by daily quizzes.
—Medico-Chirurgical College of Kansas City, Missouri, Second Annual Announcement, 1899.

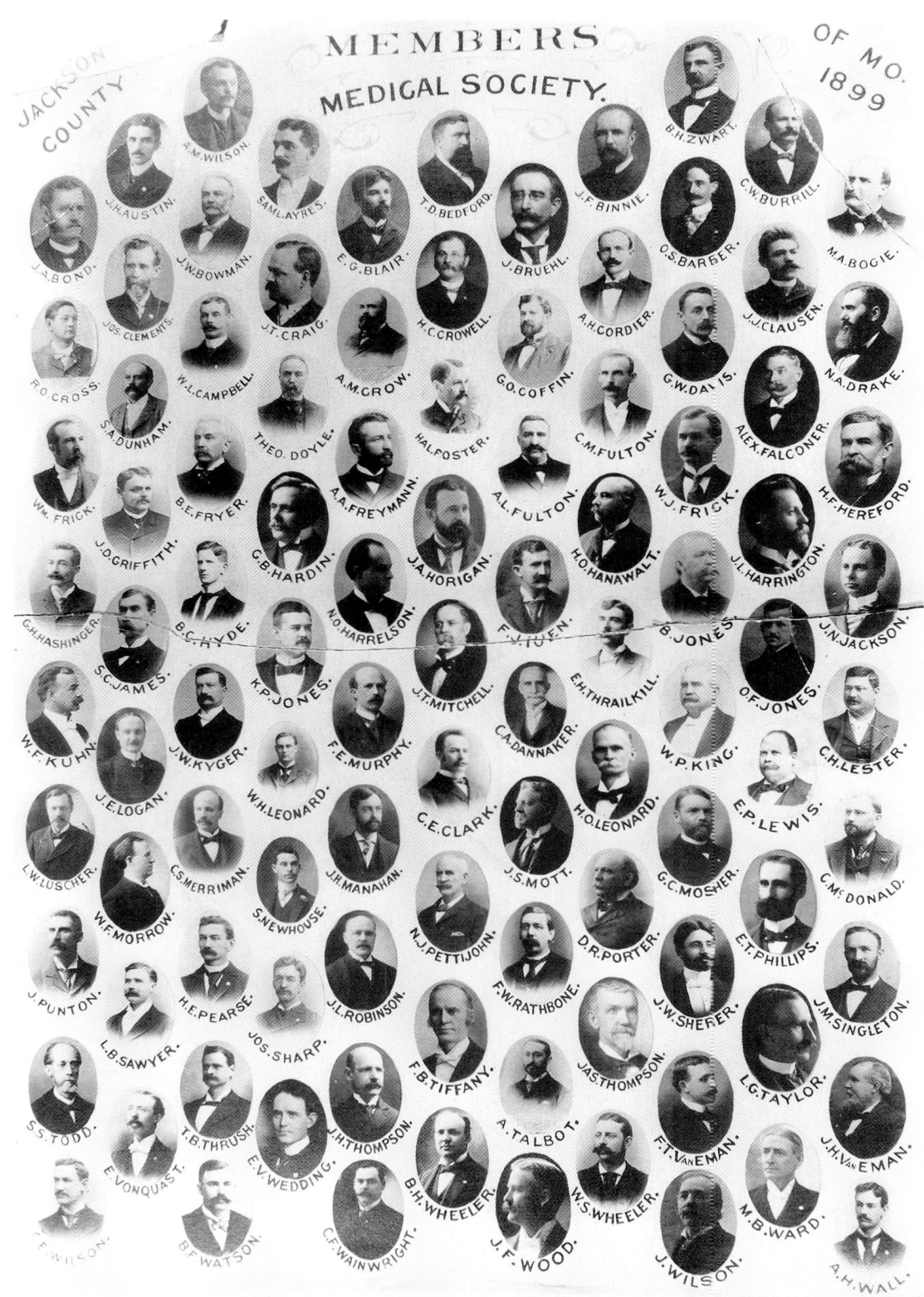

The Jackson County Medical Society in 1899. Many of these members joined the first faculty of the new University of Kansas Medical School in Rosedale.

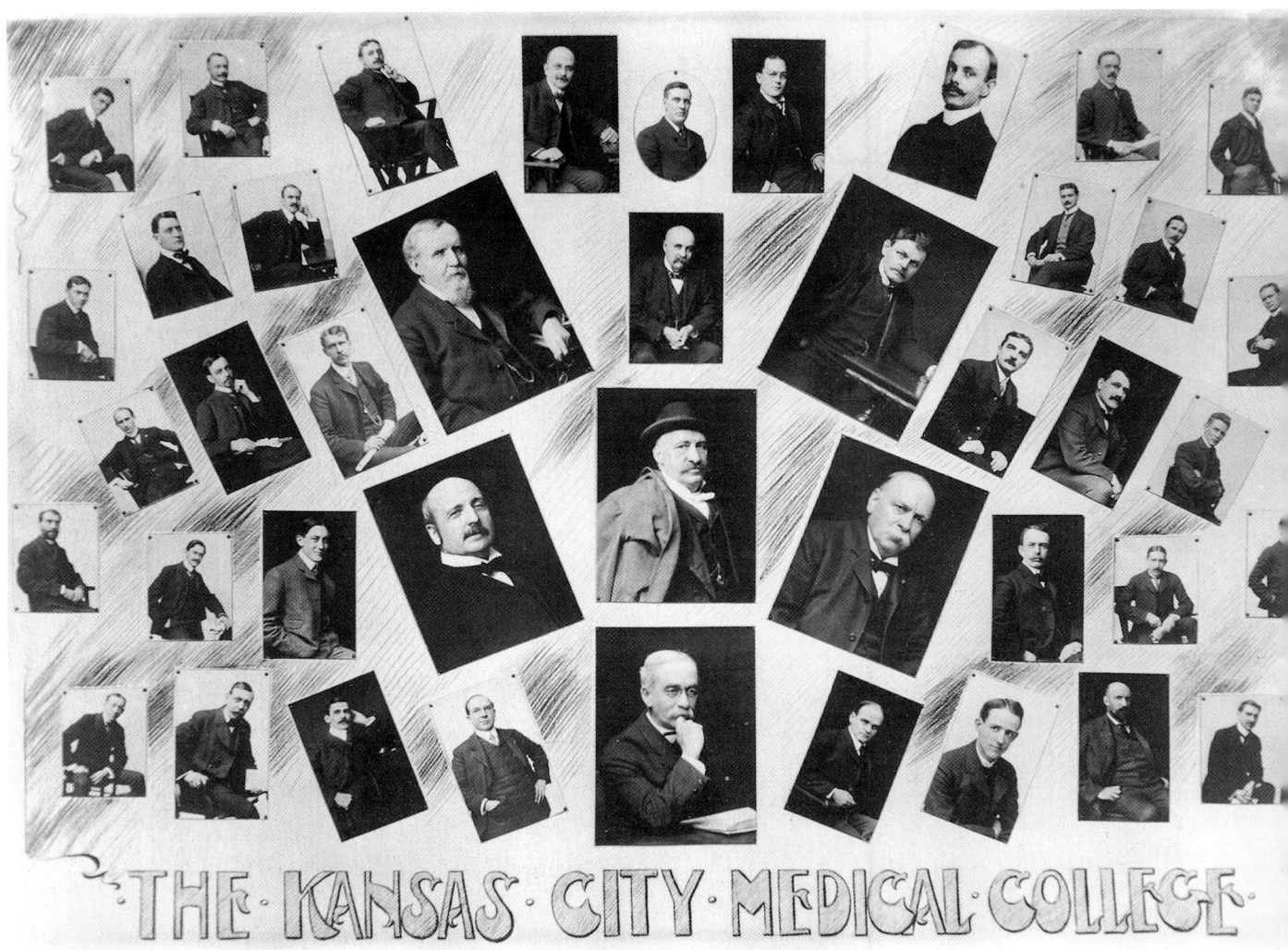

The 1902 faculty of the Kansas City Medical College.

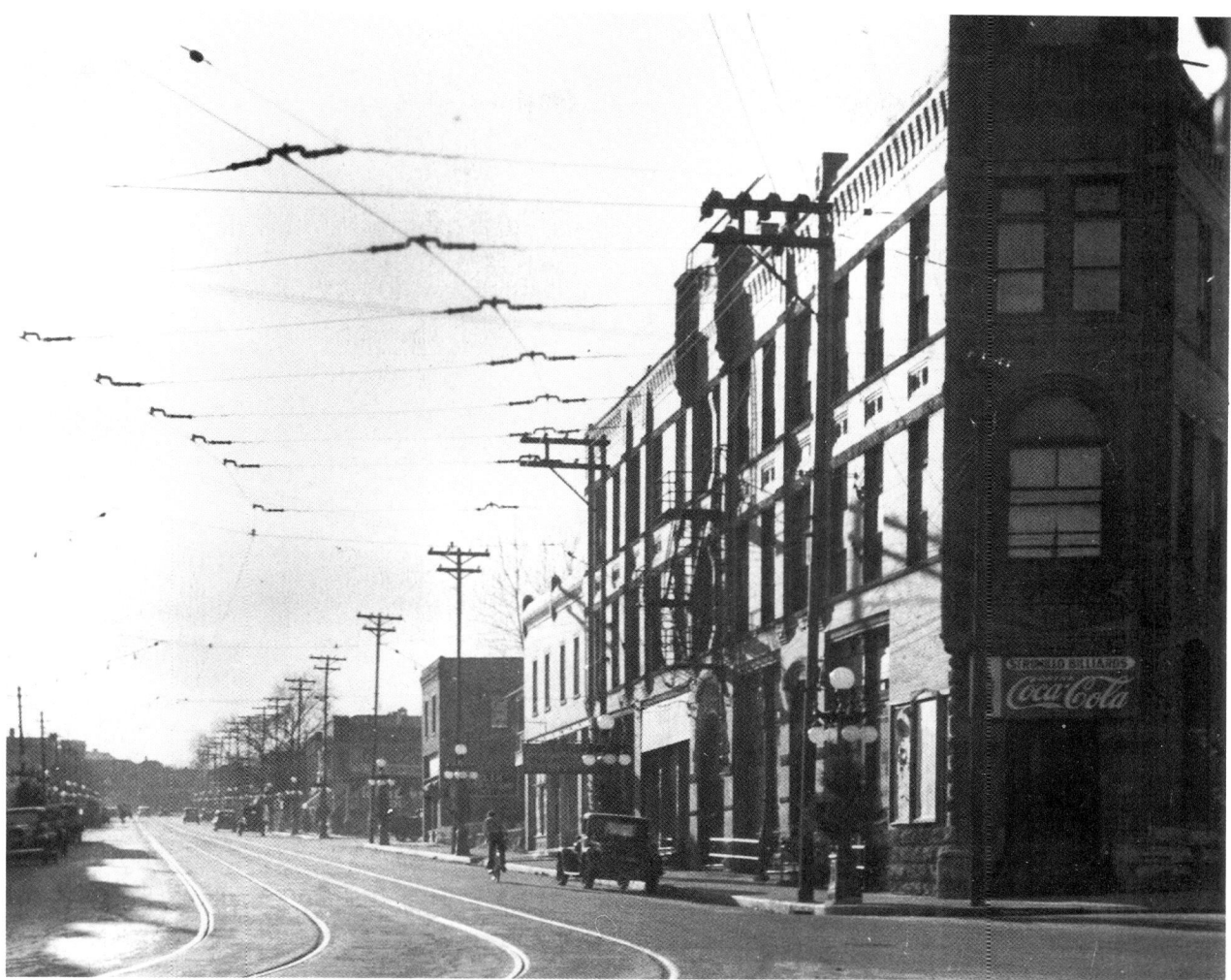

The Simpson Building at the corner of Simpson and Central avenues in Kansas City, Kansas. Originally the site of the College of Physicians and Surgeons, this building was the first home of the new University of Kansas School of Medicine from 1905 to 1906.

The College is located in its large three-story and basement building, at the corner of Central and Simpson Avenues, in Kansas City, Kansas, on the Grand View electric line of the Metropolitan Street Ry., accessible from all parts of the two Kansas Cities for one car fare, and distant a ride of only five minutes from the Union Depot. The location is high and sightly and could not be improved. It lies midway between and only a few blocks from Bethany and St. Margaret's hospitals. The College building is commodious, modern, and admirably proportioned and constructed for such use, with perfect light, space, and ventilation for the lecture rooms, laboratories, etc. Situated near the packing houses, railroad yards, and manufacturing plants, and with the homes of employees forming a city around it, the supply of clinical material is never-failing.
—The College of Physicians and Surgeons, Eleventh Annual Announcement, 1904–1905.

With the merger, Hoxie found himself facing a situation that present students and teachers would see as Utopian, but one Hoxie knew to have all the delights of the sub-basement of Dante's Purgatory. To edify his 96 students, Hoxie had a merged total of 100 faculty members. Hoping things might solve themselves through some variant of the law that has the fittest surviving, Chancellor Strong hit on the idea of having all courses elective—those professors the students neglected would gradually fade away. And so they did, but not without rancor. Profound disappointment was bound to ensue, and disappointment transmutes easily to enmity. Hoxie predicted that within three years the plan would make him the most hated physician in Kansas City. In his memoirs he concluded sadly, "And so it turned out." —Robert P. Hudson, M.D., "Hoxie's Bad Dream: Early Medical Education in Kansas," *Journal of the Kansas Medical Society*, 1970.

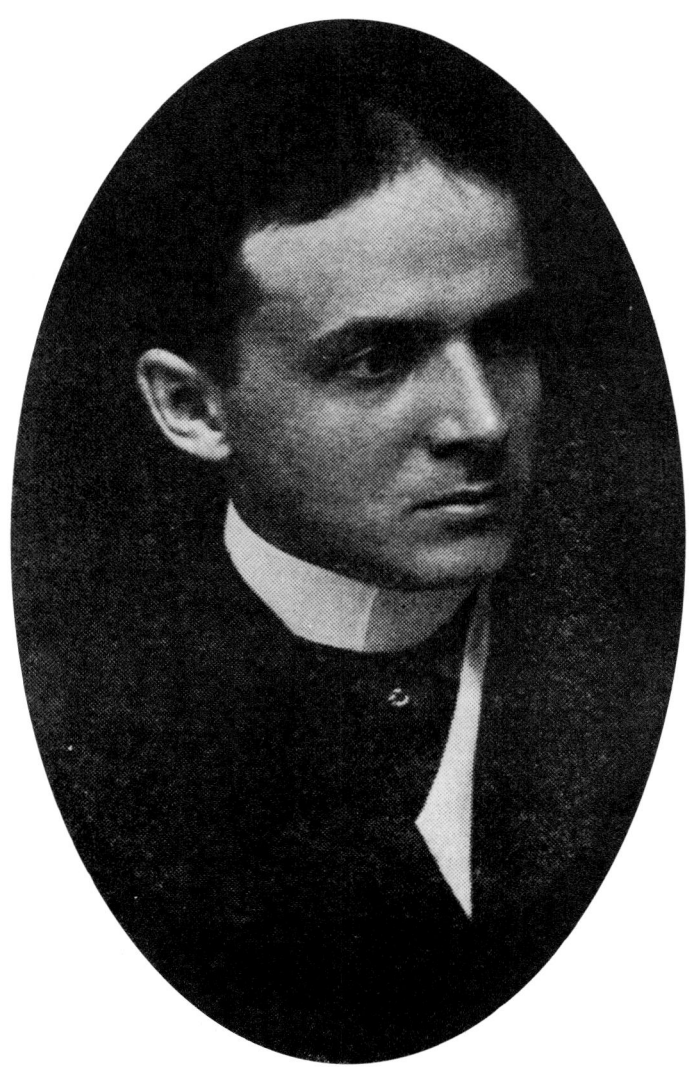

Our profession is essentially an unselfish one; and that colleague who uses it for his own aggrandizement has mistaken his calling and does his profession great harm. Therefore by the very nature of the responsibility which we assume when we seek and obtain the title, doctor of medicine, we pledge ourselves to lives of ministry and service rather than to lives of ease and self-indulgence. We are then to seek to better the health both of individuals who seek us out and of the body politic— which may then seek to rid itself of our services as of those who point out faults. To fulfill our calling will demand personal sacrifice— and that frequently for an ungrateful public. The Spirit of the Age will frequently argue—and prove—us fools for seeking a Utopia; but the Spirit of Medicine, the spirit that has animated our forerunners, bids us to be idealists, to believe in man and work for his salvation. We must therefore, if we would follow the better way, consider ourselves the priests of medicine and serve her with the devotion of the Nazarite.

For these reasons your success cannot be reckoned by the dollars you may accumulate, nor by the fame you win; but by the good you do and by the blessings which will be showered upon your memory.
—George Howard Hoxie, M.D., "The Goal," in *The School of Medicine of the University of Kansas*, 1906 (unpublished manuscript).

George Howard Hoxie, M.D., dean of the School of Medicine from 1905 to 1911.

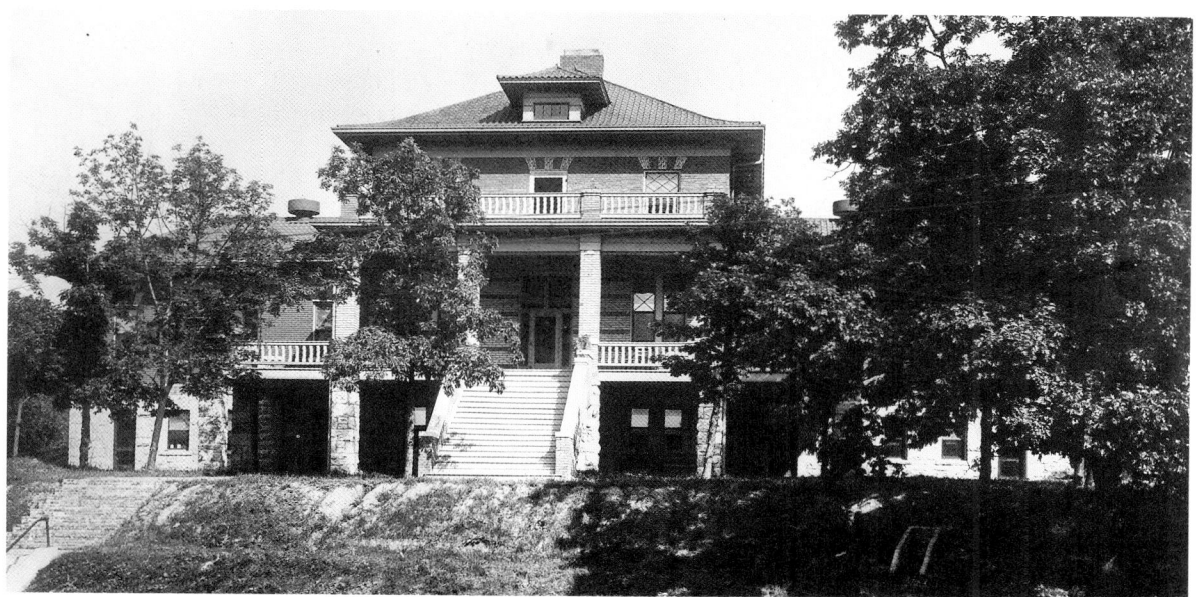

The original hospital building, completed in 1906. Named after Eleanor Taylor Bell, the building became the Training School for Nurses upon completion of a new hospital in 1911.

The tract is situated on a beautiful eminence, really a spur of a hill jutting out into the Turkey Creek Valley. While the position is lofty, the grade is so gradual that the approach from all points will be easy. The ground is covered with a fine growth of trees, which are capable of being beautified and cultivated to any extent desired. Standing at any point on the hill, the observer can see the whole of Turkey Creek Valley and the southern portion of Kansas City, Mo. No more beautiful site for a college can be found in the country.
—*Wyandotte Gazette*, December 31, 1896.

The new buildings at Rosedale are built to conform with the most advanced requirements of medical instruction. Special laboratories and facilities have been provided for investigation along various lines of medical work, so that it is now felt that the medical instruction given here compares favorably with the other schools of the University and the older medical schools of the country.
—University of Kansas Special Announcement of the Advance in the Requirements for Admission to the School of Medicine, 1906.

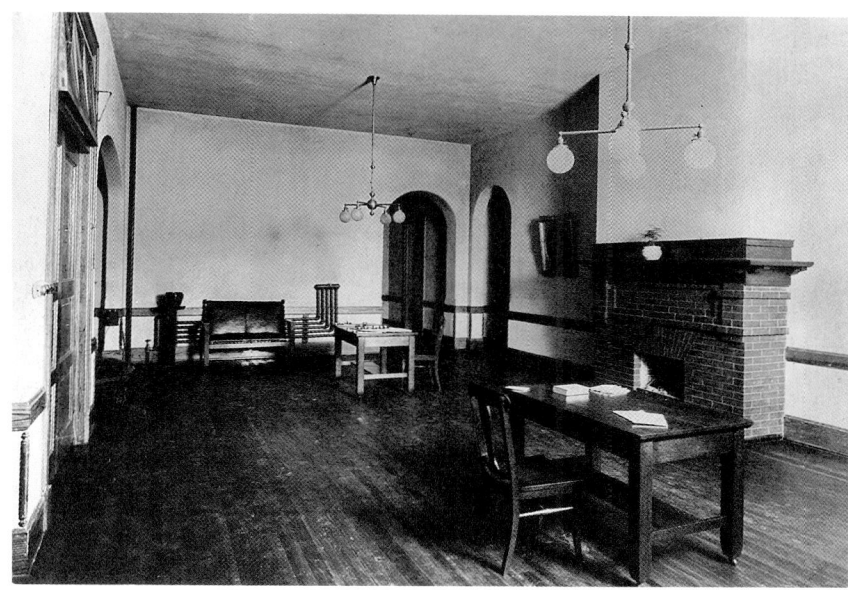

Reception area of the new Eleanor Taylor Bell Memorial Hospital in Rosedale, ca. 1907.

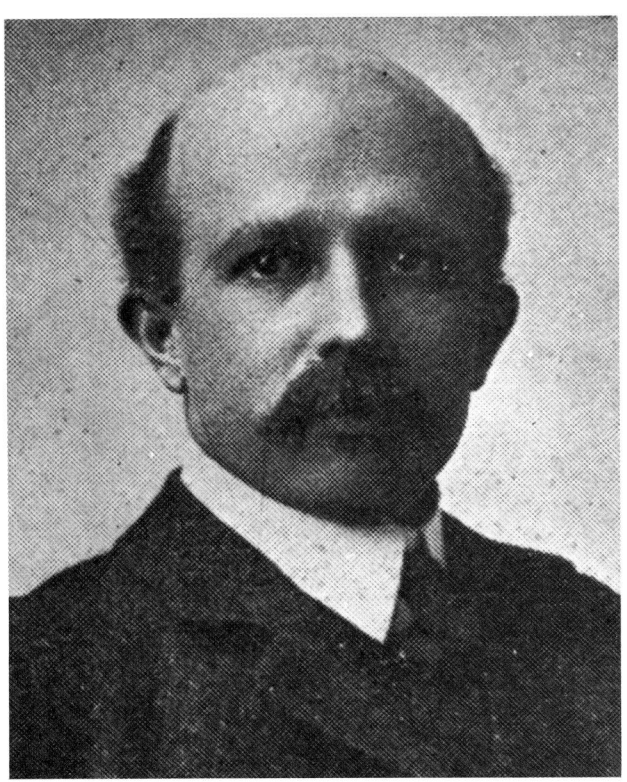

Dr. Murphy was a little below the average height; rather rotund, or should I say robin-esque, in shape; had very bright, intelligent, grey eyes; a small closely cropped mustache; was rather ruddy and definitely bald. He was a very polished gentleman with delightful manners—with much of what we often describe as Old World courtesy. He was well educated, had done postgraduate work in Germany, the Mecca of medicine at that time, and was a man of great honor and integrity.
—Ralph H. Major, M.D., *An Account of the University of Kansas School of Medicine*, 1968.

While a member of its faculty, you were its chief representative in science, the pride of your colleagues, the inspiration of your students. Your labors while here are written in its archives, in the literature of the world, in the hearts and memories of its alumni. —Certificate presented to John F. Binnie, M.D., from the University of Kansas School of Medicine, 1929.

Franklin E. Murphy, M.D., professor of internal medicine and one of the founding fathers of the medical school. Dr. Murphy was on the faculty from 1905 until his death in 1933.

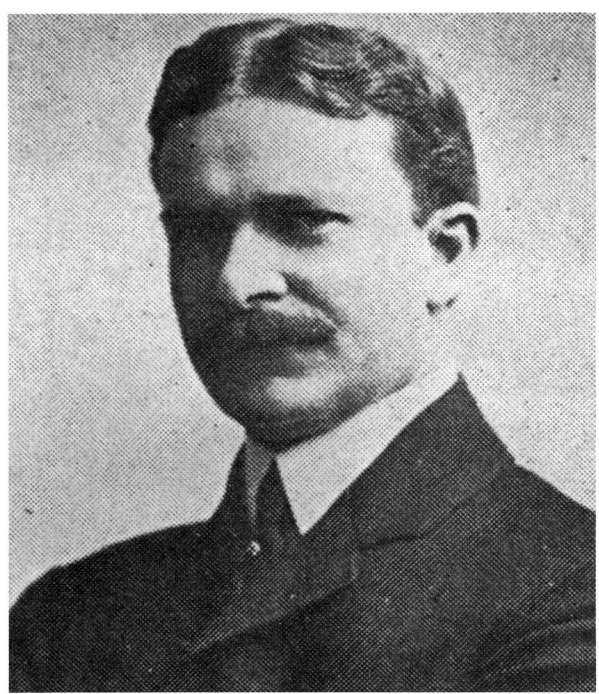

Ernest F. Robinson, M.D., professor of surgery, 1905–1909.

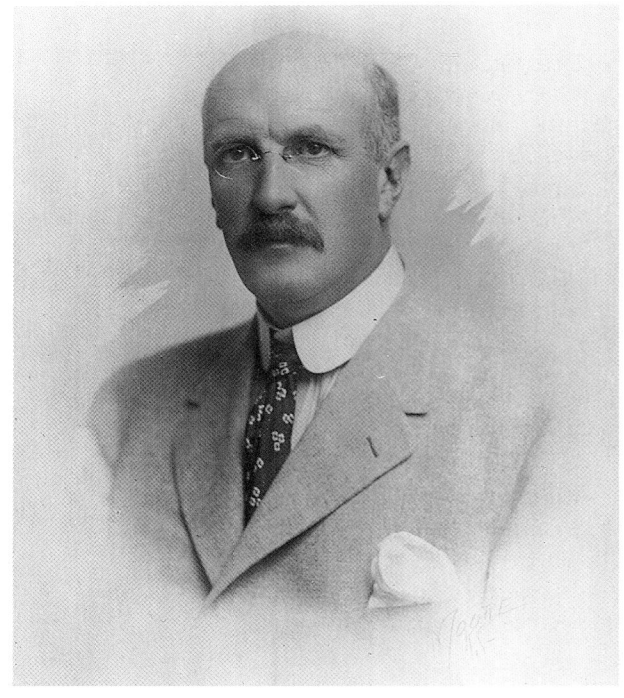

John Fairbairne Binnie, M.D., professor of surgery, 1905–1911.

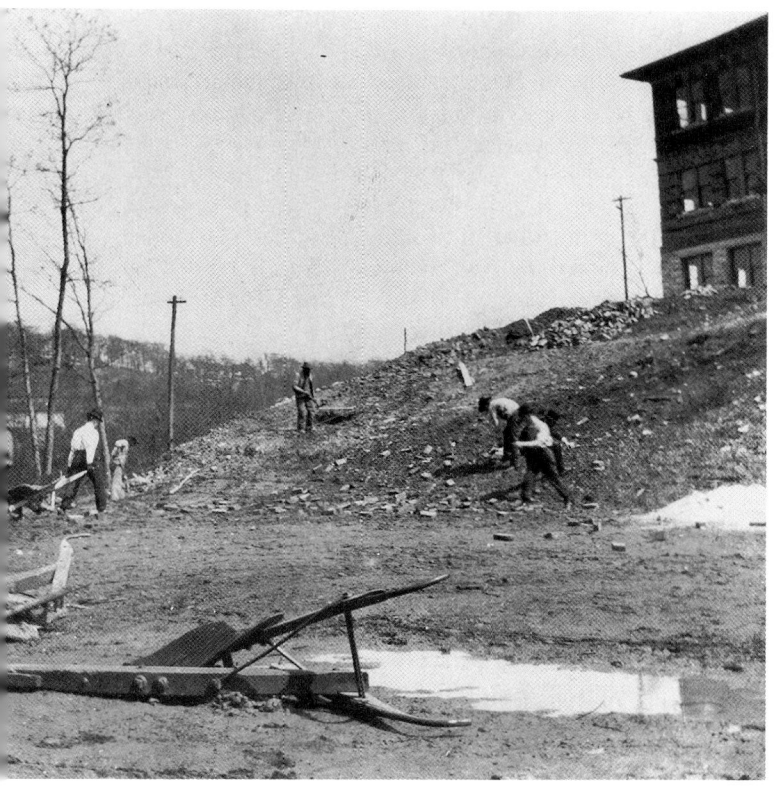

Medical students building sidewalks on Goat Hill for a legislative visit, ca. 1910.

The management of the hospital caused me more grief than the deanship. Not so much with the professional side, because we always had good nurses. Rather it was the business administration that bothered me; the hiring of lay help, the purchasing of supplies, the keeping of accounts, and all the minutiae of conducting a self-liquidating enterprise. The grounds were raw and unkempt. . . . I remember vividly the time when we were notified that a committee of the legislature was on the way to inspect us; I called on the students to help me lay brick sidewalks over the rough paths.
—George Howard Hoxie, M.D., *Reminiscences of the Beginning of the School of Medicine of the University of Kansas*, unpublished manuscript, 1940.

Two dispensaries will be maintained—one in the building formerly occupied by the Medico-chirurgical College, 914–918 Independence Avenue, Kansas City, Mo., and the other near the packinghouses in Kansas City, Kan. These two buildings will be in the centers of the two districts of Kansas City most in need of free medical attendance, and students will therefore have an unusually good opportunity to study disease in some of its worst forms. The University will make the effort to correct the evil so often charged against American medical centers—that clinical material is really wasted—by seeking to put surgery and medicine on a scientific basis, and directing its instructions to utilize the best developed methods both for the study and the treatment of the sick who come to its dispensaries for relief.
—*Bulletin of the University of Kansas*, the School of Medicine, Announcements for 1905–1906.

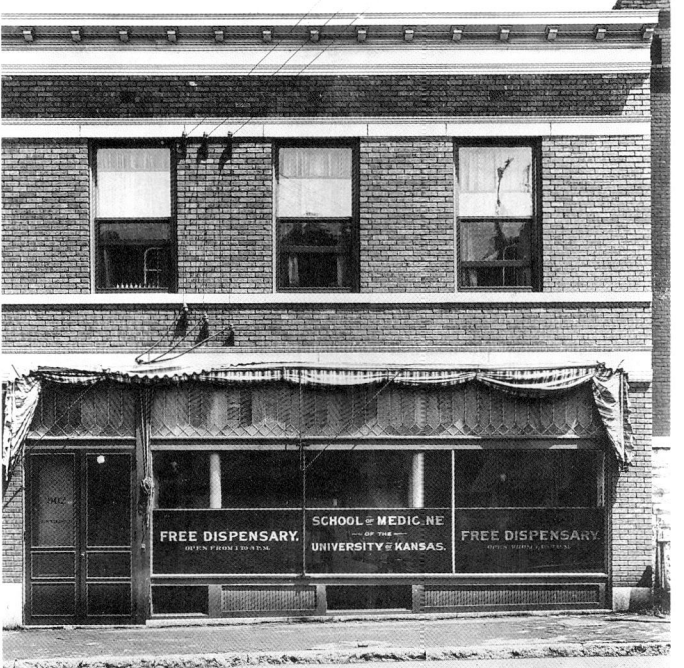

The "north-end" dispensary, located at 914 Independence Avenue in Kansas City, Missouri, ca. 1910.

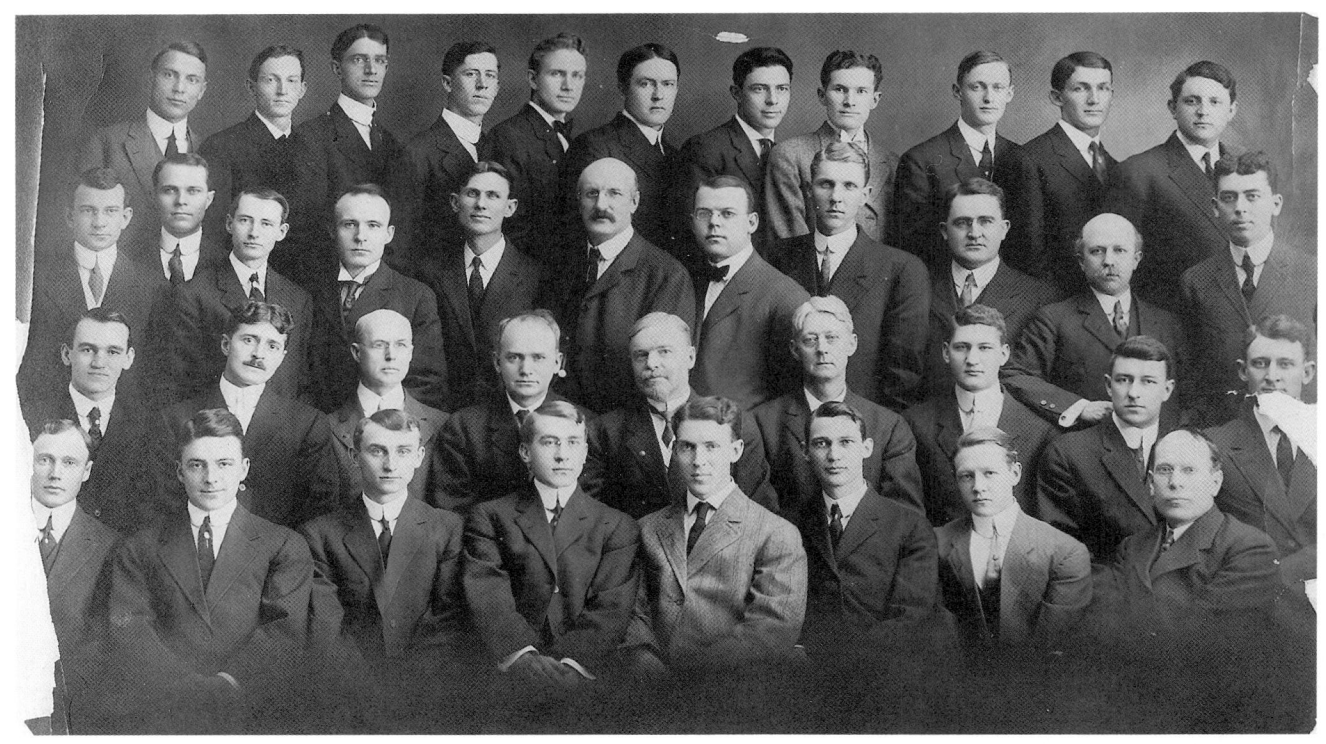

Students and faculty, ca. 1906.

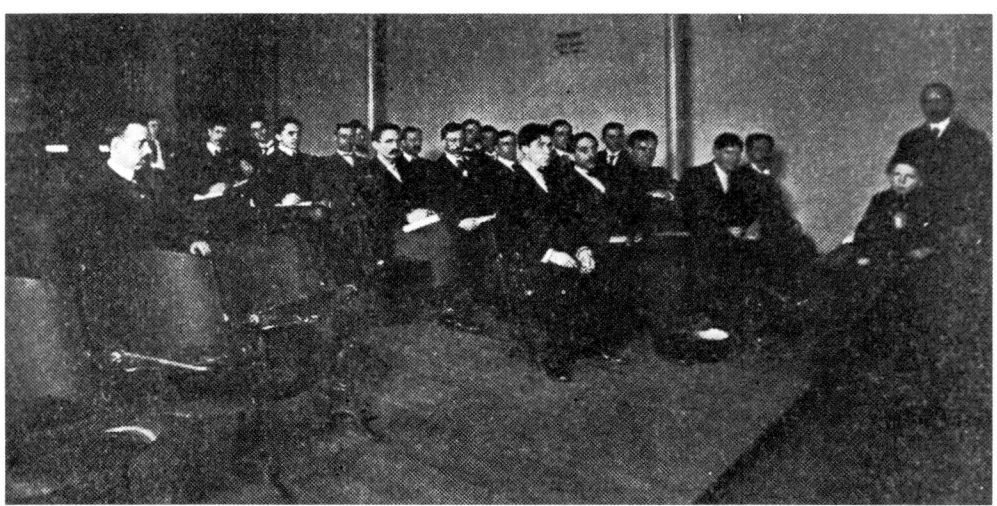

Medical class in pediatrics, ca. 1907.

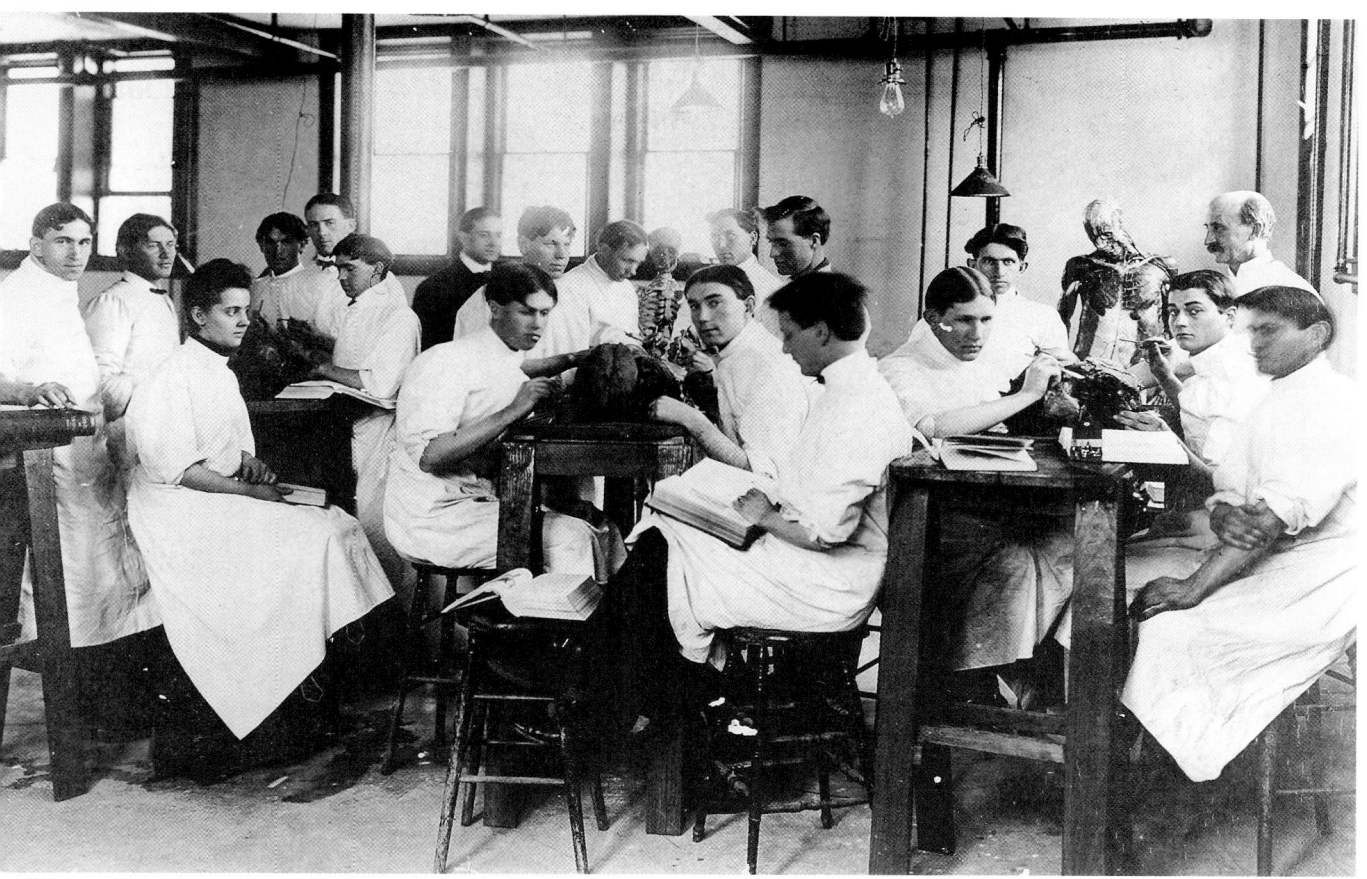

A 1907 anatomy class.

The goal of medical education and the object of medical science are one and inseparable, but they are separated from everything else in the world. The physician may be, and indeed he is, peculiarly fitted by his knowledge to advise the community on certain social problems which it must face, but as soon as he employs any but the scientific method for their solution, so soon he finds himself lost on a vast rhetorical sea, without the shadow of a compass or the vestige of a pilot. The elimination of every conventionally sentimental and altruistic consideration is the price that is paid for what comes to be at last the finest sentiment and the highest altruism—the discovery of truth.
—Logan Clendening, "The Goal of Medical Education," *The School of Medicine of the University of Kansas*, 1906.

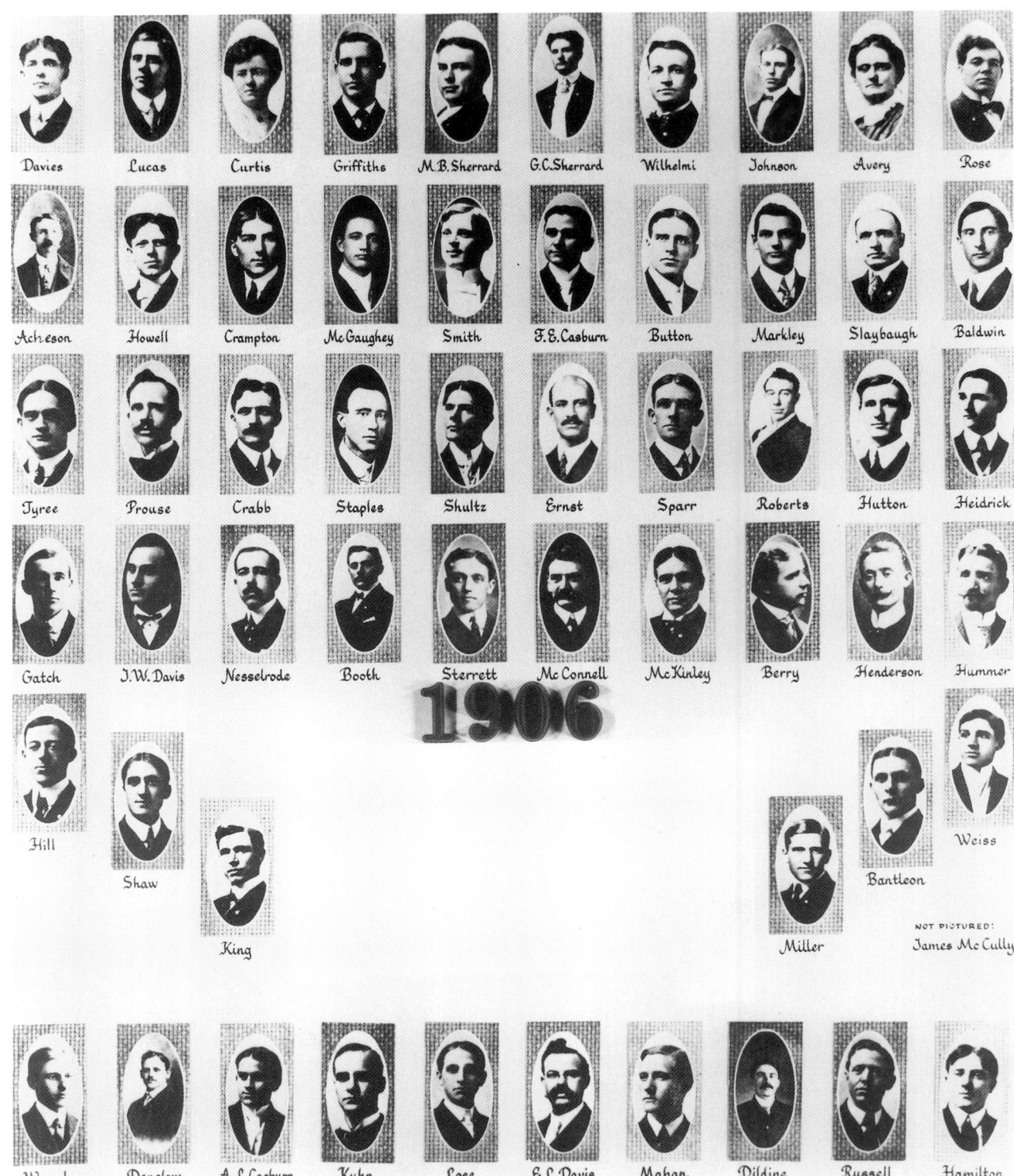

Davies | Lucas | Curtis | Griffiths | M.B.Sherrard | G.C.Sherrard | Wilhelmi | Johnson | Avery | Rose

Acheson | Howell | Crampton | McGaughey | Smith | F.E.Casburn | Button | Markley | Slaybaugh | Baldwin

Tyree | Prouse | Crabb | Staples | Shultz | Ernst | Sparr | Roberts | Hutton | Heidrick

Gatch | J.W.Davis | Nesselrode | Booth | Sterrett | McConnell | McKinley | Berry | Henderson | Hummer

1906

Hill | Shaw | King | Miller | Bantleon | Weiss

NOT PICTURED:
James McCully

Worrel | Denslow | A.L.Casburn | Kuhn | Lose | E.L.Davis | Mahan | Dildine | Russell | Hamilton

The first University of Kansas School of Medicine graduating class, 1906.

Doctorate Service

Class of 1906

School of Medicine

University of Kansas

Sunday Morning, June Third

Nineteen Hundred and Six

Eleven O'clock

Westminster Congregational Church

Thirty-Sixth and Walnut Streets

Kansas City

Class of 1906 doctorate service.

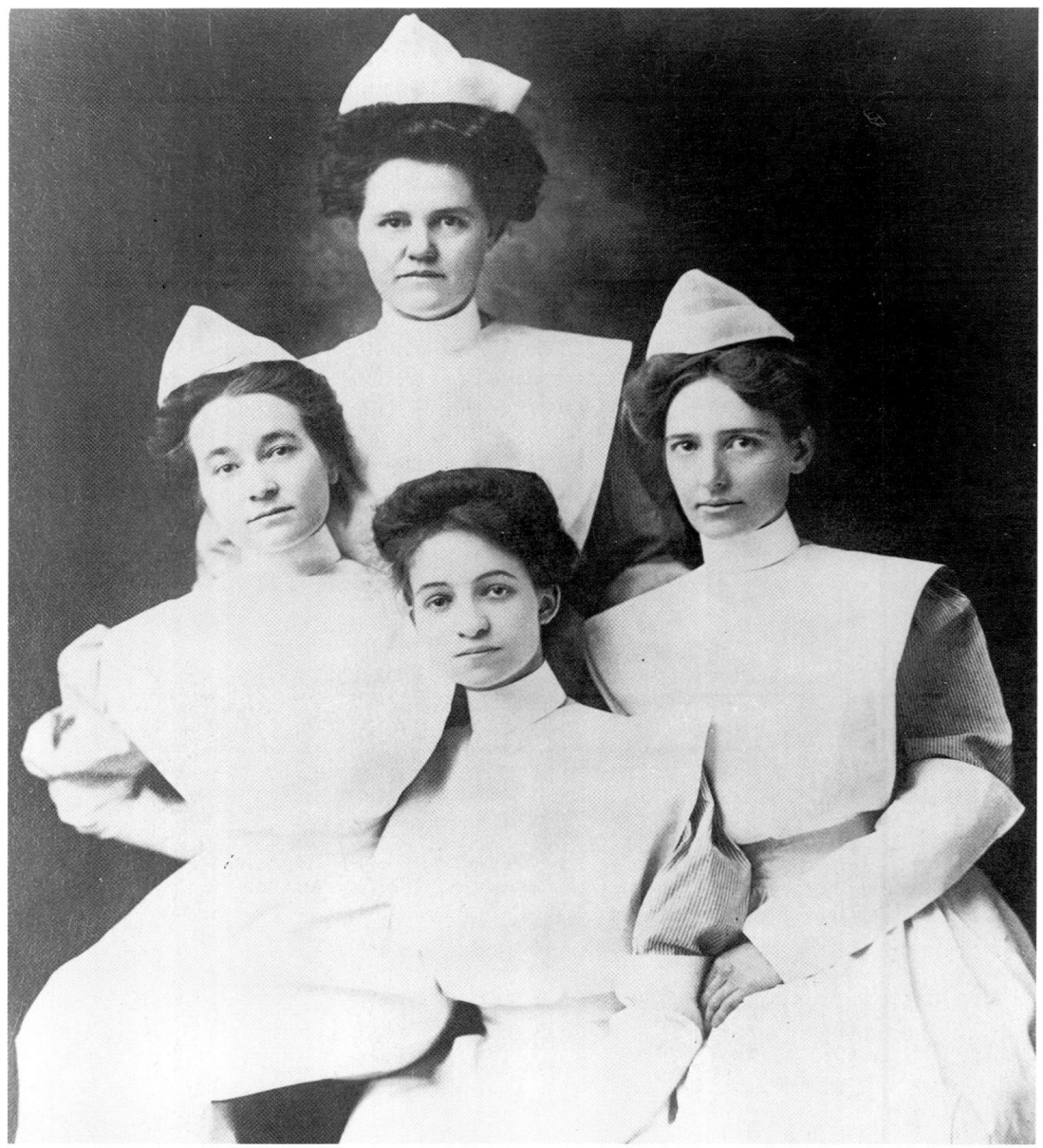

The first graduating class of the Training School for Nurses, 1909.

Here I must pause to pay my respects to the memory of Pearl Laptad of Lawrence who came down to superintend the nurses and start a nursing school. She was a graduate of Christ's Hospital, Topeka, and was a monument to its integrity and thoroughness. She literally wore herself out. The nurses under her inspiration regarded service as their aim in life, not money, not places of authority. . . .

    She did a marvelous job of initiating standards in spite of the paucity of materials and equipment. She resigned in the slump after 1908 and we had a succession of head nurses and superintendents: some good and some not so good.
—George Howard Hoxie, M.D., *Reminiscences of the Beginning of the School of Medicine of the University of Kansas*, unpublished manuscript, 1940.

You have probably noticed that recently the matter of the very existence of our School of Medicine has come up. I wish, therefore, that you should tell me frankly whether you think the state ought to give up its medical school. Shall we leave our standard of medicine and the physical welfare of our people to agencies entirely outside of our own state? Shall we withdraw from the field and allow another institution or another state to occupy one of the most strategic points in medical education to be found in this country? Shall the twenty-five hundred doctors of Kansas be entirely without recognition in the professional education of the state? —Chancellor Strong to "Dear Doctor," December 10, 1910.

And so, for the school, the years 1909-1911 were years of "marking time" for us in Rosedale. We were trying to keep the school intact until the authorities at Lawrence and Topeka could agree on a new program. We could not plan anything at our level. I did not know how much longer I must hold the fort; but I was grateful to the doctors and nurses who kept at their jobs without any promise of a worth-while future. My memories of those days are like those of a bad dream, where one set of visions merges into another without any explanation or logical sequence.

My service with the University ended with the graduation of the Class of 1911.
—George Howard Hoxie, M.D., *Reminiscences of the Beginning of the School of Medicine of the University of Kansas*, unpublished manuscript, 1940

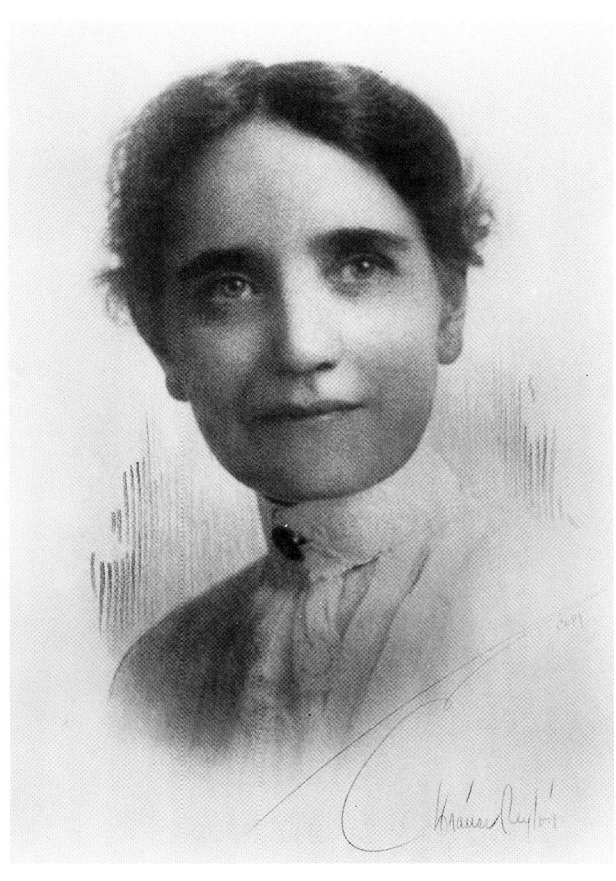

Miss Pearl Laptad, first principal and lecturer of the Training School for Nurses, 1906–1908.

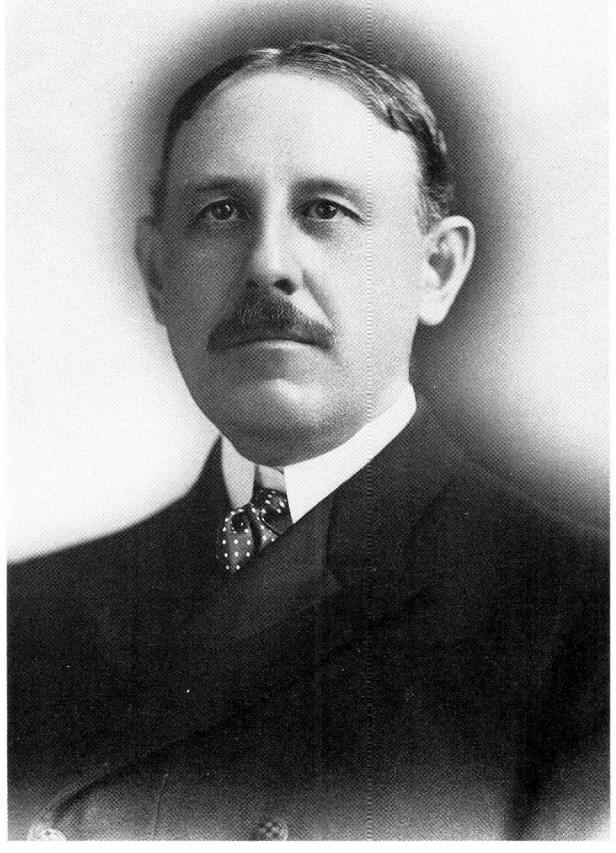

Frank Strong, chancellor of the University of Kansas from 1902 to 1920.

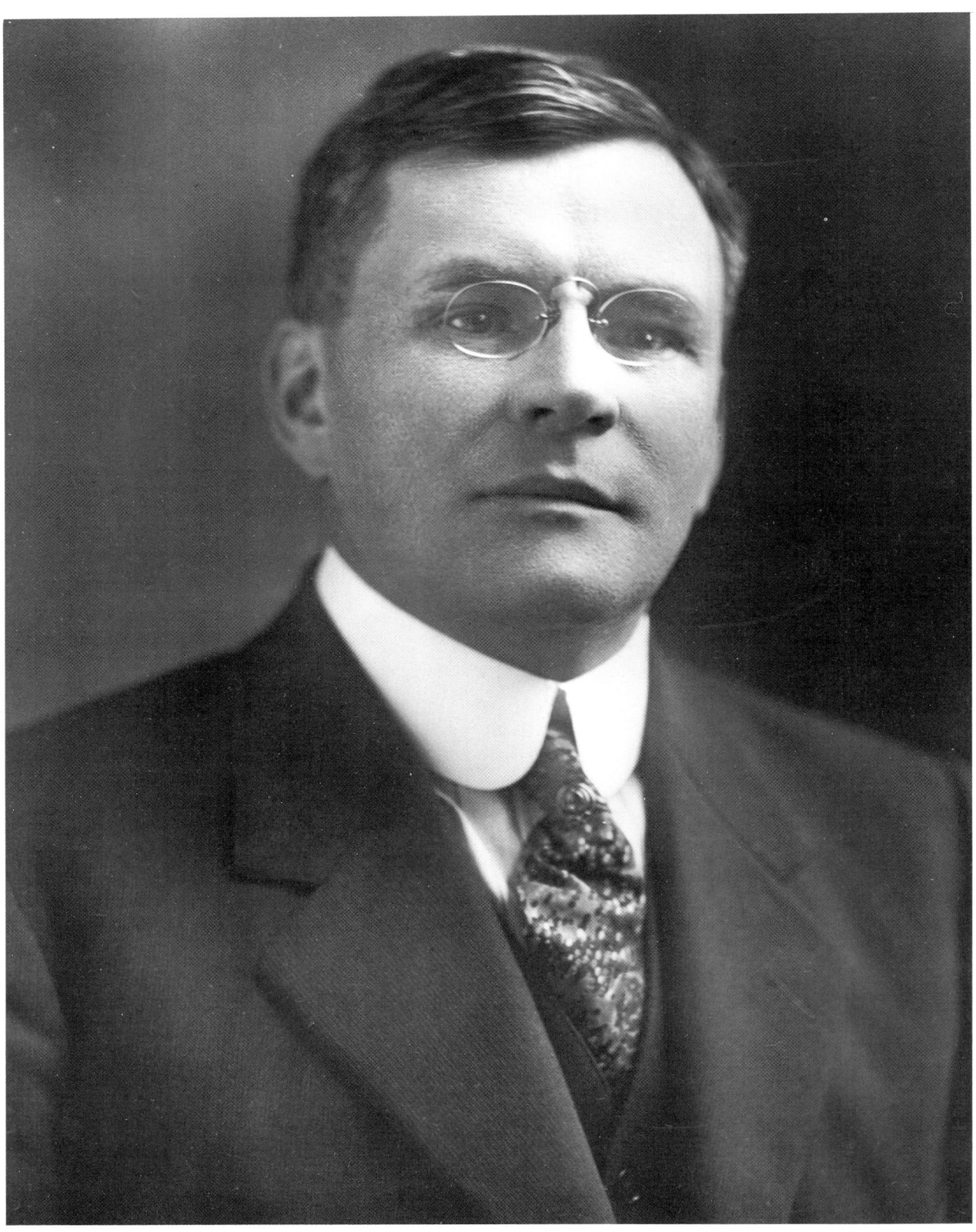

Mervin T. Sudler, M.D., dean of the University of Kansas Medical School from 1911 to 1924.

2

A Few Friends, More Enemies

The University of Kansas School of Medicine received severe criticism in Abraham Flexner's explosive and influential report of 1910, *Medical Education in the United States and Canada*. Flexner, who produced this report under the auspices of the Carnegie Foundation for the Advancement of Teaching, criticized Kansas for having what he called "two half-schools," one in Lawrence and the other in Rosedale. He believed the facilities so poor and the budget so inadequate that the University of Kansas would need "to refrain from many other projects, pending the upbuilding of a credible school of medicine." To emphasize the poor state of affairs, Flexner called the divided institution a "medical department" rather than a legitimate medical school.

Flexner's critical evaluations failed to lead to a renaissance in public medical education in Kansas, however. With powerful outside opponents, the rather forlorn Rosedale school remained in serious trouble. A state appropriation of $50,000 provided for a third building, but the legislature forced the closing of the dispensary on Independence Avenue in Kansas City, Missouri, which Flexner had described as managed in an "incredibly slipshod manner." Ironically, it was the Flexner report, in part, that saved the Rosedale Campus. The report harshly condemned conditions in most proprietary schools, especially in the anatomy laboratories, notably including the Kansas Medical College in Topeka. "The dissecting-room is indescribably filthy," Flexner observed. "It contained, in addition to necessary tables, a single, badly hacked cadaver, and was simultaneously used as a chicken yard." The Kansas Medical College eventually closed and the University of Kansas School of Medicine absorbed its alumni. Even as the future of the Rosedale campus remained in doubt, the University of Kansas gradually solidified control over public medical

education in the state. The legislature appropriated $24,000 for the construction of outpatient and laboratory facilities on the Rosedale campus, giving the school a total of four buildings. Thereafter, the political leadership of Kansas balked at further construction or improvement projects. Despite the demise of the Topeka school, interests in Wichita and Manhattan continued to entertain hopes of taking the clinical program away from Rosedale.

In 1912, a confidential letter from an American Medical Association accreditation committee to Chancellor Frank Strong strengthened the chances of the medical school remaining in the Kansas City area. The AMA committee had gained so unfavorable an impression that the members thought it fair to inform Kansas authorities in advance of a formal report. In essence, the letter to Strong—sympathetic in tone and somewhat understanding—ranked the school at the bottom of public medical schools and beneath most private medical institutions in North America and abroad. The division of the University of Kansas School of Medicine into two parts came under scathing criticism, and the two-year program at Lawrence was a target of special disparagement. The letter noted that only two of ten participating teachers had any medical training, claiming that such a situation existed nowhere else in the entire world. In comparison, Rosedale fared better. The main faults cited concerned clinical considerations, especially the small number of beds and consequently few patients at Bell Hospital. This difficulty proved fairly easy to solve. The medical school successfully negotiated an agreement that added the 365-bed St. Margaret's Hospital in Kansas City, Kansas, as a teaching hospital. This and other changes mollified the AMA and the medical school retained its accreditation, even though it continued to operate the two-year program in Lawrence. The best way to reach St. Margaret's from Rosedale, however, meant traveling the long way around through Kansas City, Missouri. The medical school could not seem to escape its Missouri connection.

As the clinical program took shape in Rosedale, a dedicated faculty made up almost entirely of Missouri physicians gradually evolved. These medical school instructors received only nominal compensation, if any, for performing teaching and clinical responsibilities. Two founding fathers, Robert Schauffler, M.D., and Franklin E. Murphy, M.D., came from the Kansas City Medical College. John F. Binnie, M.D., a graduate of the University of Aberdeen in Scotland, was a surgeon and the author of a standard handbook, *Manual of Operative Surgery*. Marshall A. Barber, M.D., professor of bacteriology, had achieved an international reputation (the renowned Robert Koch of Germany found his work impressive) for perfecting a capillary pipette capable of isolating a single bacterium. Ralph H. Major, M.D., a William Jewell College graduate trained in medicine in Germany, began his tenure, first as an anatomy teacher, which, with a short break, spanned four decades. Distinguished pathologist and researcher Arthur E. Hertzler, M.D., surgeon and researcher Thomas G. Orr, M.D., nose and throat specialist Sam Roberts, M.D., obstetrics and gynecology professor Don Carlos Guffey, M.D., and clinical professor of medicine Peter T. Bohan, M.D., were among those who played significant roles in the formation of the school.

Three other pioneers died young. William T. Fitzsimons, M.D., the victim of a German bombing raid, was the first American military officer killed in World War I. Walter Sutton, M.D., an associate professor of surgery also famous for his contribution to genetics—the Sutton-Boveri hypothesis—served in and survived the war unscathed, only to die not long afterwards of acute appendicitis. S. Milo Hinch, R.N., the Supervisor of Nurses and Superintendent of Bell Hospital, died suddenly of anaphylactic shock, but not before she had secured high standards of education for Kansas nurses.

Although the Rosedale campus had begun to establish traditions of excellence, the number of students declined after those absorbed from the old proprietary schools completed their medical training. In 1915, only thirty-one medical and twenty-four nursing students graduated. The downward trend gradually was reversed, but not before it provided more ammunition for the enemies of the Rosedale location.

After Dean George Hoxie resigned, Chancellor Frank Strong tried to strengthen the medical school's political position by appointing Samuel J. Crumbine, M.D., as dean. Crumbine, who had been a frontier physician in western Kansas, was the able and energetic secretary of the Kansas State Board of Health in Topeka. His well-publicized "Swat the Fly" campaign, which promoted public involvement in the eradication of disease-bearing flies, and his crusade against unsanitary public drinking cups had made him one of the most visible men in Kansas. While critics charged that he was an empire builder who unfairly and over-zealously enforced the pure food and drug laws, Crumbine had many friends in the legislature. On the surface, his appointment seemed a good one; he remained at his health post in Topeka and, in addition, received no salary as dean. In all but name, Mervin Sudler, M.D., the associate dean, ran the medical school. Crumbine's role was to lend credibility and to handle legislative relations.

This arrangement, with Crumbine as the titular head and Sudler as the chief operating officer, lasted until 1921, when Crumbine's political opponents forced his resignation from the medical school post, although he lasted for three more years as secretary of the Board of Health. He then left Kansas for New York, where he achieved an international reputation in public health—one of many people once associated with the medical school who gained fame and fortune elsewhere.

The Rosedale site remained a problem. "From time to time, committees from the legislature would visit the Medical School," Dr. Major recalled. "After they had climbed to the top of 'Goat Hill,' getting rather dyspneic in the process, had stood on its heights, and looked out over the dreary expanse of rocky and hilly real estate, the legislators seemed rather silent and subdued when we talked about covering these hills with new buildings." At one point, the legislature appropriated seed money to build a large hospital. A rather bizarre proposal called for constructing a new Bell Hospital on a high bluff above Goat Hill, using elevators to connect the various parts of the school. The obvious solution was to locate a better site. In 1920 that option became a distinct possibility when the Rosedale city government and a consortium of medical school physicians purchased (for $32,000) a relatively level section of land known as the Kern tract and presented it to the state for a new campus. This tract was also in Rosedale, at 39th and Rainbow Boulevard, less than a mile straight south of Goat Hill. In 1922, Rosedale was annexed by Kansas City, Kansas, strengthening the medical school's political position.

After a hard fight, the legislature appropriated $235,000 to build a classroom and teaching hospital at 39th and Rainbow. The new structure opened in what is now Kansas City, Kansas, in 1924, but what should have been a joyous time soon turned sour. A bitter controversy followed in August when Governor Jonathan Davis fired Sudler over patronage matters; one charge against him was that the faculty contained too many Missouri physicians. So, even with a new building, in what should have been the brightest hour of its young life, the University of Kansas School of Medicine continued to face an uncertain future.

The photographs are a continuation of those in the first chapter, illustrating student and faculty activities, as well as the general condition of the original medical school. The views of the interior and exterior of the Rosedale campus radiate a strong sense of impermanency. Still, the medical students appear more earnest, and, perhaps, more serious and qualified than their proprietary school predecessors. Faculty members seem carefully posed, befitting their positions as prominent members of the medical community. The wartime photos of Sutton and Fitzsimons are especially poignant. Pictures of the school may be the equivalent of a thousand words, but they fail, except in a very general sense, to convey the controversies and frustrations that characterized the first two decades of the University of Kansas School of Medicine's existence. Yet, the photographs of the construction of the new facility at 39th and Rainbow provide a sharp contrast with the rather unpleasant-appearing Rosedale site—a break with past practices and the promise of a new start. Unfortunately, for every problem solved, additional problems would continue to plague the development of a public medical school in Kansas.

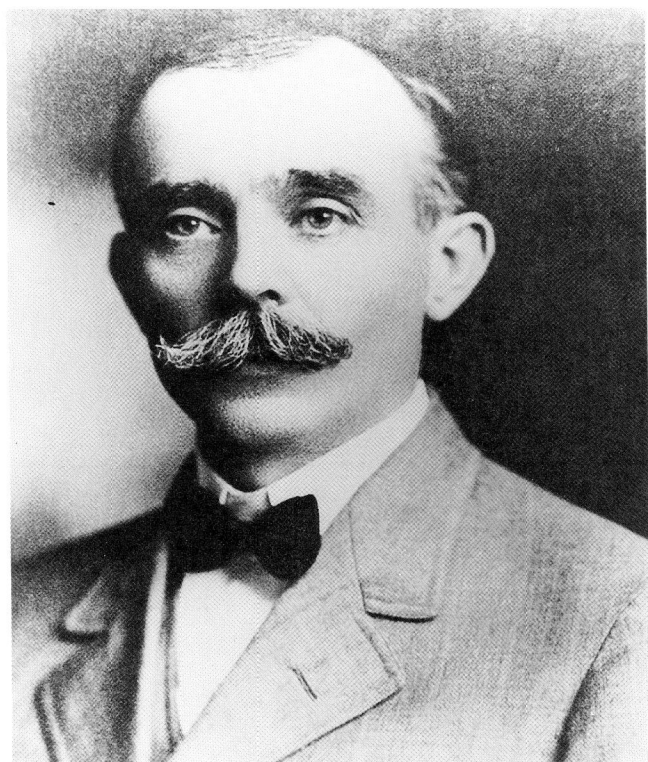

Samuel Jay Crumbine, M.D., titular dean, 1911–1919. Dr. Crumbine moved the state of Kansas into the forefront of public health issues.

The elevation of Dr. S. J. Crumbine to be the executive head of the medical school of the University of Kansas is a commendable move in the direction of bringing the work of the university and the state health department into a more effective co-operation. Doctor Crumbine has thoroughly established his efficiency as secretary of the Health Board of Kansas. He has applied the practical ideas to the methods and operation of the department that have made it a factor in the life of the state.

The medical department of the university should be the medical school for all Kansas. The state health board should operate with it, utilizing all the knowledge gained in the conduct of the school for the benefit of the public health. Doctor Crumbine is the man to make such a policy effective, as his work on the health board has demonstrated.
—"The Right Policy," *Kansas City Star*, 1911.

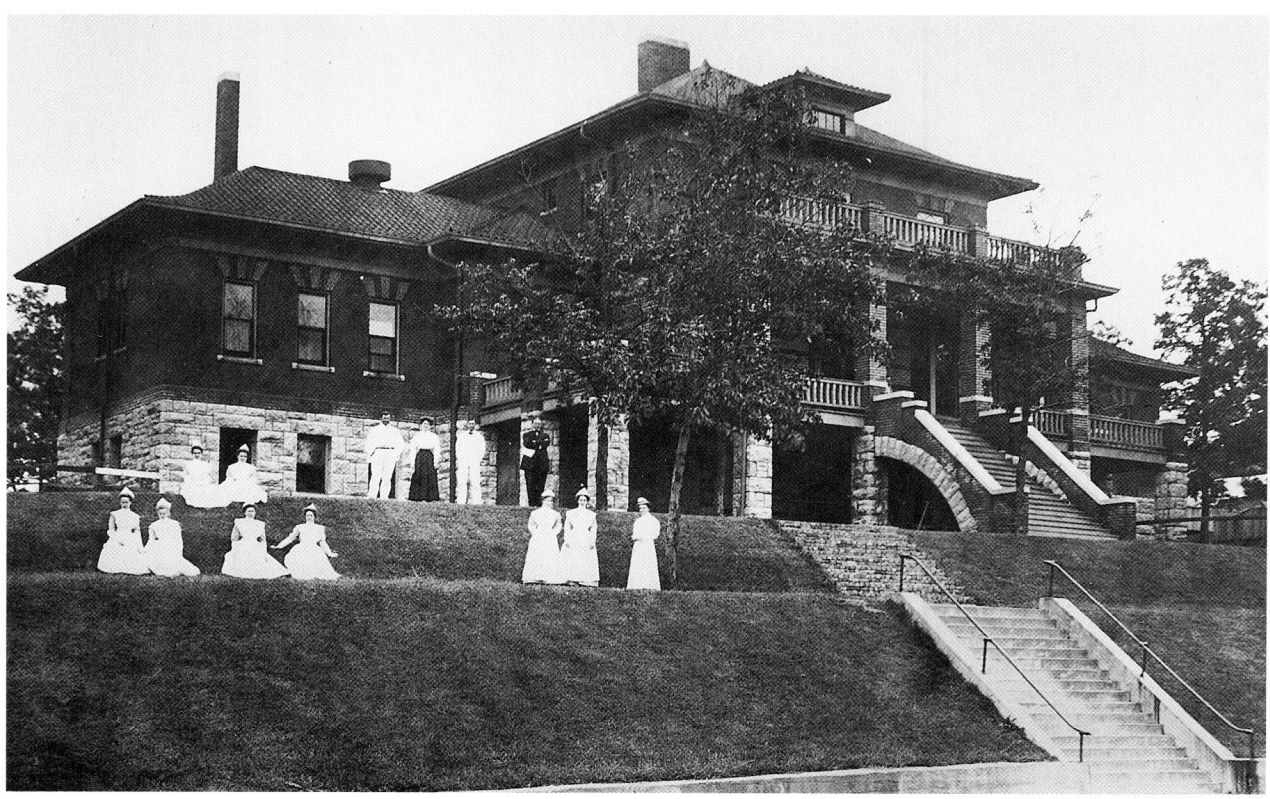

Nursing students posing on the campus in 1912.

The legislature meeting this winter will decide by its appropriation whether the medical profession will be the only profession without any provision for training and education, in the educational system of the state, or whether it will possess a school under the control of the State University with sufficient resources to meet the demands of decent medical education. And the University cannot conduct a medical school on the old haphazard plan that has been in vogue in the proprietary schools. Only University methods as recognized by the American Medical Association and the Carnegie Foundation can be used.

Whether the legislature will act favorably on the question or not, depends on the medical profession of the state. If the profession wants such an institution then it must make this want felt throughout the state and especially through the members of the legislature representing the various counties. The advice of the entire profession has been asked in making these plans. And, in fact, the directing and controlling influence lies with it. And while the school has accomplished much in the past, its future success now depends largely on the support and approval of the profession of the state.—"Will Medicine Be the Only Profession without a School Supported by the State?" *Kansas Medical Journal*, January 1911.

The plans for the school and hospital in Kansas City, Kas., contemplate a hospital for Kansas City, Kas., Wyandotte County and the whole state of Kansas, where persons will be treated and cared for at actual cost.

The principal reason for having the school in Kansas City, Kas., is that there are in large cities more persons of small means who will be treated by the school clinics than there are in the towns further out state. While these persons will get the best and most scientific medical treatment in a modern hospital, the medical students will be observing and studying their cases.
—Newspaper account, January 6, 1911.

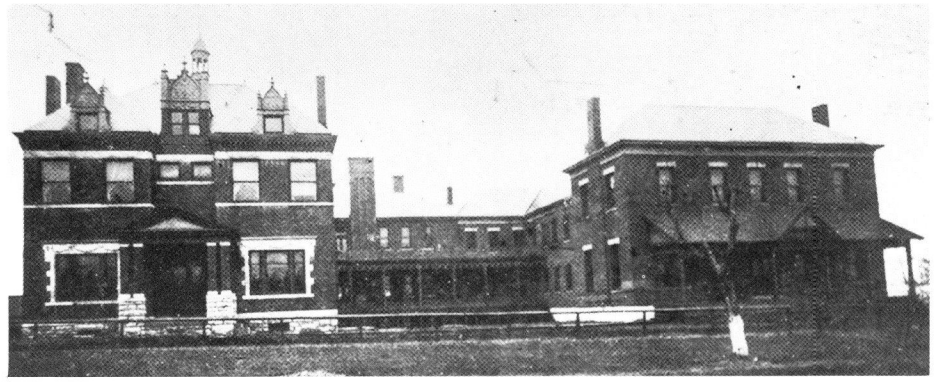

A 1909 view of Kansas City General Hospital, which served as a training facility for University of Kansas School of Medicine interns.

Medical knowledge has increased in the last half century by leaps and bounds, and with this increase medical education has become more complex. Laboratory studies have increased in number and importance, making the cost of instruction much greater. This has been so great that the colleges organized and maintained for individual profit have disappeared, and only such institutions as have adequate support from the state or private endowment may hope to survive. Meanwhile, this wider scope has assumed such importance that the training of physicians is only a part of the work. However, that there is a demand in Kansas for this education of physicians by the University is shown by the increasing number of requests from various communities of the state for young physicians, and by an entering class of fifty students in September, 1913. It is now the only recognized School of Medicine in the State of Kansas.
—"The Training of Physicians," *Bulletin of the University of Kansas*, October 1, 1914.

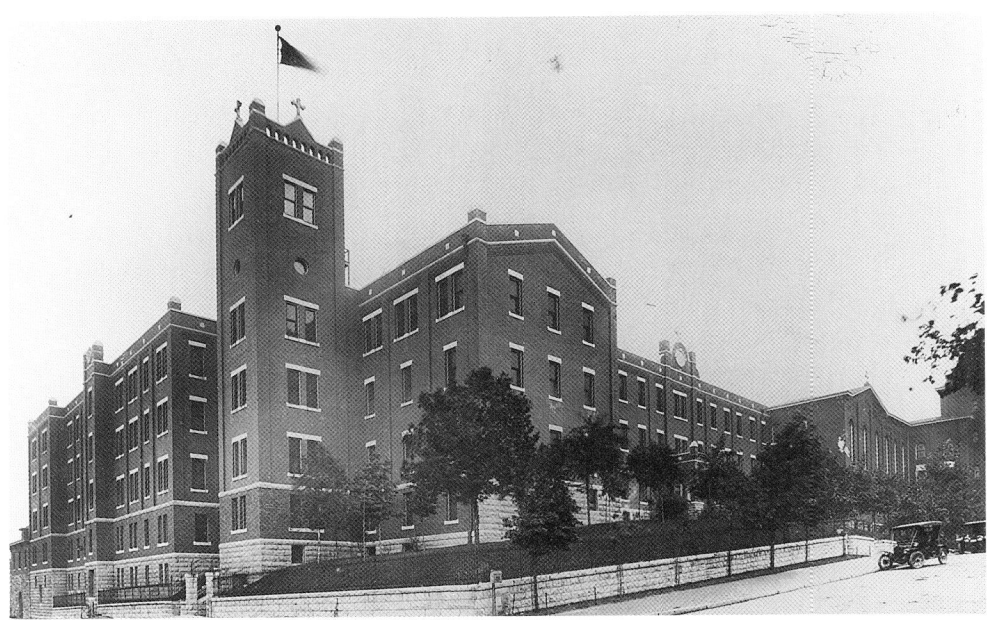

St. Margaret's Hospital was also used as a clinical training facility for the medical school. At the time (ca. 1910) St. Margaret's would not allow women medical students or interns to train there, so they were sent to General Hospital in Kansas City, Missouri.

Miss S. Milo Hinch, a Canadian maiden lady and a graduate of the New York Hospital, was Supervisor of Nurses and Superintendent of the Bell Memorial Hospital. She was a rather large woman of middle age, amply proportioned but not obese, quite incisive and positive in her statements, and regarded as a strict disciplinarian. However, she had a fund of dry humor and was a very interesting conversationalist.

Miss Hinch set a high standard of education for her nurses, and, while they had a certain awe of her, mingled at times with a touch of fear, I never heard a nurse whom she had trained speak of her except in terms of deepest respect and gratitude for the excellent training she had received from Miss Hinch.
—Ralph H. Major, M.D., *An Account of the University of Kansas School of Medicine*, 1968.

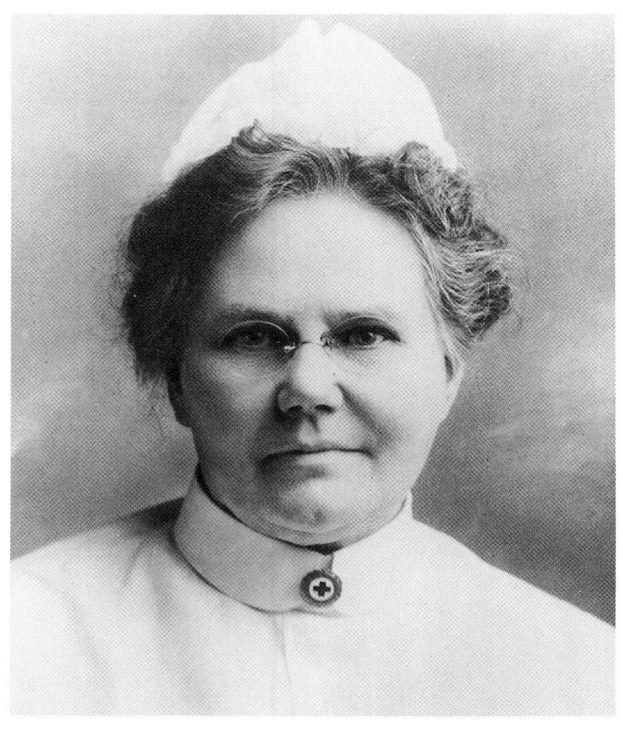

S. Milo Hinch, R.N., was supervisor of nurses and superintendent of Bell Memorial Hospital from 1914 to 1920.

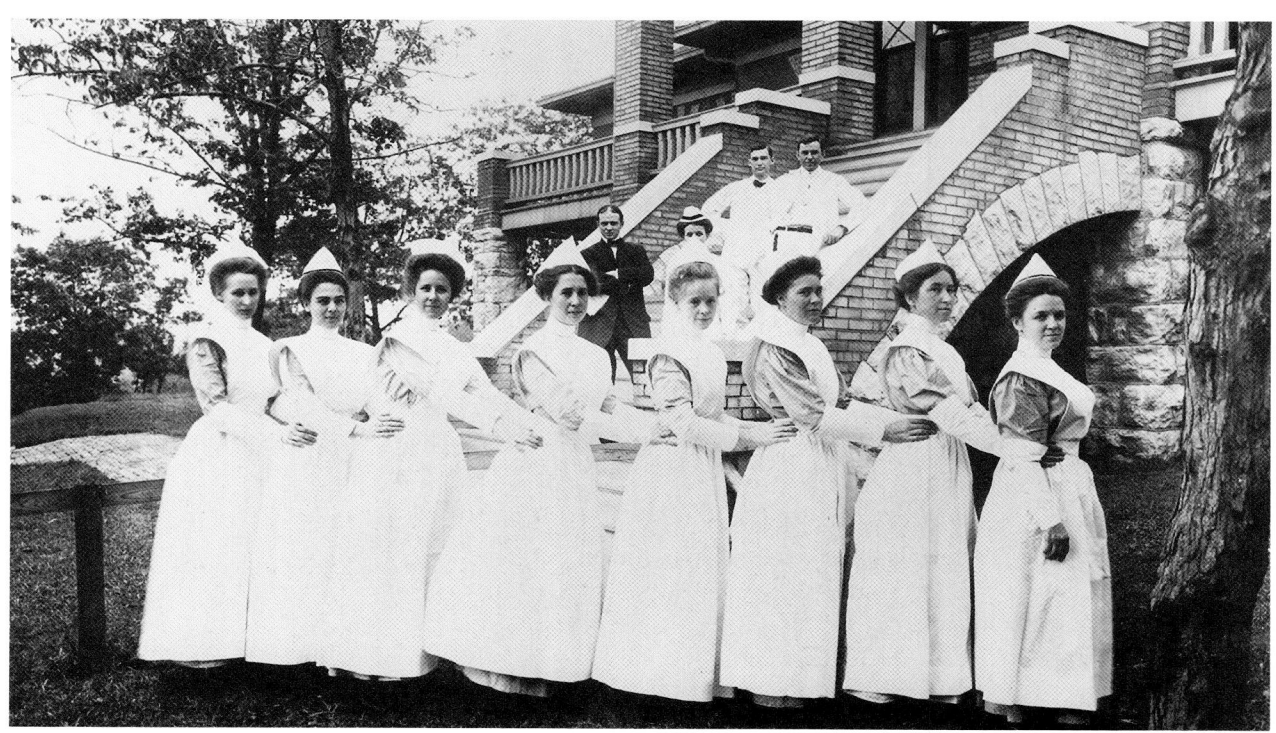

Students of the Training School for Nurses, 1912.

The Training School for Nurses: Women of good character between the ages of twenty and thirty are eligible for admission. Those with a high-school education are given preference. Those who are accepted are accepted with the understanding that they must spend a probationary period of three months in the school, during which time they will receive board, laundry and lodging, but no other compensation. During the remainder of the course an allowance of $7 a month is given to cover the expense of uniforms, books and instruments.

A young woman who wishes to enter the school must make formal application to the supervisor of nurses of the Bell Memorial Hospital, Rosedale. With this application should be sent letters showing what educational advantages she has enjoyed, testifying to her good moral character, and to her good health.—*Bulletin of the University of Kansas*, October 1, 1914.

The Bell Memorial Hospital
requests the honor of your presence at the
Graduating Exercises
of the
Nurses of the Training School
on Friday evening, April the thirteenth
one thousand nine hundred and seventeen
at eight o'clock
New Dispensary Building
Rosedale, Kansas

Graduation announcement for the Training School for Nurses, 1917.

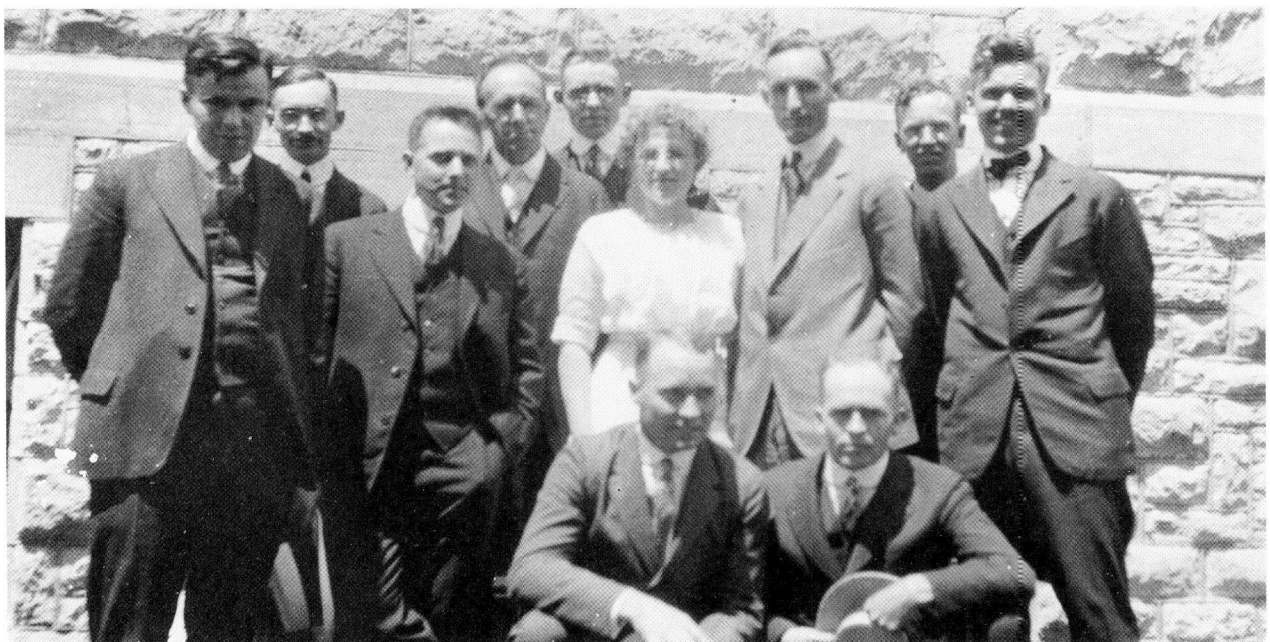

The medical class of 1916.

I think I have said to you all that is necessary in the argument for Topeka, except this one practical suggestion that the Kansas Legislature will not make an appropriation for an institution to be located practically in Missouri. All modern methods and modern men which you desire to bring to the service of Kansas City could be brought to Topeka. No one would object in the least and all will give hearty co-operation.

Here is a city of 100,000 on one hand and a city of 50,000 on the other. You are a stranger to the conditions here. . . . I think the same argument has operated in the minds of various Kansas physicians who have voted on the subject. The merit of the question, I think is that the rabble of Packing Houses in Kansas City will not support a Medical College. Whereas, the citizenship of Kansas will do so, if given an opportunity.—W. S. Lindsay, dean, Kansas Medical College, to Mervin T. Sudler, M.D., January 25, 1911.

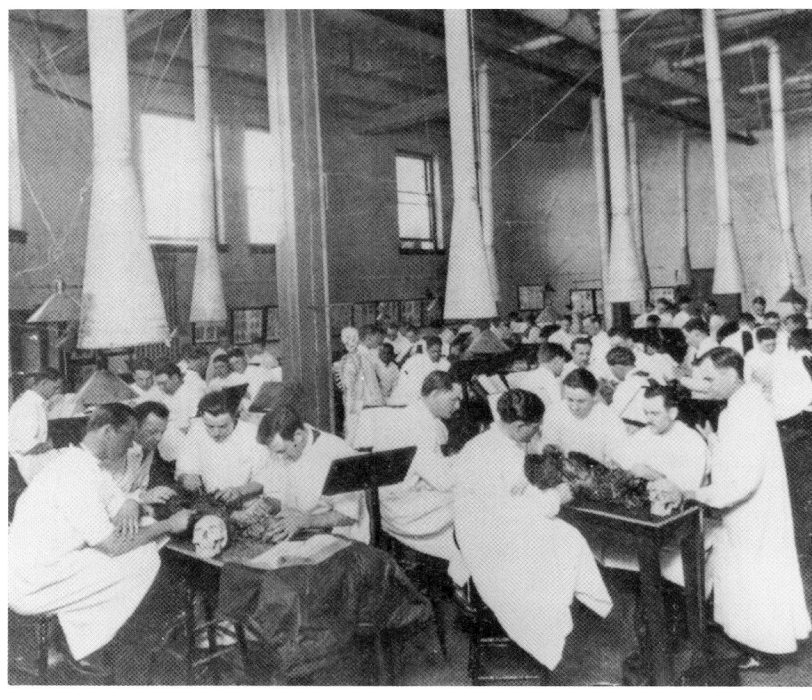

A medical school anatomy class, ca. 1920.

Practically all of our faculty and everyone who has worked here agree that there is not a better opportunity in the United States to develop a medical school than there is right here. In fact, I do not believe that any other institution can show the results for the facilities and the amount of money invested. We have always been a Class "A" institution; though we have often been on "the edge," so to speak.

When you remember that the school of medicine of the University of Kansas stood ninth in point of attendance and sixteenth in point of income, I think that speaks for itself. However, I feel sure that we cannot maintain our present work unless the new hospital is under construction or authorized, with the inspection coming in this winter. All of the members of the faculty felt very strongly that at the last legislature the State should decide to either support a Class "A" institution or discontinue the school. —Mervin T. Sudler, M.D., associate dean, University of Kansas School of Medicine, to Dr. Huffman, October 1, 1919.

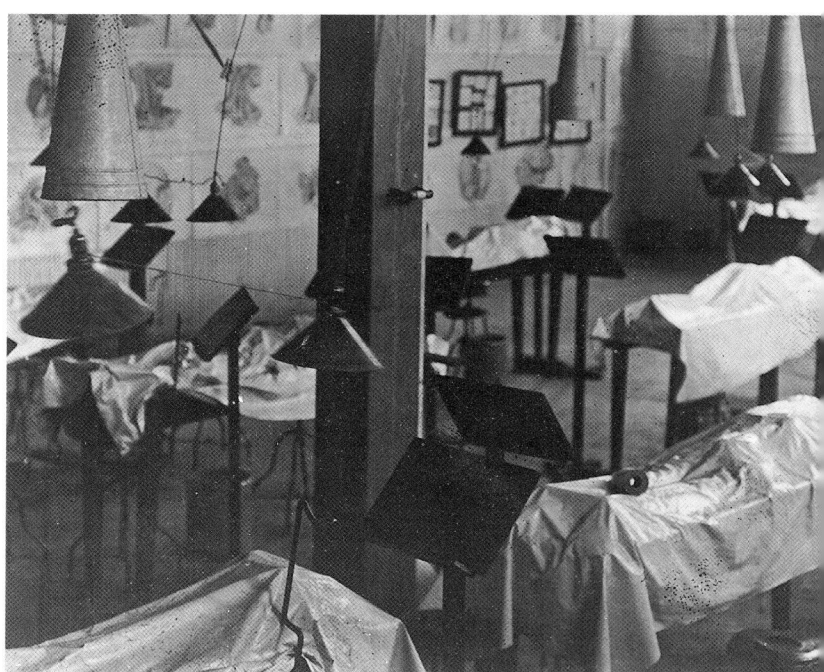

Laboratory and dissecting room.

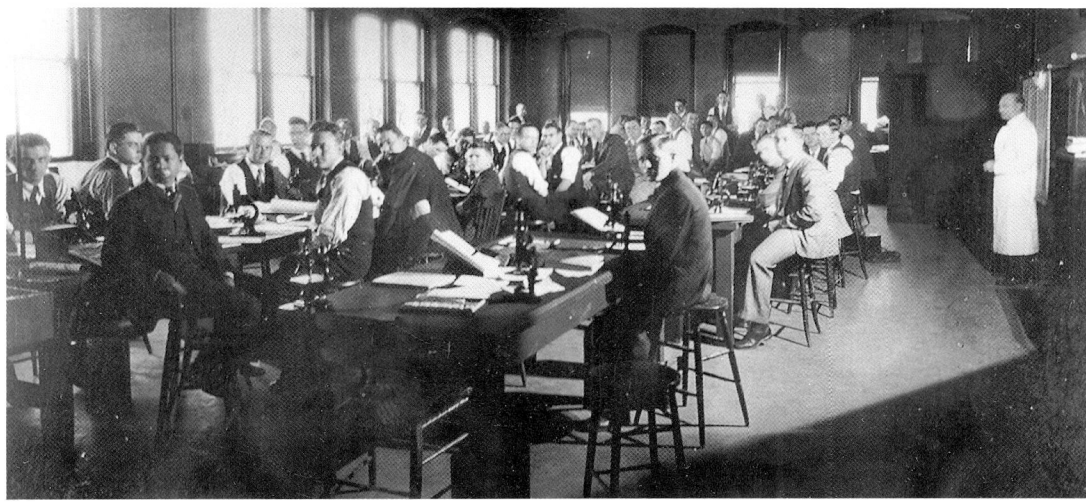

Students in a laboratory class, early 1920s.

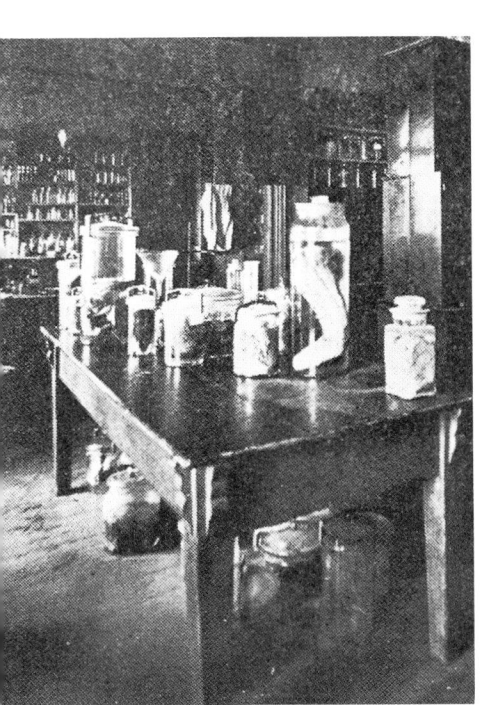

Pathology laboratory and museum, ca. 1920.

During the past year the work has been difficult for a number of reasons: More space is needed both for the hospital and the dispensary. The hospital especially needs acommodations for patients suffering from contagious diseases and tuberculosis. So far, it has been impossible to install any X-ray equipment; and this is urgently needed. No adequate roadway has been provided from the street through the grounds belonging to the institution, and at times it has been necessary to carry patients upstairs for about thirty feet in order that they might enter the hospital. The work of the out-patient department has suffered from the same cause. It is essential that adjoining property be acquired and that the grading and paving necessary to provide an easy approach be done as soon as possible. —"Report of the Work of the Bell Memorial Hospital at Rosedale, Kansas," *Bulletin of the University of Kansas*, December 1, 1912.

At the end of the laboratory there were a number of cases with open shelves upon which rested glass jars containing pathological specimens. This museum of pathological anatomy . . . was, as I found out later, an excellent collection. It had, however, been neglected . . . and now many jars were empty, others had lost their tops and were half filled with fluid out of which protruded drying and disintegrating specimens.

But what disturbed me particularly was the rubbish which had accumulated on the floor in heaps—broken test tubes, dried up specimens, empty cardboard boxes, waste paper, and just plain dirt. . . . When I asked about the janitor service, I learned that the janitor lived in a room on the basement floor, but, as he had a bad heart and could not climb the stairs, Dr. Sudler didn't have the heart to ask him to come up to the second floor. When I saw the poor fellow later, trying to go up the stairs to the first floor, puffing with each step and as blue as a baby with congenital heart disease, I understood Dr. Sudler's compassion and also realized that the pathological department would have to be its own janitor.—Ralph H. Major, M.D., *An Account of the University of Kansas School of Medicine*, 1968.

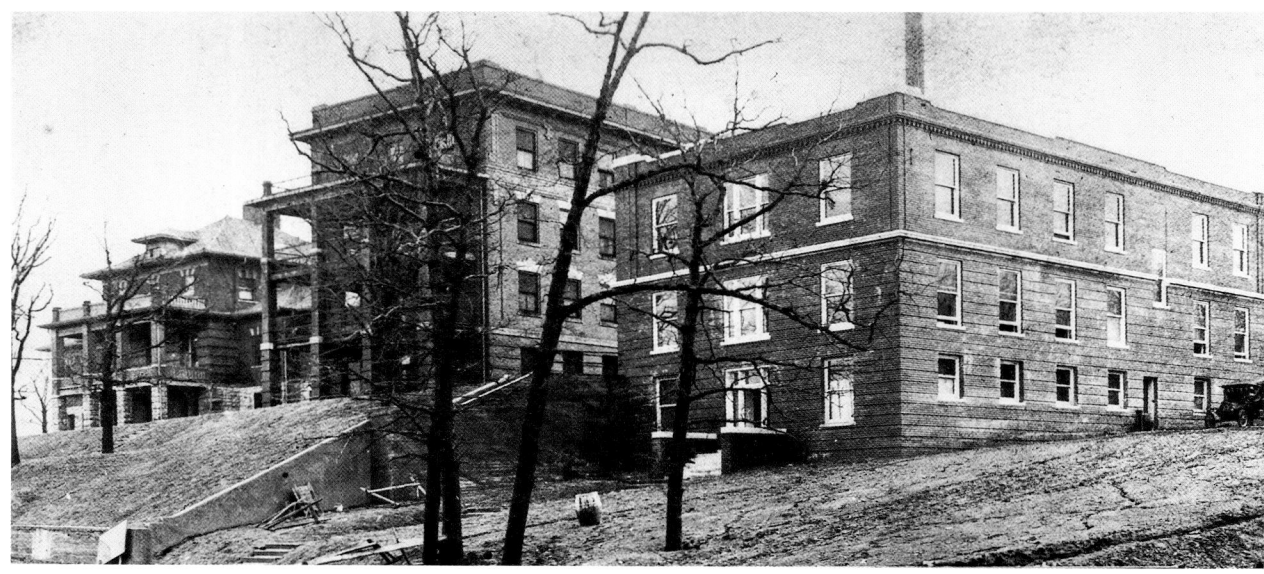

The completed Goat Hill campus of the University of Kansas School of Medicine, 1916.

It is with the deepest regret I learn that the Commercial Club of Topeka will ask this legislature to remove the medical school from Rosedale to Topeka.

Several years ago I gave a large portion of my property to the State with the assurance that the school and the hospital would be located on it, there to remain for all time. I did this through a desire to do something to help advance my profession and also that I might erect a living monument to the memory of my wife, Eleanor Taylor Bell.

My home was made on Kansas soil several years before Kansas was given a place among the States of our Union, and so great was my faith in her people that I gave deed in fee simple to my lands and thousands of dollars of my money so that the State might do the thing I so much desired.

The chancellor and the board of regents of the university assured me that my gifts would be held sacred for the purpose given.

The legislature accepted my property and have sold it and given deeds to it and have taken my money and spent it, and even though I now be reimbursed, to take it away will be a great disappointment to me—a complete shattering of my early and lifelong ambition—and, coming as it does in the ninety-third year of my life, with my body feeble and my mind having lost largely of its former power of concentration, I feel it as a great blow.

Knowing that I am nearing the other side, I earnestly ask that the legislature of 1913 finally and for all time to come to settle the question of the location of the medical school that I may, with an unshaken faith in the people of my state, die in peace. And as my last request I ask that the appropriation for the medical school this year be granted.

Because of my feebleness I have asked my son-in-law, L. H. Rose, to represent me. Please write him and, through him, let me know what you will do for me.

—Simeon Bishop Bell, M.D., to the Kansas State Legislature, January 10, 1913.

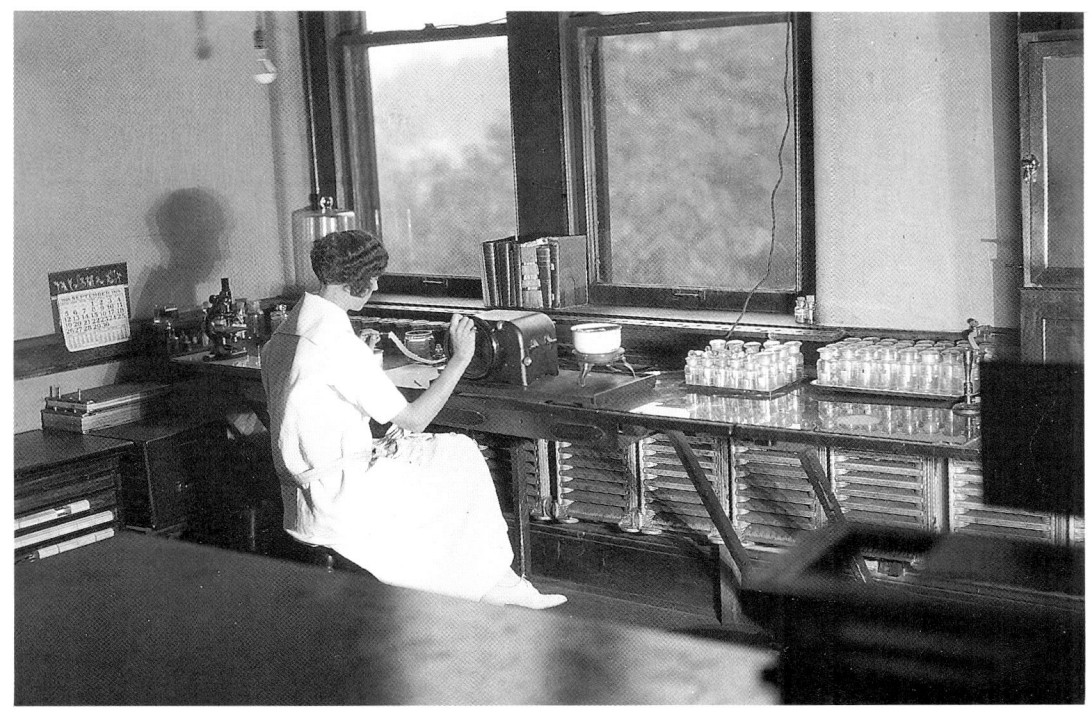

A laboratory assistant at work, early 1920s.

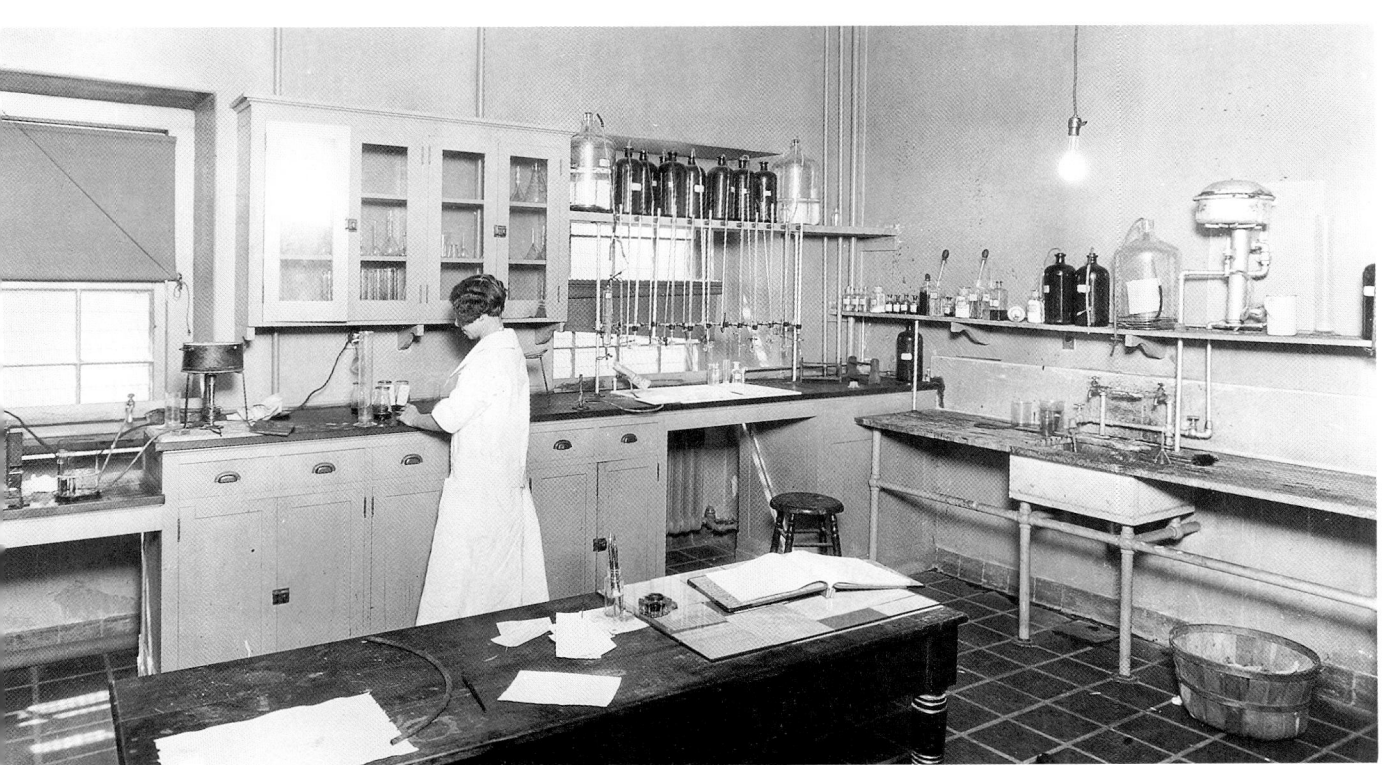

A laboratory in Eleanor Taylor Bell Hospital, ca. 1923.

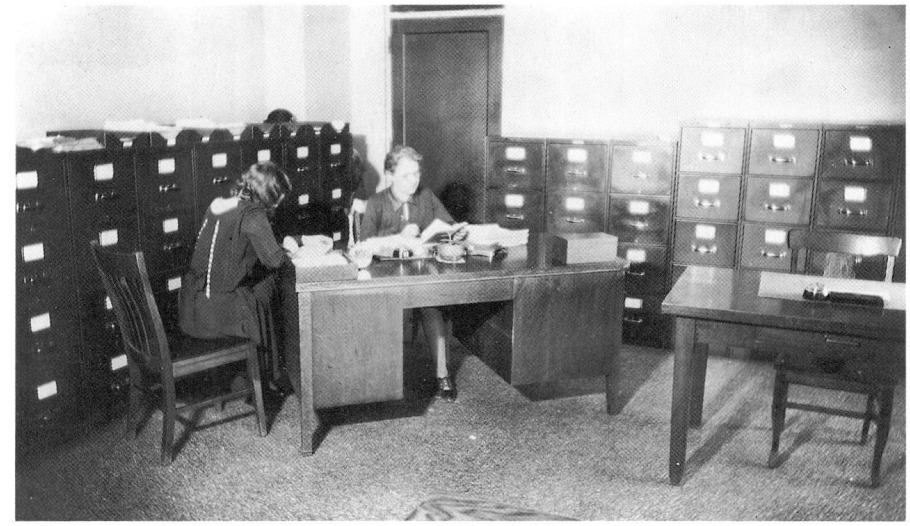

The medical records room in the early 1920s.

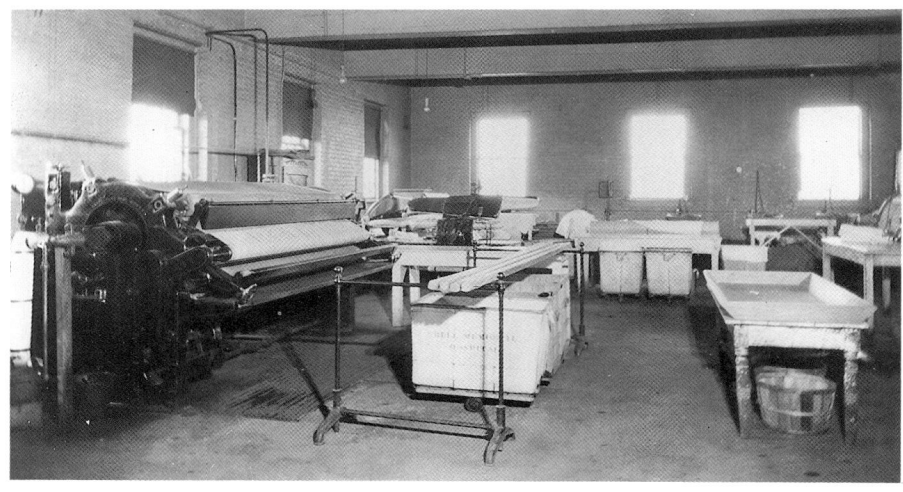

A 1920s view of the hospital's laundry facility.

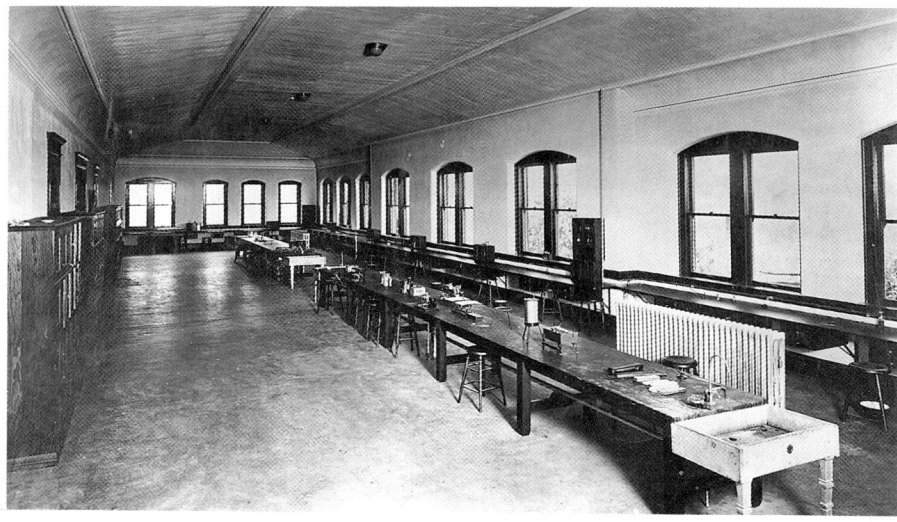

The interior of the general laboratory for clinical pathology, ca. 1918.

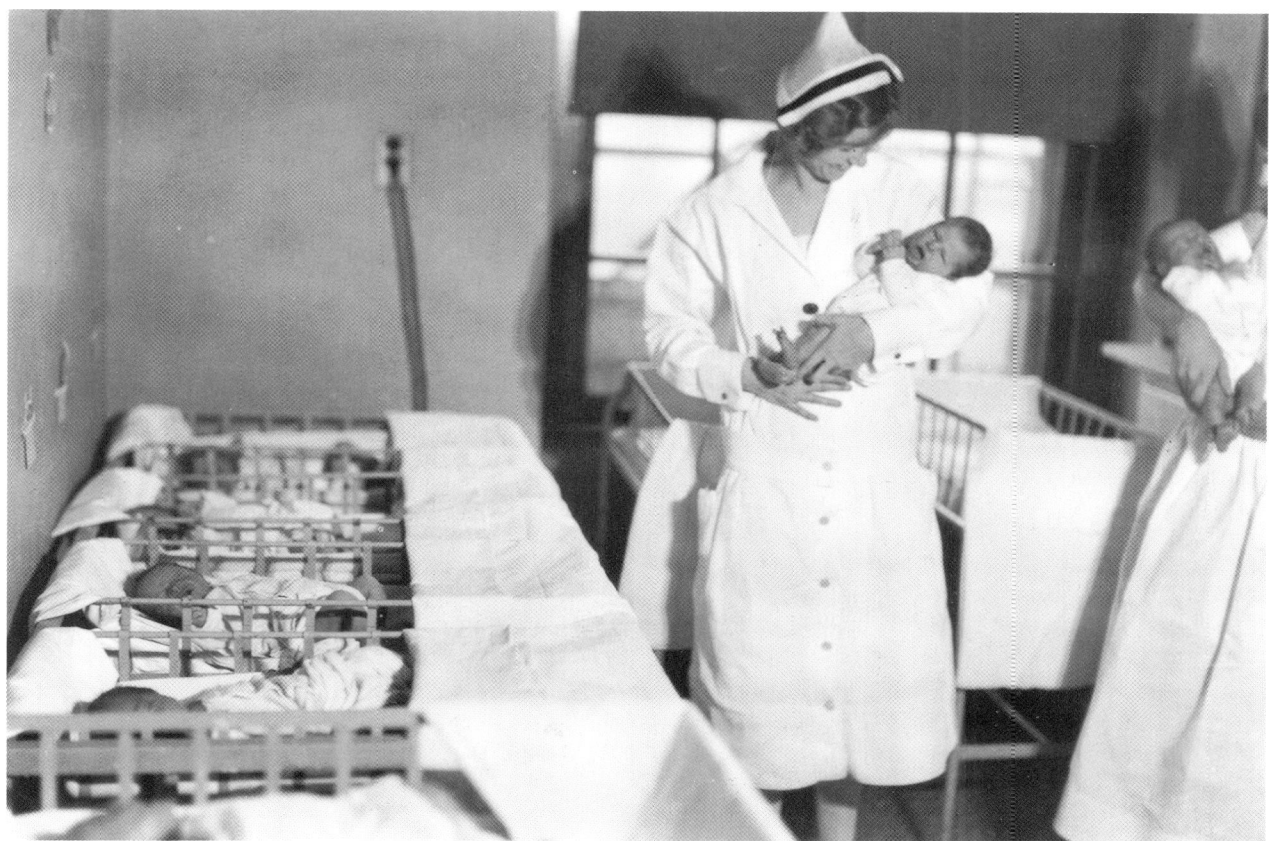

The hospital nursery, ca. 1922.

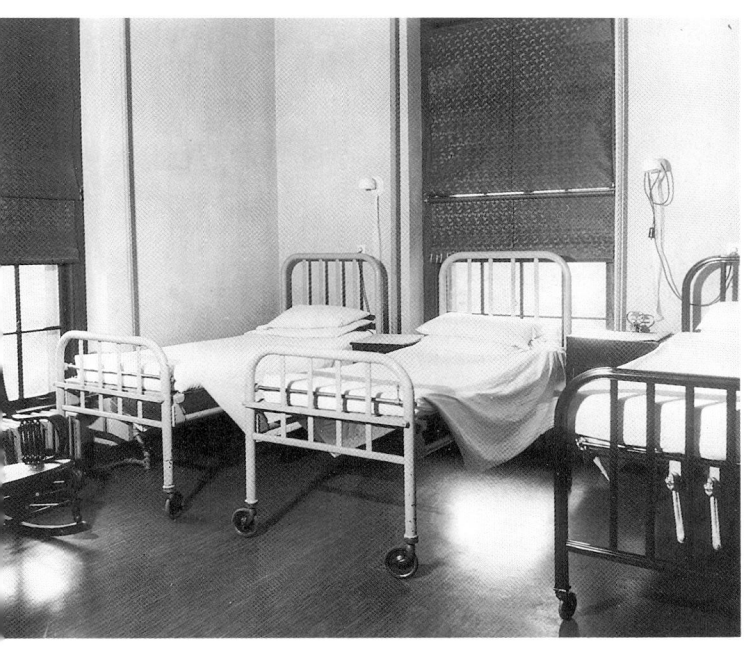

The pediatrics ward in 1920.

As I have told you on a number of occasions, I have never seen a better opportunity for the development of a medical school than there is here. We have more students than we can properly take care of. Our hospital is continually overflowing in spite of the unattractiveness of the acommodations in comparison with those of other institutions. The National Government, as you know, has asked that the medical school be kept intact and running; and as far as I know this is the only institution maintained by the State of Kansas of which the Government has made this request.

Because of the lack of support of the institution by the State, the medical school has had to stand still, which means that it is losing step. . . . This lack of support in view of the national emergency and the needs of the people at present seems criminal.
—Mervin T. Sudler, M.D., to Chancellor Lindley, March 11, 1918.

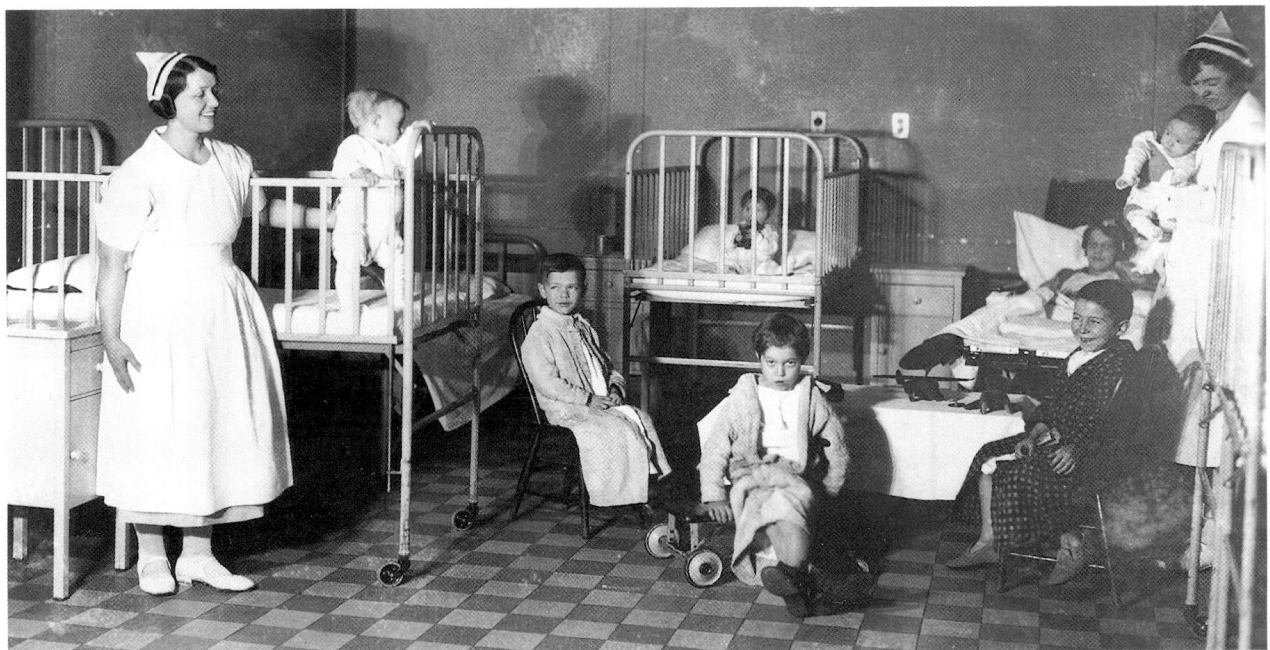

Student nurses with pediatric patients, ca. 1924.

There is going to be a medical school somewhere in Kansas. . . . Wyandotte County can have it. Rosedale can have it. But the thing she must do is to obtain the necessary money to buy the land, or else the proposition is lost to her forever.

If Wyandotte County purchases land, there will grow up on that hill, where the present Bell Memorial Hospital is located, one of the greatest medical schools in the West.
—"Appeal by Governor Allen," *Kansas City Times,* November 14, 1919.

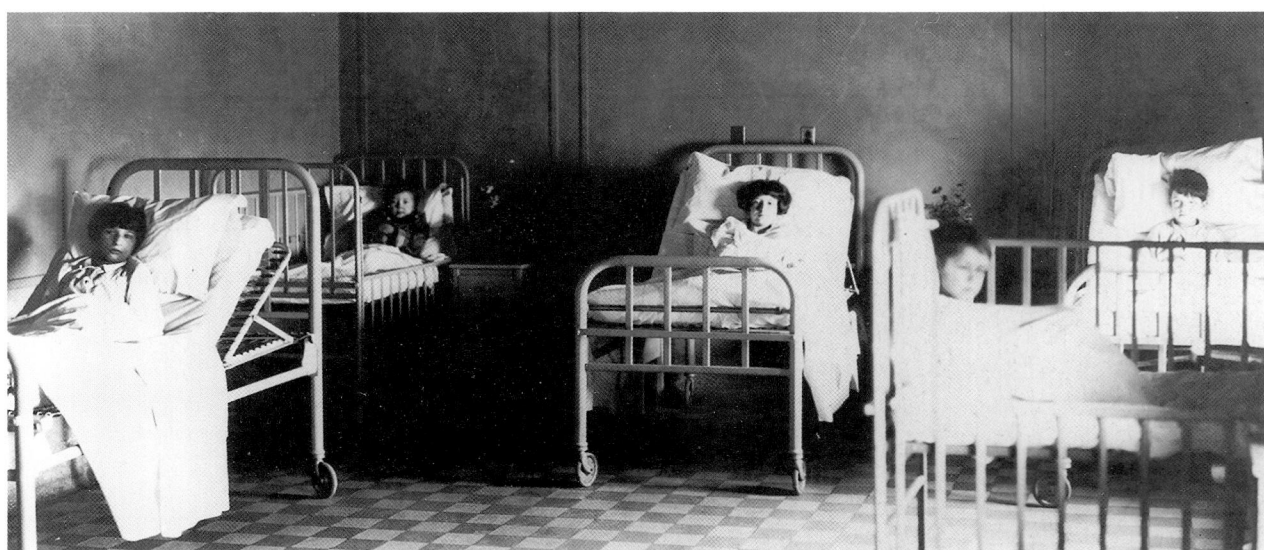

A corner of the Children's Ward in Bell Memorial Hospital, 1920s.

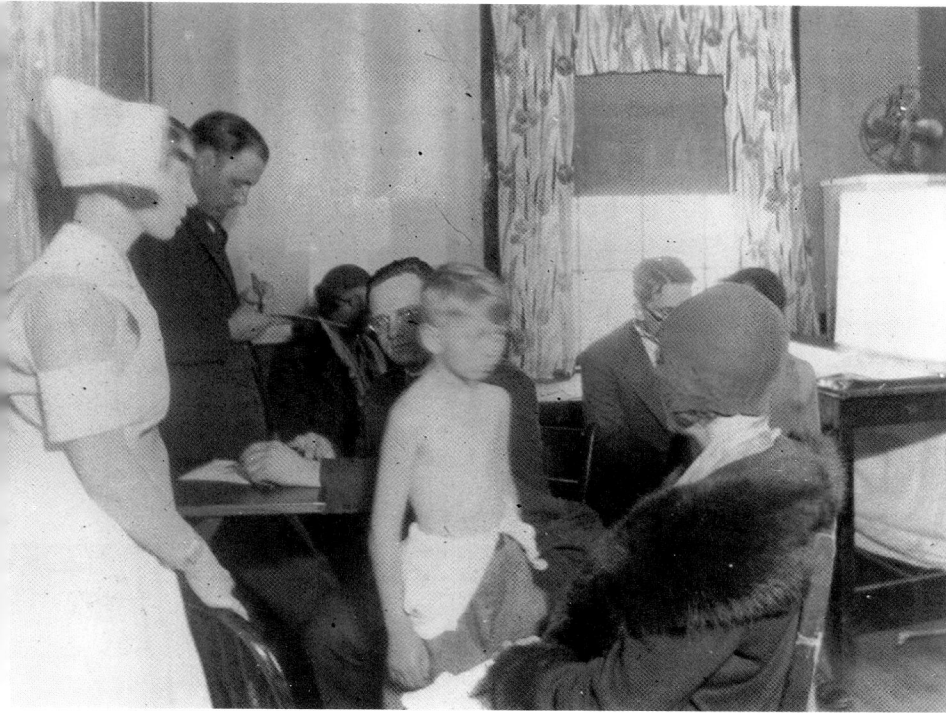

Patients in the pediatric clinic, early 1920s.

There are poor persons—men, women, and children—in every community suffering from curable diseases, needing only the right treatment to make them comfortable, perhaps well, and even self-supporting. Unless state aid or private charity be extended to these unfortunates their diseases will run their courses.

Our social organization has many defects. Men are born with unequal intelligence, ability and worldly goods, receive unequal education, and therefore the best that social justice has yet done places and leaves most of the wealth in the hands of a few. —"Report of the Medical Work of the University of Kansas," *Bulletin of the University of Kansas,* November 1, 1916.

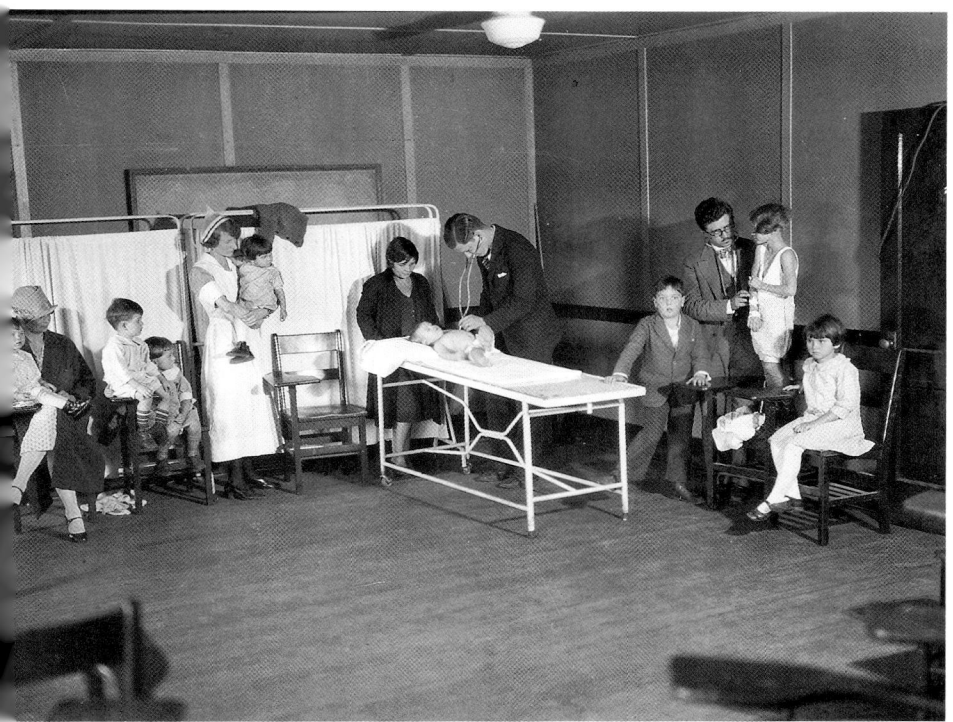

A doctor examining children in the pediatric clinic.

Kansas City, Kansas, has neither a tuberculosis sanitorium nor a quarantine hospital for contagious diseases. No person, no matter how rich nor how poor can avail themselves of hospital care in Kansas City, Kansas, if they are suffering with diptheria, small pox, measles, scarlet fever or kindred diseases. Often we cannot properly quarantine people, as for instance, in a rooming house, because of no hospital facilities, and thus the public health is endangered.

The student at Kansas University does not have access to any contagious work while in school. . . . The students surely need that work.—*Kansas City Kansan,* June 8, 1920.

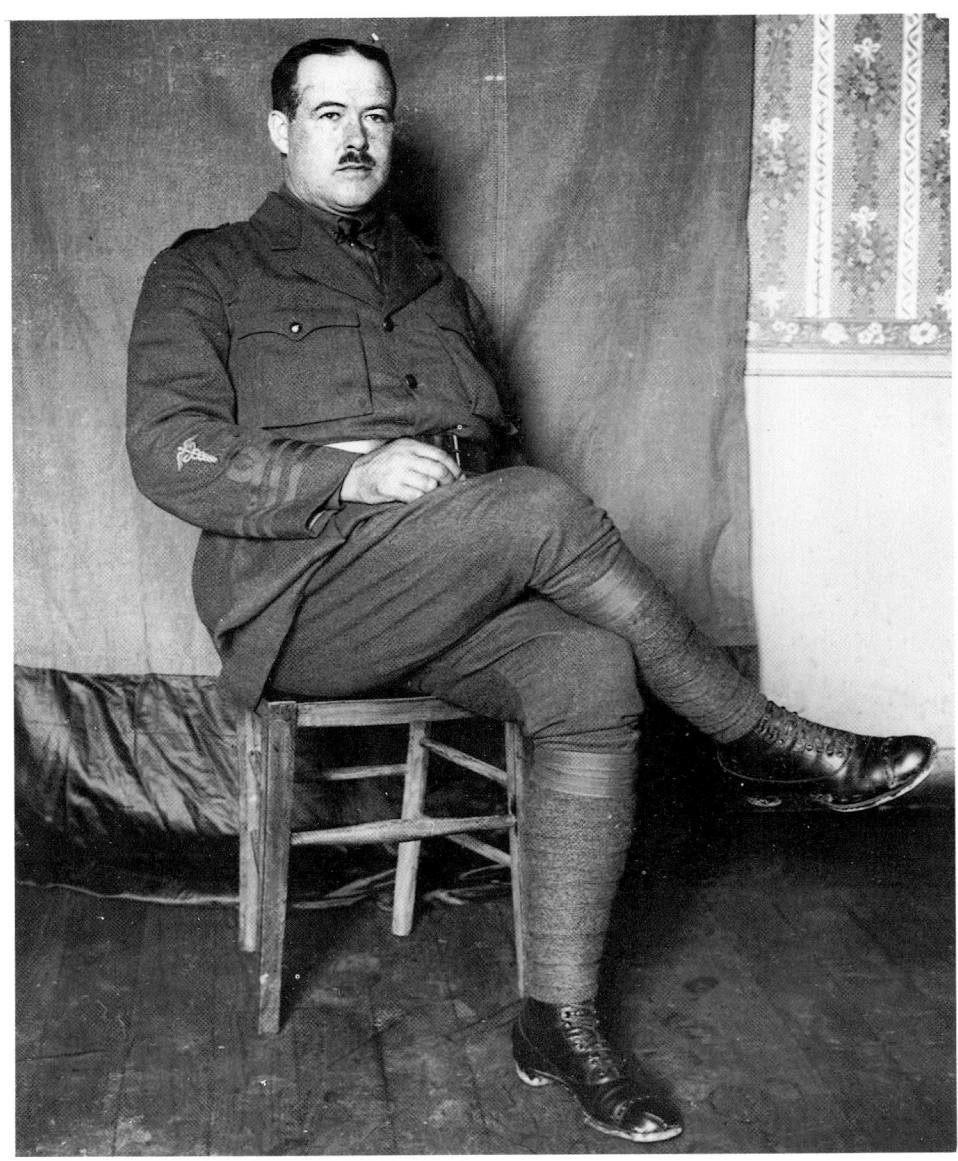

Walter S. Sutton, M.D., in military uniform.

Dr. Walter Stanborough Sutton was assistant professor of surgery at the University of Kansas from 1909 until his death in 1916. . . . His paper, "The Chromosomes in Heredity" published in April, 1903, is one of the major landmarks in biomedical literature. For six months during 1915, he was on military leave, a member of the surgical staff of the Mrs. Harry Payne Whitney Unit of the American Ambulance Hospital in France. He became an expert in war surgery. His inventive ability produced instruments capable of localizing foreign bodies such as bullets and shell fragments with a fluoroscopic x-ray screen. His method was the first of three systems of x-ray localization to be taught every military roentgenologist during World War I.

His publications were limited—because his brilliant career was cut short by his death at 39 from a ruptured appendix.—*Bulletin, the University of Kansas School of Medicine and Medical Center*, February 1965.

On the day Walter Sutton entered the University of Kansas, he was a marked man. His fellow students, as well as the Faculty who had the profound privilege of having him in their classes, recognized him as unusual in the degree in which he possessed a number of admirable traits. . . . So, it was in the most natural way that the University came to regard him as an extraordinary student. His University expected much of him, and he never disappointed it.—*Emporia Gazette*, November 13, 1916.

To most of us the great war has seemed a long distance away and the hideous frightfulness of it all only penetrates our consciousness dimly—"The blood of men runs not red ten thousand miles away." We are told that men are giving their lives to the cause of liberty and justice but these are men whom we have never seen and to whom we had no personal tie. The death of the first American army officer in France changed this and brought home keenly to the University of Kansas that the liberty of our country was again in jeopardy and that men were giving their all in order that democracy might live; and the future of a free country be safe-guarded. The old truth that war takes its death toll from the youngest, most promising, and best has again been emphasized. To those of us who bade goodbye to Dr. Fitzsimons only a short time previously when he left his work in the School of Medicine, the news of his death on the night of September 4, 1917, when the Harvard unit in France was bombed by airplanes, brings the realization of the immense sacrifice which war extracts from a country.
—Associate Dean Mervin T. Sudler, M.D., in *Graduate Magazine*, vol. 16, 1917–1918.

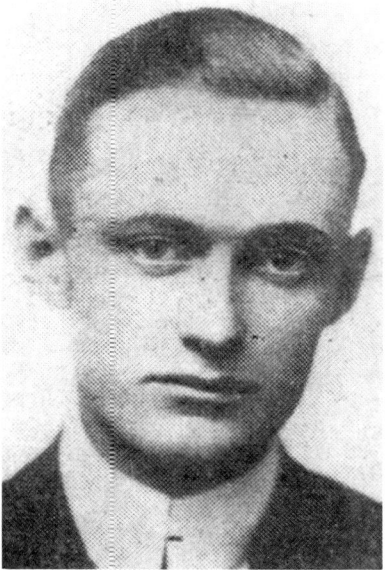

The first American officer killed by enemy action during World War I, William T. Fitzsimons, M.D., was both a graduate and faculty member of the University of Kansas School of Medicine.

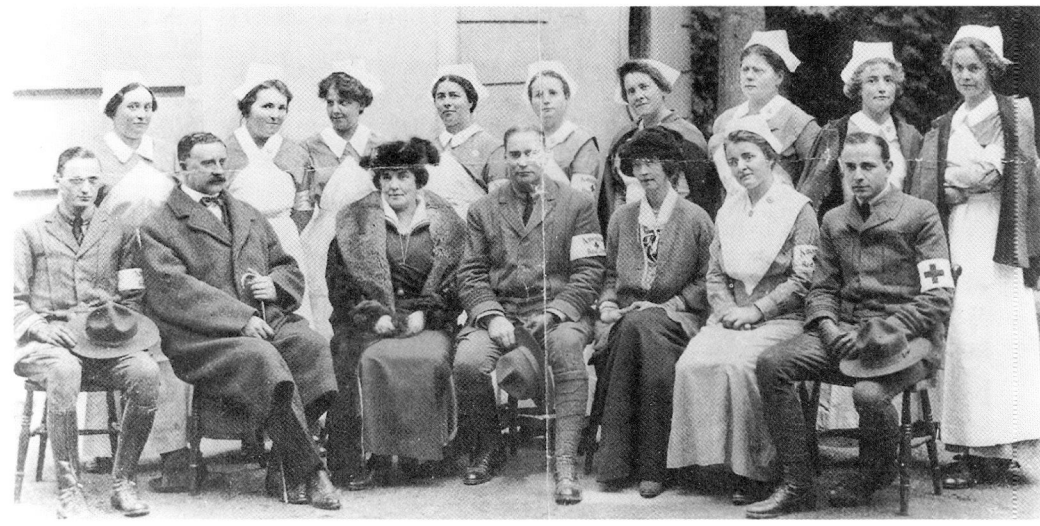

Dr. William T. Fitzsimons (left front) with his military hospital unit in England, 1917.

The legislature, from our point of view, was composed of a few friends, more enemies, and then the great mass of indifferents. The Governor of the state, at the time of my introduction to state politics, was rather friendly to the school; his successor was definitely hostile, proposing on one occasion that the state abolish the Medical School and subsidize the medical students, sending them out of the state to get their medical education. Later, after the rather reluctant state legislature had passed a very modest appropriation bill for the Medical School, the Governor, in a public statement, said that he was signing the appropriation bill with no enthusiasm and that he would like to veto the appropriation for the Medical School but could not do so without vetoing the appropriation for the entire University.
—Ralph H. Major, M.D., *An Account of the University of Kansas School of Medicine*, 1968.

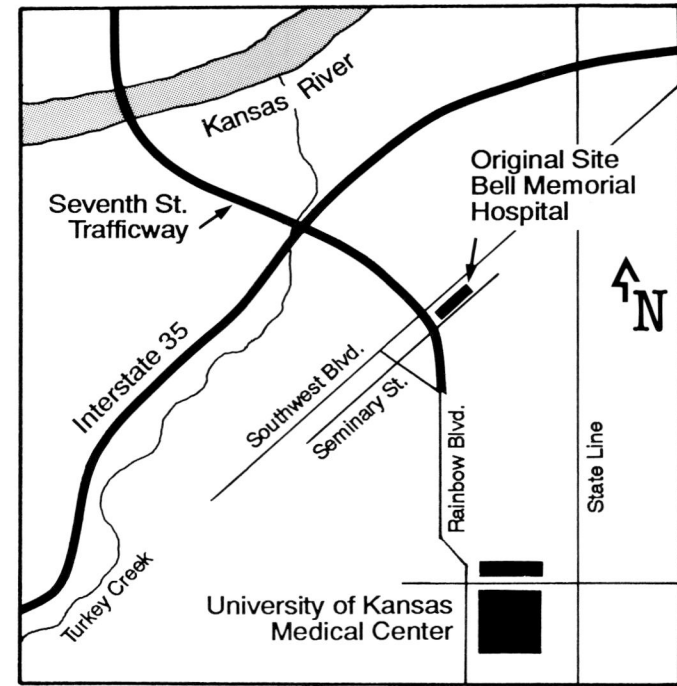

The citizens of Rosedale have caught the vision of a great medical school, a Kansas institution, to be erected and maintained permanently in Wyandotte County. And the little town, unaided as yet by Wyandotte County or the Kansas City, Kas., Chamber of Commerce, is going in to save the medical school with a determination and a punch that argue well for the raising of $35,000 for additional lands on which the state may spend $200,000 available for additional buildings to the present Bell Memorial Hospital.
—"Good for Rosedale," *Kansas City Times*, November 15, 1919.

Kansas is witnessing the spectacle of its state university being used as a political plum tree for "deserving Democrats." The Dean of the medical school, Dr. M. T. Sudler, whose name has been linked indelibly with the state medical school and with Bell Memorial hospital as the man who built the school and hospital, has been dismissed because Governor Davis has a Democratic politician who must be "taken care of."
—*Kansas City Star*, July 24, 1924.

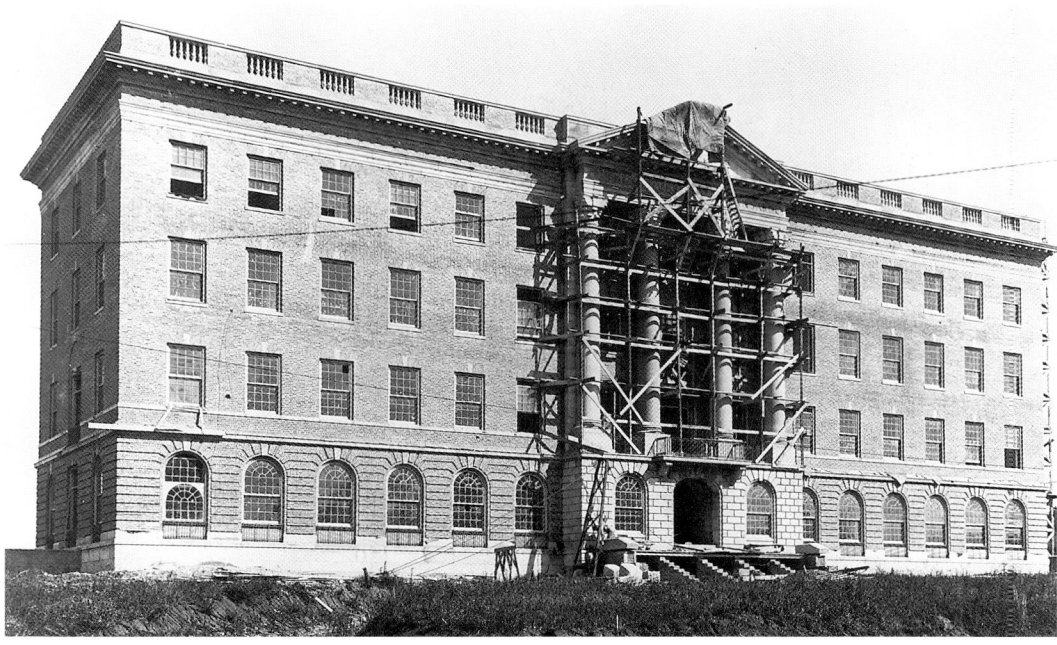

The new University of Kansas School of Medicine and Bell Memorial Hospital nearing completion in 1923.

The University of Kansas, according to reports, has for years been subject to injurious political influence and recent evidence supports these reports. Several months ago the Governor went over the head of Chancellor Lindley and "fired" Dr. Mervin T. Sudler, the dean of the medical school. More recently (Dec. 27, 1924) the Governor peremptorily "removed" the Chancellor himself—but an injunction has been granted to prevent it. . . .

The teaching plant at Kansas City is just now in its worst plight so far as lack of concentration is concerned. Its clinical building with the laboratories and library is at Rosedale, while the center of teaching at present is at the new Bell Hospital, one mile further south, in Kansas City, Kansas. Some clinical teaching is done at St. Margaret's Hospital some four miles away as the crow flies, but several more before one can get there either by automobile or street cars.
—Association of American Medical Colleges Inspection Report, December 4 and 5, 1924.

I also appreciate your good opinion about my pioneering work in the medical school. All I can say is that I gave all I had in the way of planning and effort for eighteen years to try to develop it. It was a case of making "bricks without straw" and when I was dismissed without reaching my cherished goal of a teacher of surgery I did my best to forget that part of my life. . . .

If I had realized just how long and how much pioneering it would require I would certainly have been too frightened to undertake it.
—Mervin T. Sudler, M.D., to Harry R. Wahl, M.D., July 17, 1948.

Mervin Sudler did more than develop the medical school. He blew the breath of life into it on numerous occasions when the last spark of life had apparently fled. He also gathered about him a group of energetic enthusiastic young men, whom he inspired with his enthusiasm for high standards in medical education and his determination that the University of Kansas School of Medicine should not perish from this earth.
—Ralph H. Major, M.D., "Mervin Tubman Sudler, 1875–1956," unpublished eulogy.

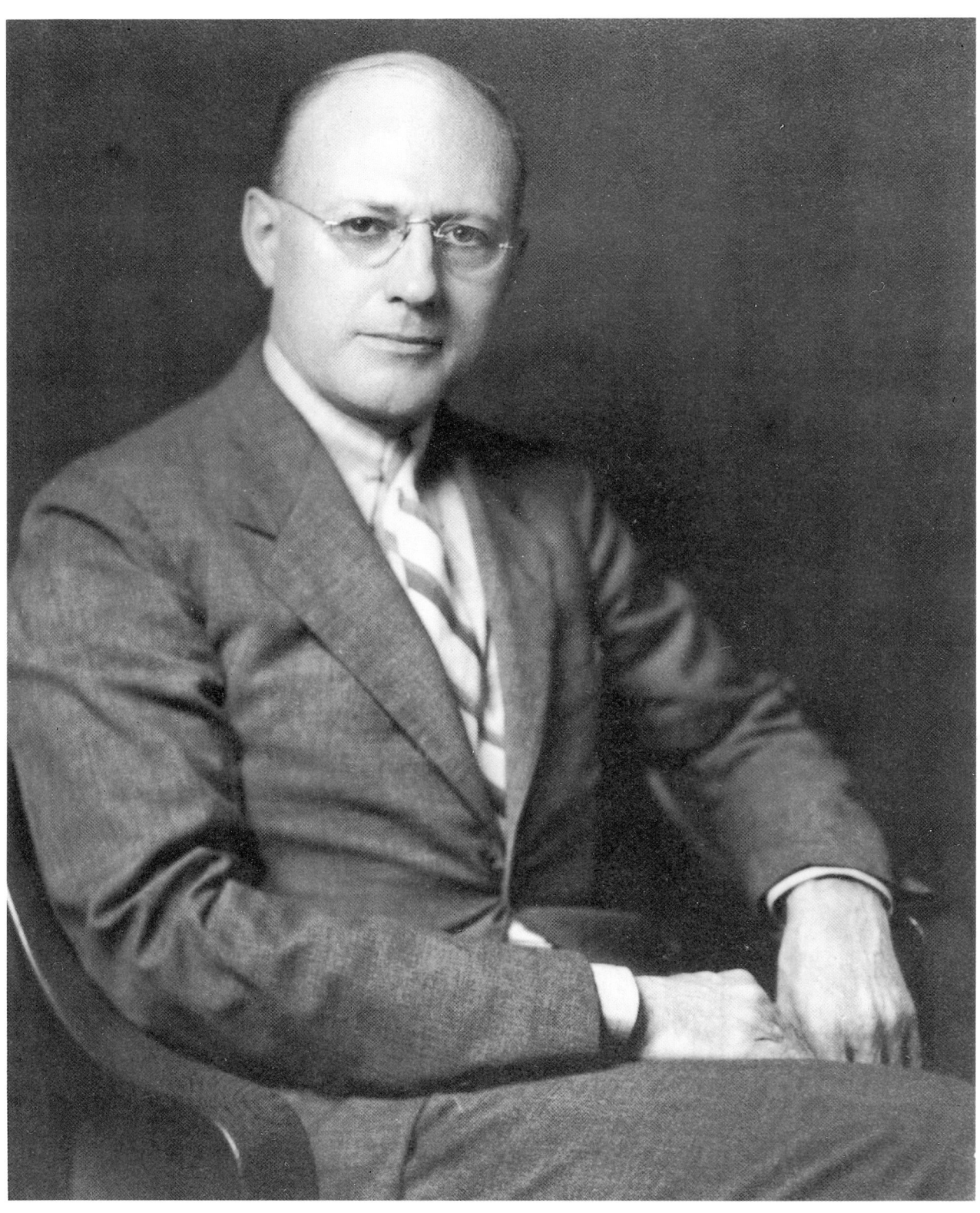

Harry Roswell Wahl, M.D., acting dean of the School of Medicine from 1924 to 1927, who also served as dean from 1927 to 1948.

3

Years of Struggle

The abrupt removal of Mervin Sudler, M.D., as dean of the University of Kansas School of Medicine indicated the institution's weak political position in Kansas. The faculty rose to Sudler's defense, pointing out what they considered the obvious injustices involved, but no massive public outrage followed. After all, most of the faculty protesters lived and practiced medicine on the Missouri side of the state line. Naturally, replacing Sudler proved difficult. Several candidates either turned down the position or made unacceptable preconditions before a faculty member, Harry Roswell Wahl, M.D., reluctantly became acting dean. Wahl, a professor of pathology interested in genetics, held both bachelor's and master's degrees from the University of Wisconsin at Madison and a medical degree from Johns Hopkins University. He had certain political and public relations skills that served him well. Early in his acting deanship he successfully averted the patronage appointment of a former cigar store clerk as superintendent of Bell Hospital by making the position an unpaid one and taking the job himself. In addition, Wahl continued to chair the Department of Pathology. No one could argue that he lacked energy. In 1927, after Governor Jonathan Davis (who had fired Sudler) had been soundly defeated for reelection and political conditions affecting the medical school had temporarily settled down, Wahl became dean, a position he would hold over the next two decades—the "Wahl Years."

Wahl placed an emphasis on stability, eschewing any attempt at dramatic progress. In addition to entrenched political opposition in Kansas, Wahl continued to face the problem of running a divided institution. On the University of Kansas campus in Lawrence, several different buildings and departments housed preclinical courses. The Goat Hill campus included the pathology and pharmacology departments, plus a medical library. On Rainbow

Boulevard, the new Bell Memorial Hospital contained over 120 beds. Originally planned as an administration building, it was not a true hospital, having minimal room for clinical facilities. A temporary wood and pasteboard structure, used as a combination outpatient department and dispensary, adjoined the north side of the hospital. Another temporary building, often referred to as the "barracks," functioned as a segregated "Negro Ward," serving black inpatients and outpatients. There were, however, no black physicians on staff or black nursing or medical students on campus. Research facilities on the Rainbow Boulevard campus were minimal—the only small laboratory was directly above the furnace room of Bell Hospital—until Dean Wahl converted a modest wooden structure constructed as a gymnasium into a research building.

The legislature appropriated $300,000 for an additional ward and for a nurses' home, Hinch Hall, but soon the Great Depression caused state funding to dry up. Attempts to obtain private support had failed. The General Education Board of the Rockefeller Foundation, on the advice of Abraham Flexner, refused the school funds because of its political problems and multiple locations. "Well, I've seen medical schools divided into two campuses, but never before into three," Flexner told school officials. "As you know, we do not favor divided schools and will not support their building projects."

Wahl presided over what amounted to a permanent austerity program. His critics charged that he should have been more assertive in dealing with the legislature. They ignored his role in engineering a 1929 legislative action that separated the medical school's budget appropriation from that of the Lawrence campus. The new arrangement paid immediate dividends when the legislature appropriated $10,000 for the purchase of radium for the x-ray department, but inadequate state resources remained a continual problem.

In the depths of the Great Depression the school experienced a 25 percent budget cut. Wahl did not aggressively approach the legislature for funds, nor did he actively solicit the public when he failed to obtain needed finances. In return, the state's political leaders, possibly recalling the Mervin Sudler firing debacle, virtually left Wahl alone to direct the school as he saw fit. Perhaps matters would have worked out differently if the controversial Milford, Kansas, "goat gland" rejuvenation doctor, John R. Brinkley—considered a fraud and a quack by most licensed Kansas physicians—had won when he ran as an independent candidate for governor in 1932. After an autopsy report on one of his patients conducted at the medical school indicated possible malpractice, Brinkley sharply questioned the quality of the staff.

Wahl gradually settled in as leader, working long hours and undertaking additional duties without complaint. Wahl once said of his appointment, "I only accepted the position from the feeling on the part of the faculty that I was the one man who could carry the institution through these trying times, especially since I was more of a neutral-type person engaged in full-time scientific work with no clinical aspirations." He was not an autocrat, but a man who sought the help of committees and the advice of trusted friends. Wahl continued to teach and to do research. He appeared a reluctant administrator, one without either driving ambition or an overriding vision. If he entertained a goal, it was simply to keep the school open. In short, he presided over a holding operation.

Conditions in the medical school were in keeping with Wahl's conservative approach. Day after day, he dealt with the realities imposed by the sorry condition of the Kansas state treasury; getting by with less became a habit. Old medical equipment remained in use long after it should have been replaced. Housekeeping facilities looked like a scene from the London of Charles Dickens. The kitchen had a variety of sanitation problems; on one occasion a serious food poisoning outbreak affected both staff and patients, temporarily disrupting operations. During an epidemic of poliomyelitis in 1937, the school could not afford to purchase the expensive forerunner of the "iron lung." So Wahl, assisted by technicians, improvised prefabricated units for less than $300 each.

A willingness to save money coupled with the training of medical personnel to meet the needs of Kansas helped raise the prestige of the institution. Few citizens of the Sunflower State realized how low the University of Kansas School of Medicine ranked among medical schools in the United States. Even so, the school gradually became an accepted part of the University of Kansas. Wahl, with his low-key approach, carried on as best he could. "During a period of ubiquitous shortages, he held together a small cadre of dedicated and excellent physician-educators," his biographer, Helen M. Sims, observed. "His quiet, diligent approach to administrative responsibilities and his rapport with all constituents raised the quality of medical education and placed the institution in a good position to take advantage of the period of rapid growth during the years after World War II."

All through the 1930s progress was painfully slow. Wahl successfully established a small full-time faculty of able and dedicated physicians who combined their clinical and teaching responsibilities with research, primarily in anatomy, microbiology, physiology, chemistry, and pathology. Thomas G. Orr, M.D., wrote a standard text on surgery. Others, notably Ralph H. Major, M.D., made significant contributions through scholarly publications and presentations. Still, basic medical research remained a minor activity; the combination of insufficient laboratory facilities and inadequate funding made important discoveries unlikely. The best-known faculty member was Logan Clendening. Considered a "society doctor" by some detractors, Clendening wrote a nationally syndicated news column on medicine intended for a general audience. The unpaid physicians of the medical school who augmented the full-time faculty included some of the best physicians in the Kansas City area, but few were researchers. Under these circumstances, the University of Kansas School of Medicine progressed slowly as a teaching and clinical institution. As time passed, the school seemed increasingly out of date.

Although the photographs from this period reflect the slow growth of the medical school and its grim circumstances, there were signs of progress. The most visible signs were new buildings—one, the Eaton Ward (or "Colored Ward"), a brick structure erected in the late 1930s with combinations of state, private, and federal money, replaced the notoriously inadequate and hazardous barracks. In 1938, before completion of the Eaton Ward, the first black medical student, Edward V. Williams, was admitted to complete his clinical years at the medical school. The argument was made that the construction of a few new structures, such as the Connecting Corridor, kept the University of Kansas School of Medicine in Kansas City. But the physical plant, even with obvious improvements such as the new Clinic Building and Children's Pavilion, remained modest in appearance when measured against those of medical schools outside Kansas.

In terms of medical education, Kansas provided many services superior to those of the old proprietary schools, but beyond the establishment of basic programs, much remained to be accomplished. As American medical education progressed toward the mid-twentieth century, the proprietary era faded into the distant past. The new challenge would be creating state supported medical schools that not only performed the traditional healing functions, but also produced qualified medical personnel and conducted significant research.

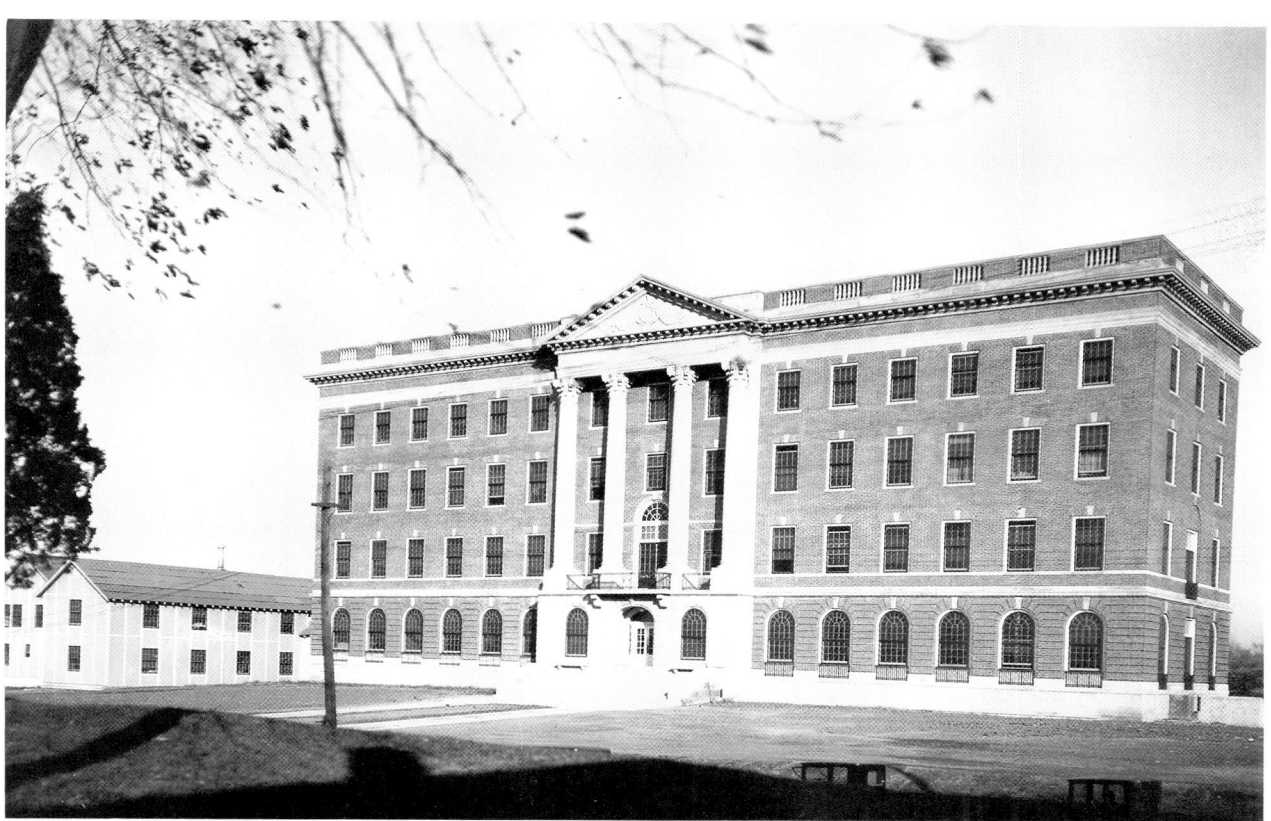

The new medical school facility and temporary "barracks" shortly after completion in 1924.

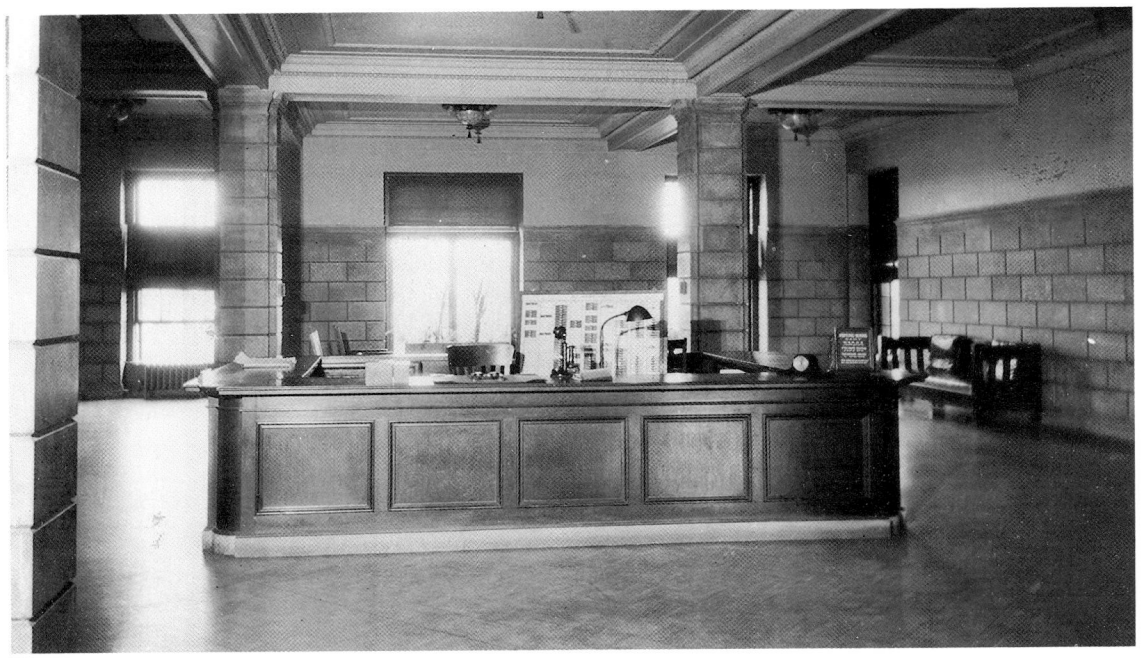

The reception area in the new Bell Memorial Hospital, ca. 1930.

In 1924, we moved to the new site. The main, or administration building, was complete as was the power plant. It had already become evident that there was no provision for Negro patients or for an outpatient department. To remedy this defect, a temporary structure of wood and celotex board was constructed to the north of the main hospital building. One wing of this building was the outpatient department, the other housed the Negro patients. This flimsy, make-shift, fire trap was erected with the idea that it was only a temporary expedient, to be removed in two years—when the legislature met again to present us with a permanent building to replace it. It was torn down some 25 years later!
—Ralph H. Major, M.D., *An Account of the University of Kansas School of Medicine*, 1968.

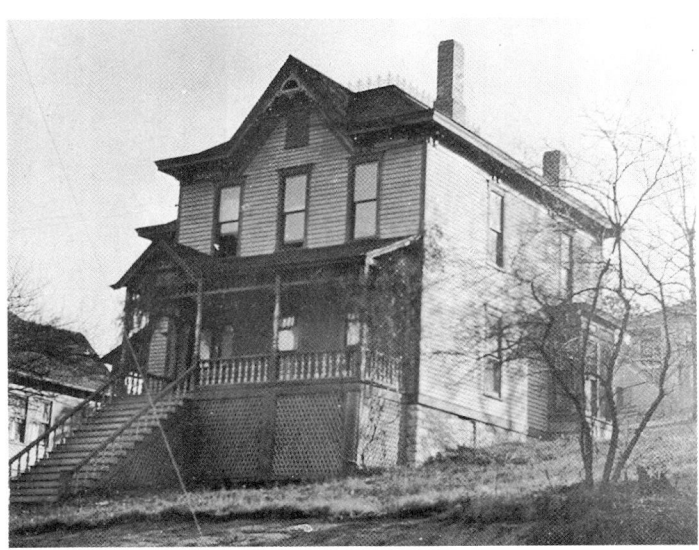

The student nurses' dormitory prior to the completion of Hinch Hall in 1928.

The Training School for Nurses is vitally connected with every teaching hospital, and the efficiency of the latter bears an intimate relation to the character of the nurses, and their training. In spite of the most unfavorable environment, the Nurse's Training School has struggled on with surprising vitality, due to the unselfish devotion of a few nurses. Without provision for instruction, with a home that was cramped, crowded and unsanitary, and with the absence of any provision for recreation, it is a wonder that any nurses at all were induced to take the training. With the movement up to the new hospital, the situation has not improved. There is at present no home for the nurses. They are scattered about in five separate houses, one five blocks away from the hospital, a condition which taxes the morale of these hard-working young women. At present there is no place where they can get together and have the social life that is such an essential part of young women. If we are to retain these nurses, and obtain new recruits to keep the hospital going, a modern nurses' home, adequate provision for instruction, and sufficient assistance are imperative. If this is done, there will no longer be the danger of a shortage of nurses, which we are being compelled to contend with at present.—"University of Kansas School of Medicine Biennial Report, 1922–1924."

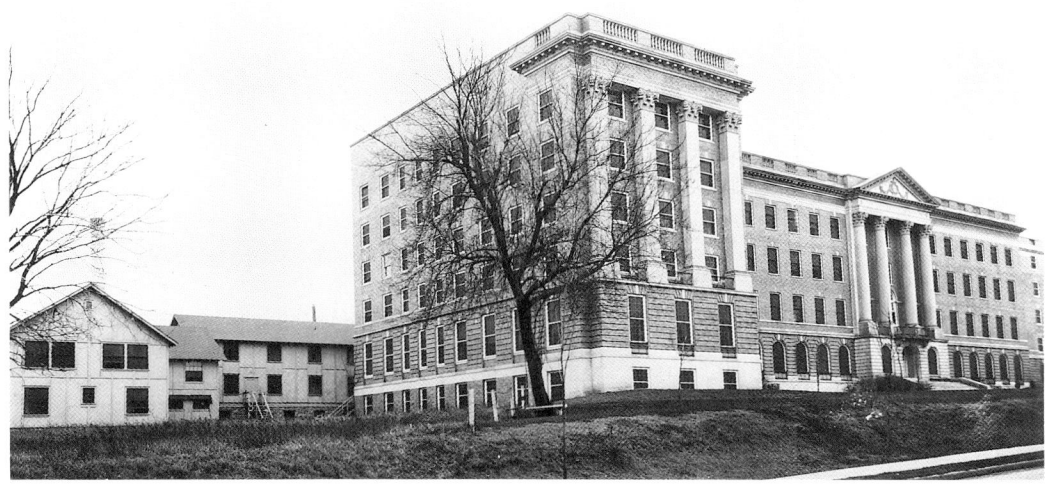

The "barracks," Hinch Hall, and Bell Memorial Hospital, 1933.

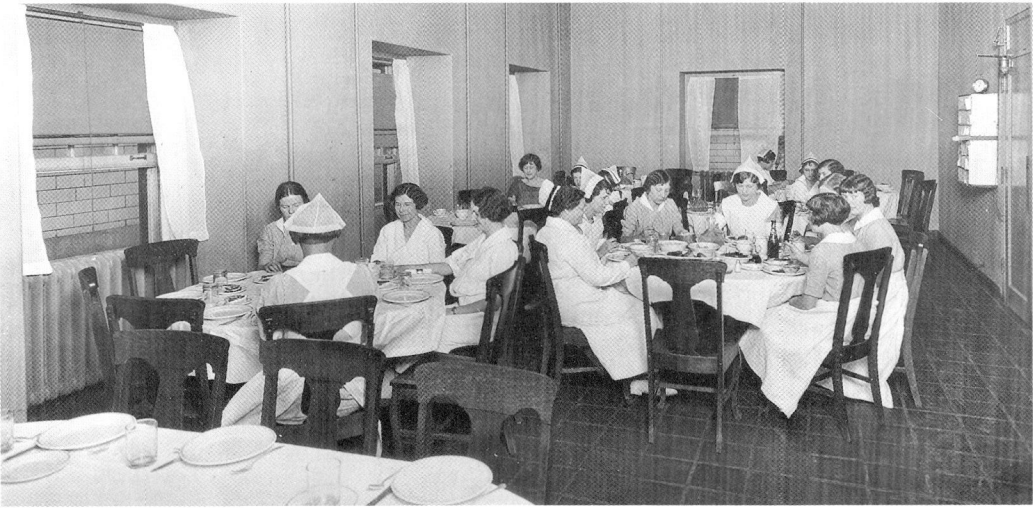

The student nurses' dining room in Hinch Hall, early 1930s.

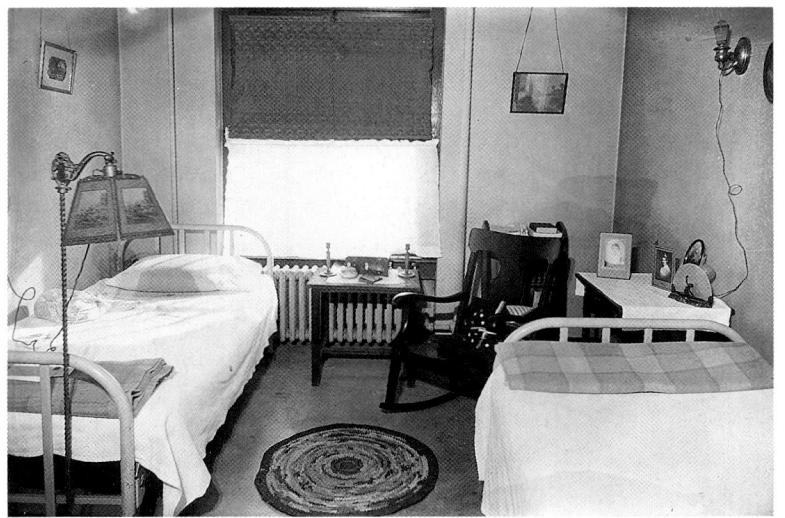

Nursing students' room in Hinch Hall, 1931.

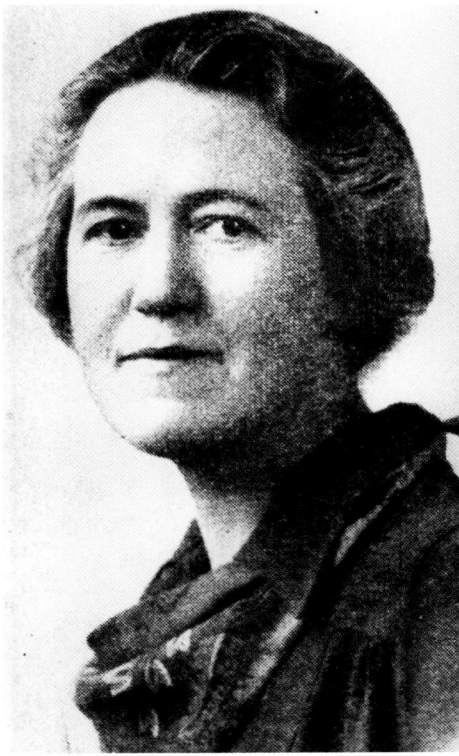

The school of nursing is one of the best in the middle west. There are many more applicants than can be admitted. Only girls with the highest qualifications can be admitted. The school of nursing offers a five and one-half year combined course to high school graduates, and at the end of this period the nurses receive a bachelor's degree in addition to their certificate of nursing. In 1938 there were 93 student nurses in the hospital.
—Ralph H. Major, M.D., Report, 1938.

Hennrietta Froehlke, R.N., superintendent of the School of Nursing, 1927–1949.

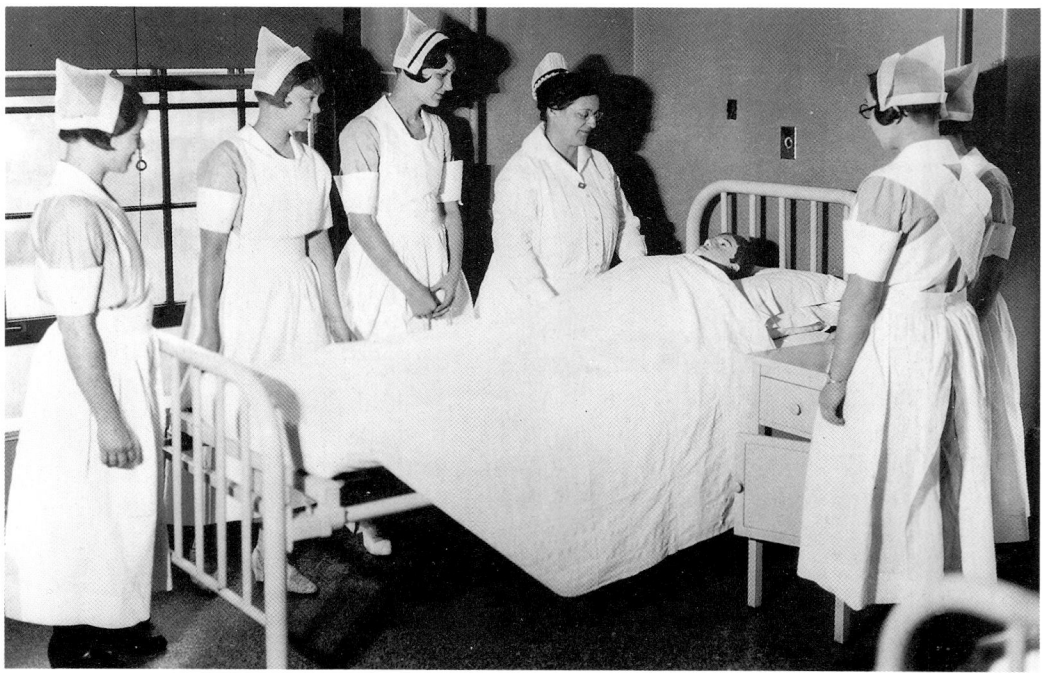

Student nurses in training, September 1930.

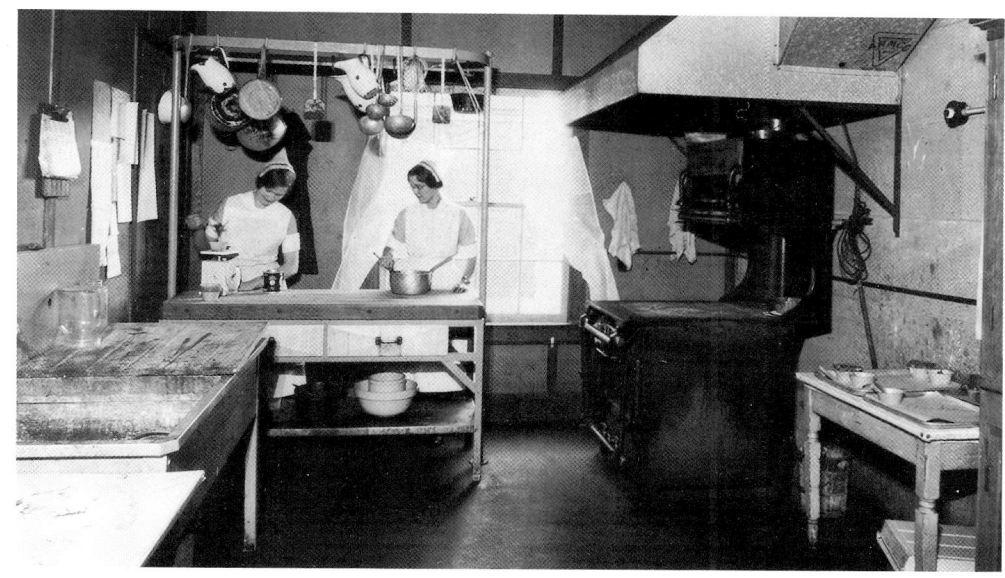

Nursing students at work in the diet kitchen, 1930.

In 1932 the first nurse was granted a degree. At first there were few degree students for in the minds of most people in Kansas nursing had no place in a University. It cost money and there was little money during the depression years. These first students were not well accepted by some personnel. There were those who feared that they were being over educated and others who were concerned that "those" students would slight some of the tasks usually done by nursing students of that time. Gradually this attitude toward them changed.
—Sara A. Patterson, R.N., "Out of Our Past," unpublished manuscript, 1966.

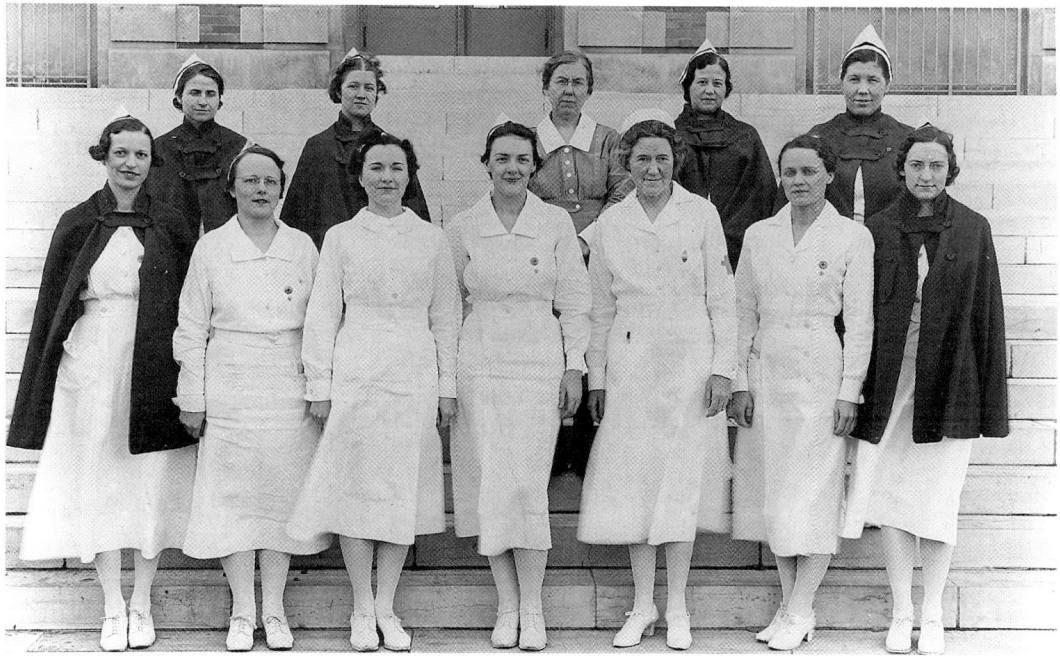

Nurses of Sigma Theta Tau, 1938.

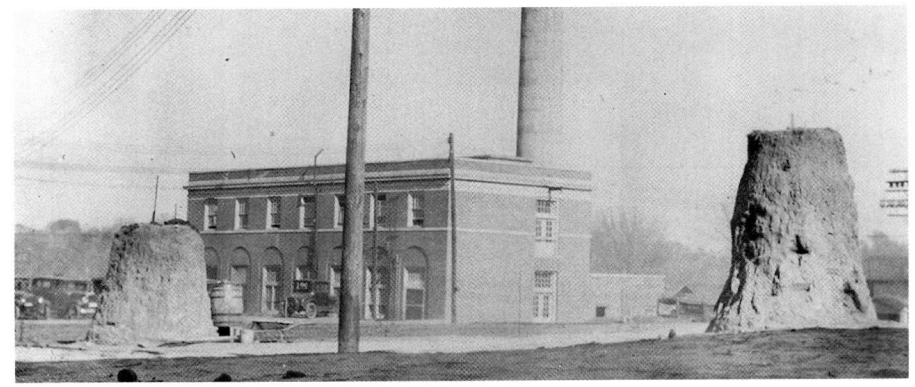

A Works Progress Administration grading project near the power plant, November 17, 1934.

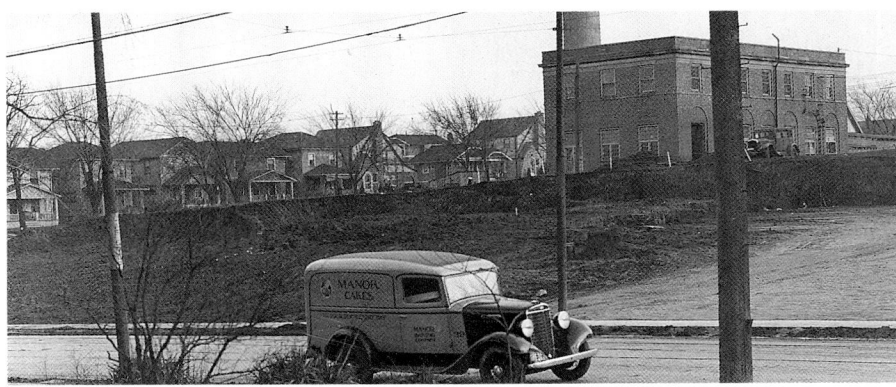

More W.P.A. grading, January 11, 1935.

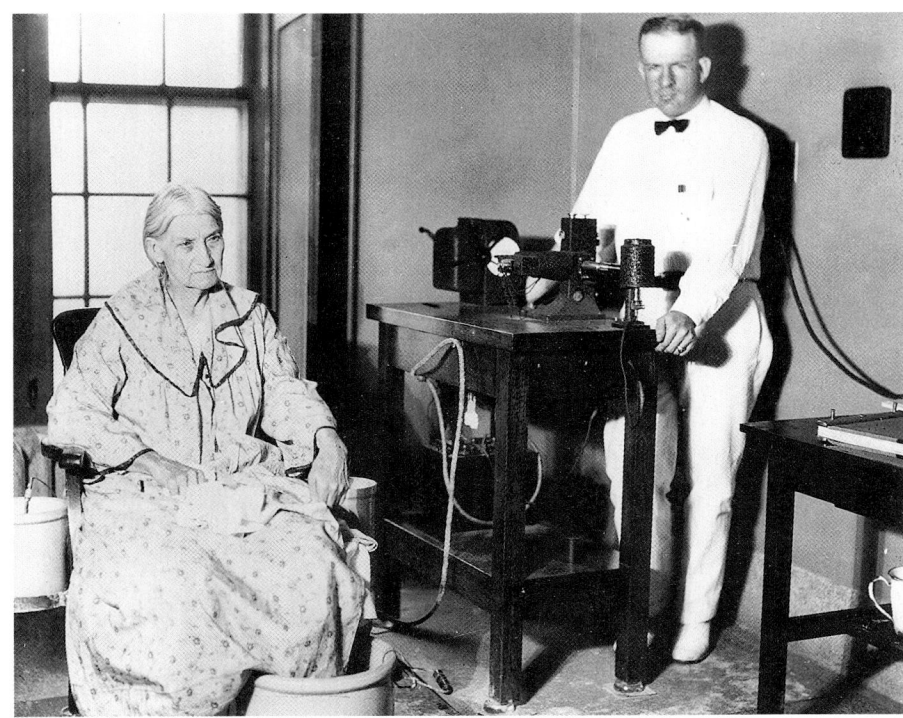

A patient receiving an electrocardiograph, 1926.

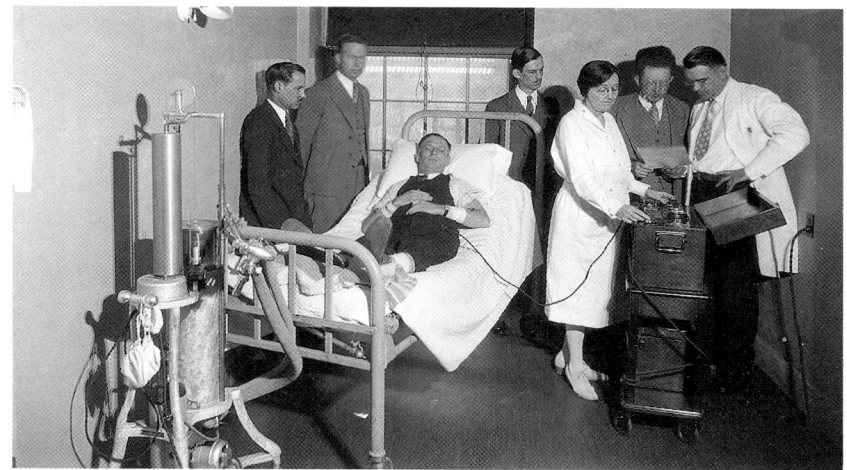

An electrocardiogram
demonstration, 1931.

The charges for x-ray work to Dispensary and clinical patients are $1.50 for each plate, dental films 50¢ (10 films for a complete set), x-ray treatments 50¢, and fluoroscopic examinations $1.50. . . .

Charges for x-ray work may be waived if the physician will make a written statement on the requisition card that this work is done for scientific purposes, and not especially for the patient's welfare.—House Order #6, Harry R. Wahl, M.D., 1925.

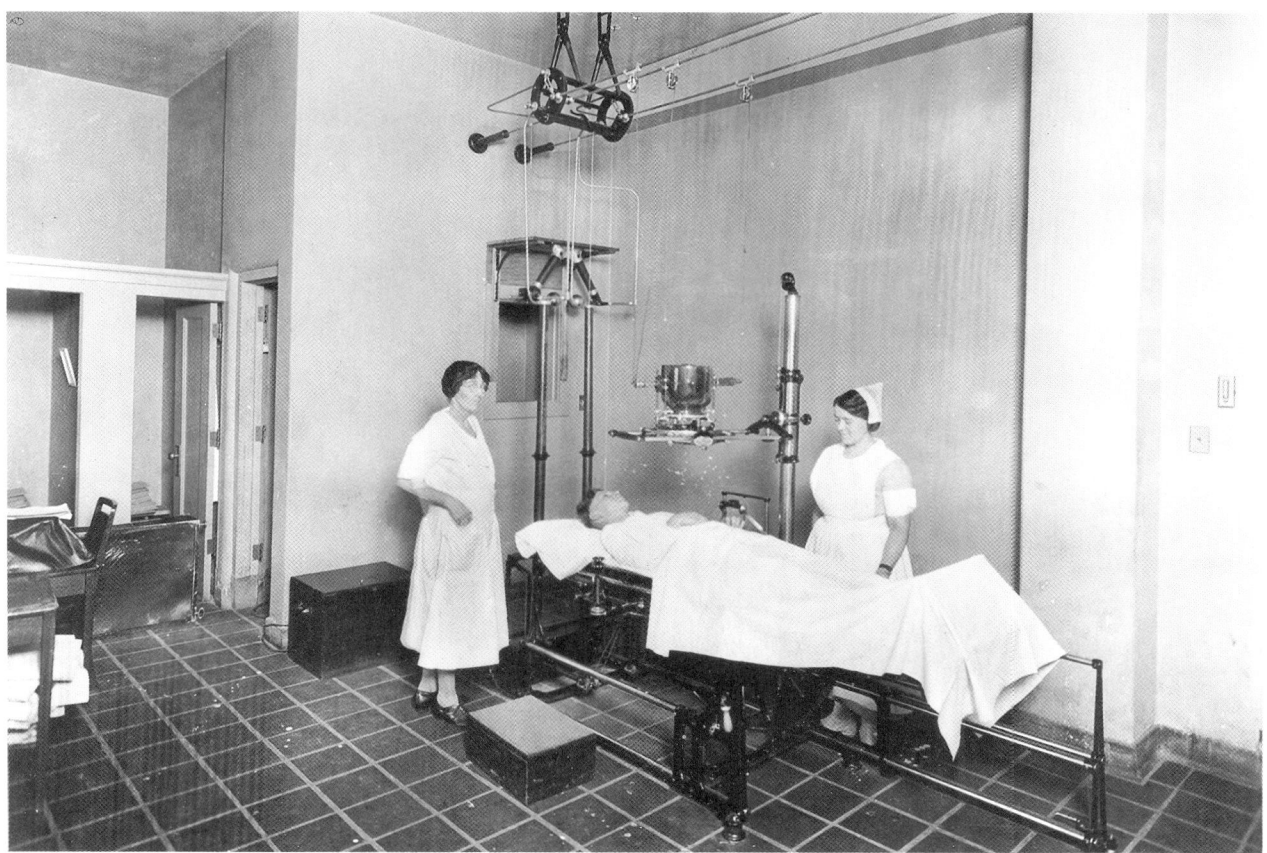

A patient in the x-ray room of the late 1920s.

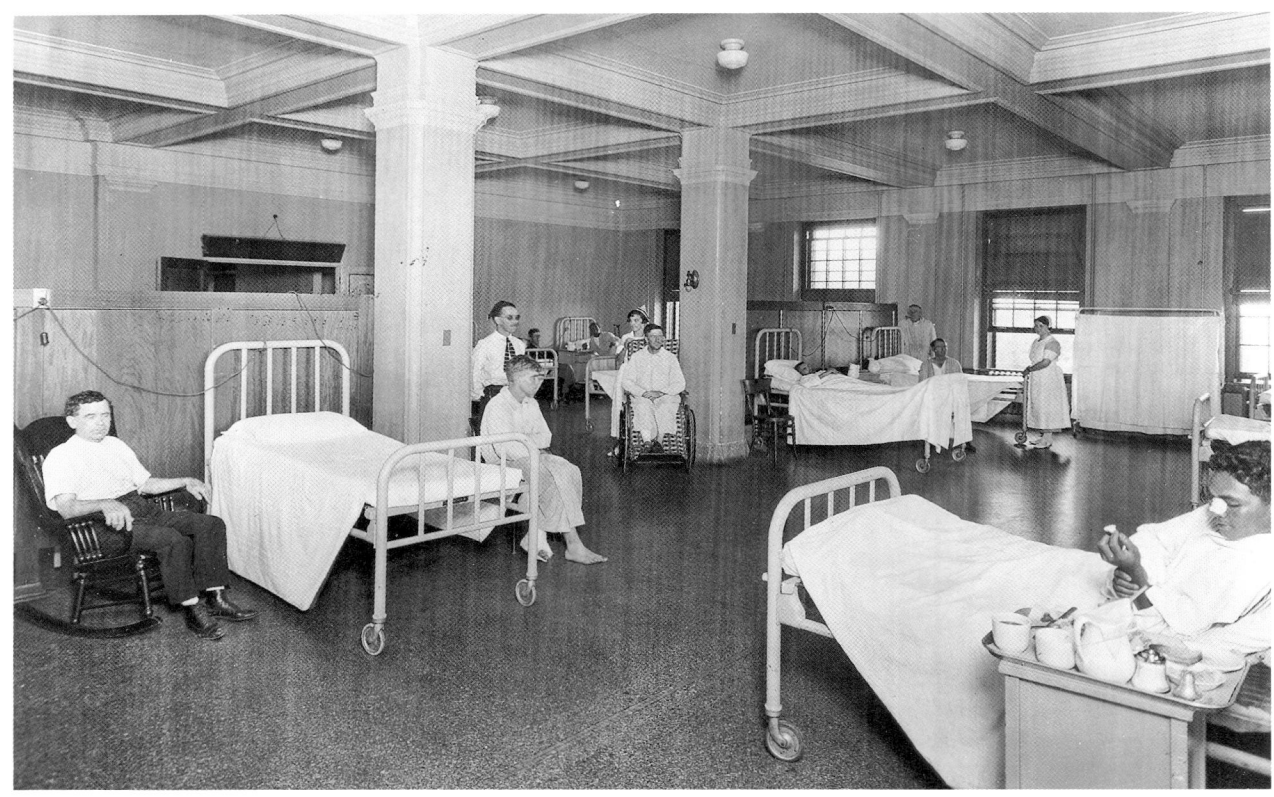

Student nurses with patients in the men's ward of Bell Memorial Hospital.

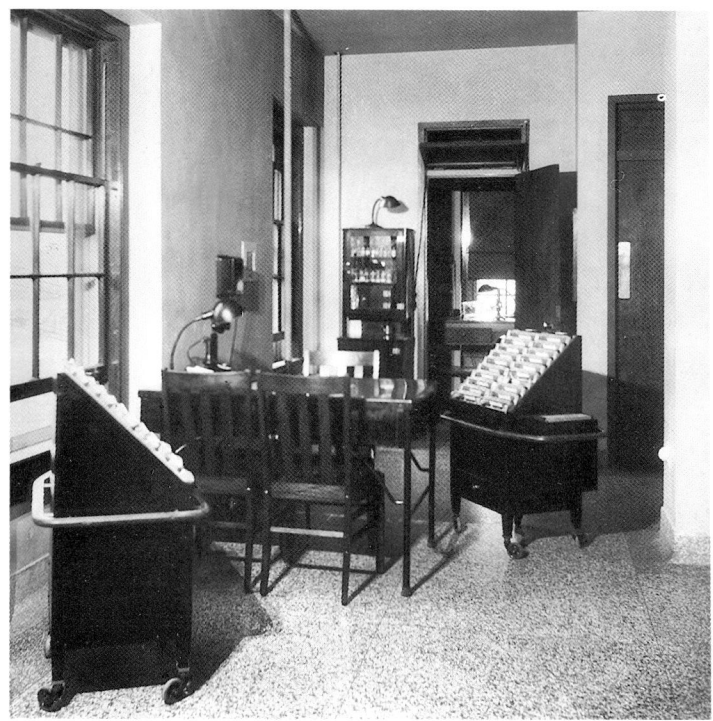

A nurses' station, late 1920s.

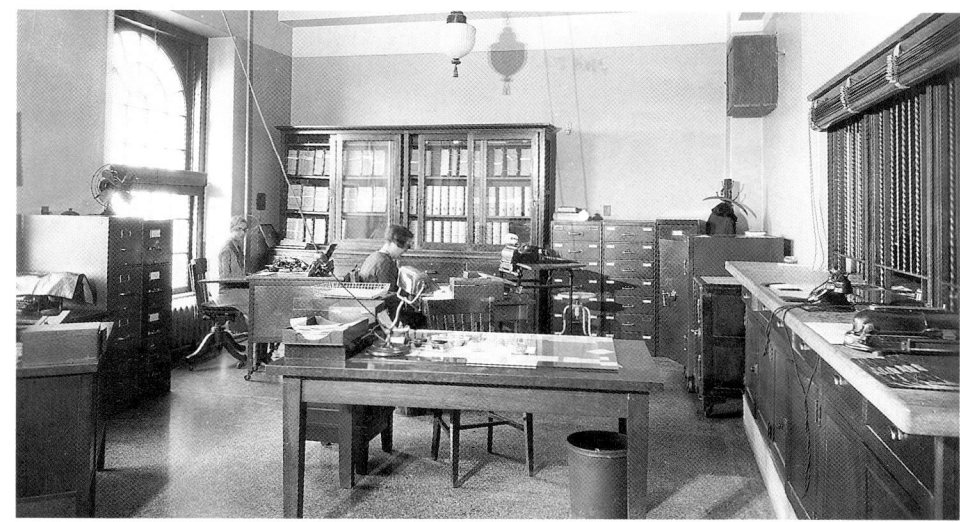

Telephone operator
and switchboard on
the second floor of Bell
Hospital, 1931.

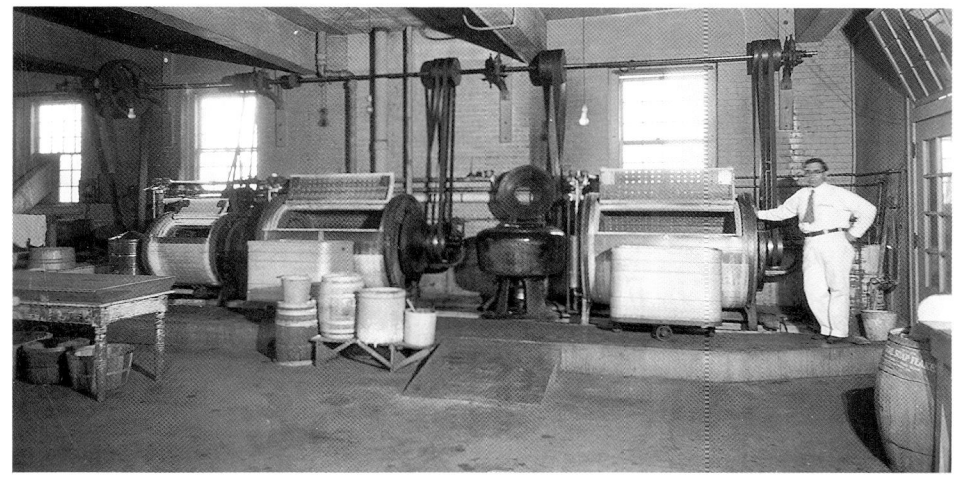

The laundry in 1931.

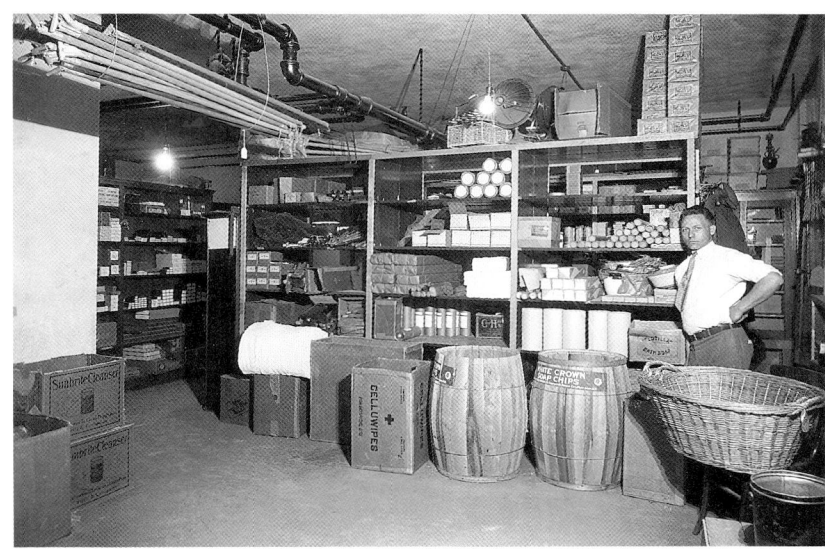

The medical school's
storeroom, 1930.

About four o'clock last Saturday afternoon Miss
Robert, one of our senior nurses, who was on duty in
the dispensary, had just come back to the dispensary
from a trip to the laboratory where she had left some
specimens, when she heard a crackling noise upstairs. She went over to the stairway to see what the
noise was and there saw the whole upper floor a
mass of flames.

The damage done involved considerable char-
ring of floor and walls of four of the dispensary
rooms on the second floor and the greater portion
of the waiting room. The rest of the floor was badly
scorched. No damage was done to the first floor
except that which may be due to some of the water
leaking through the ceiling. Approximately $1000
worth of equipment was either damaged or de-
stroyed by the fire. . . . The inner surface of the
roof was burned but the flames did not get into
the outside. We were very much surprised that
this material did not burn faster than it did.
—H. R. Wahl, M.D., to the chancellor,
June 27, 1927.

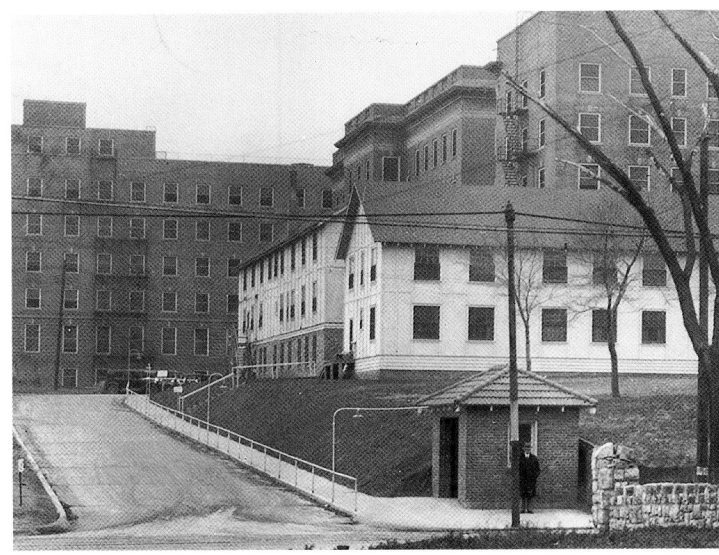

The 39th Street entrance to the dispensary
and medical school, 1930s.

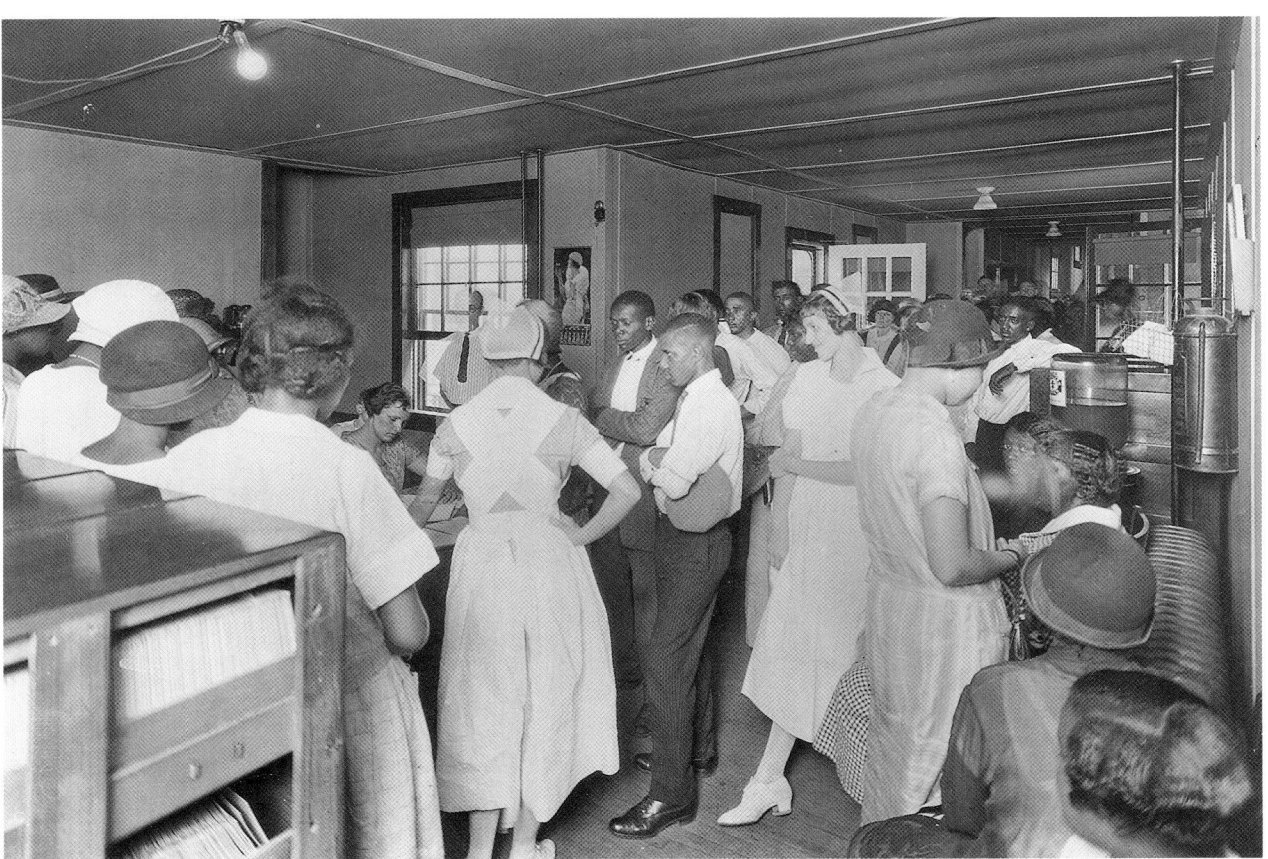

A scene in the outpatient clinic, ca. 1925.

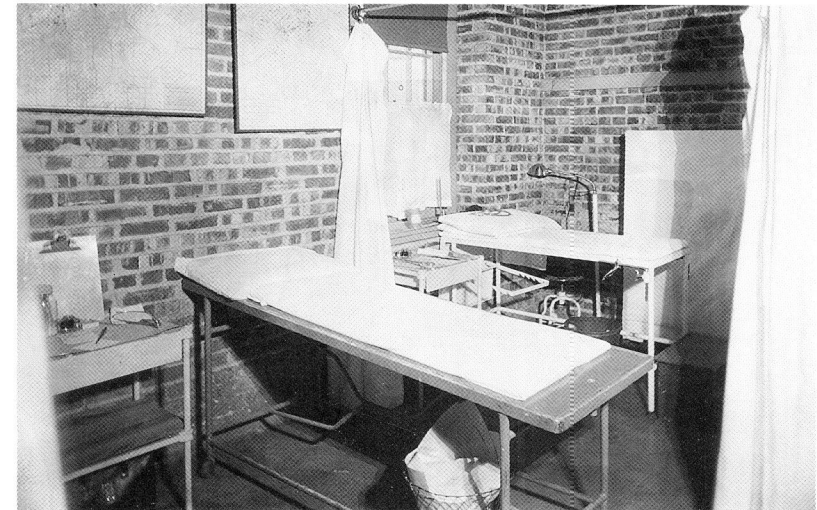

An interior view of the "barracks," 1931.

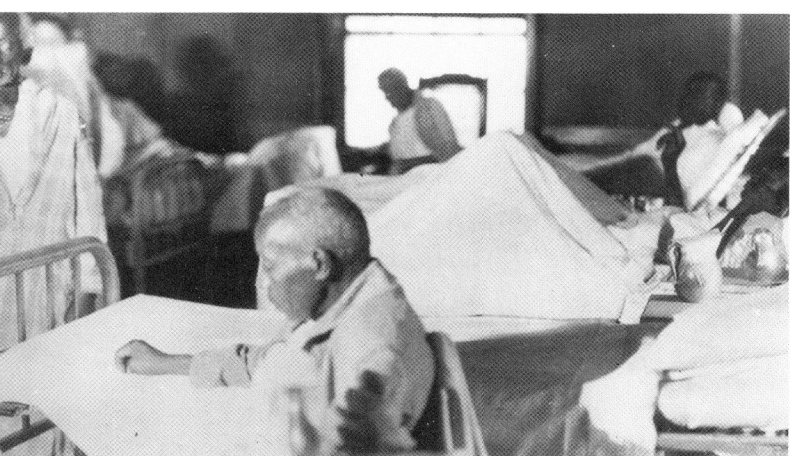

The quarters in the Dispensary are cramped. This building is a temporary frame building which is not designed to be used for more than three or four years. It is already showing signs of wear after two years of use. In this building often 150 to 200 individuals are crowded together at one time, interfering both with the proper care of the patients and the efficient instruction of the students. The clinic has not grown much in the past year because of limited physical facilities.—Biennial Budget Requests for the Years 1927–1928, 1928–1929.

Colored Ward, ca. 1925.

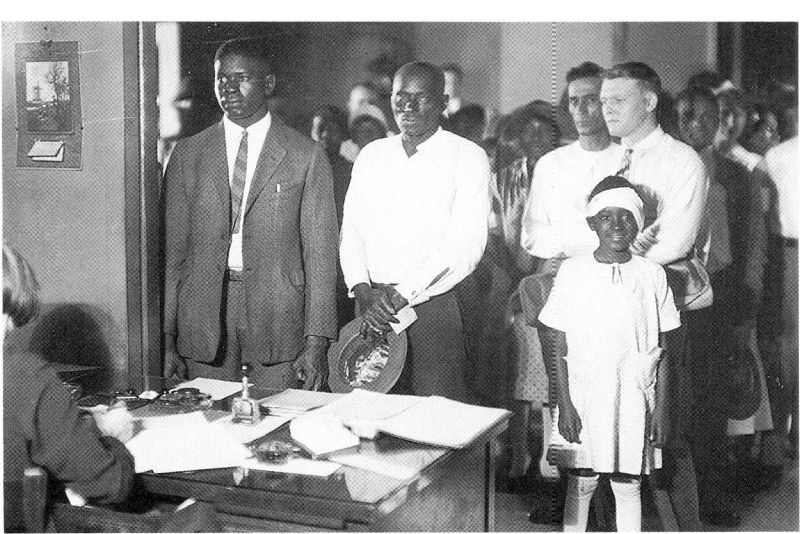

A crowd of patients waits in the dispensary, September 22, 1926.

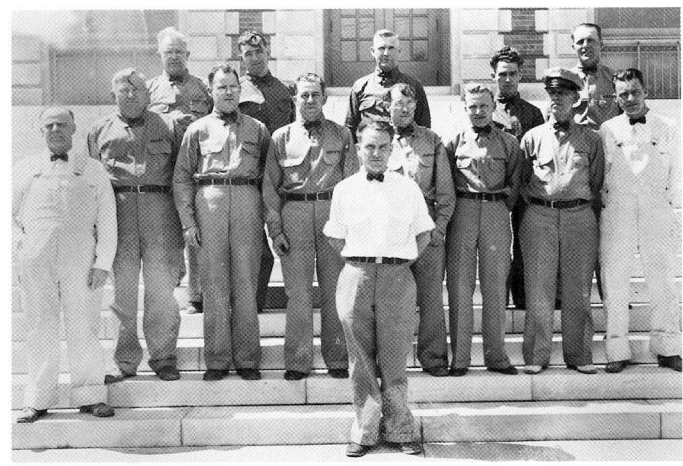

Frank Applegate, superintendent of Buildings and Grounds, with his crew, 1935.

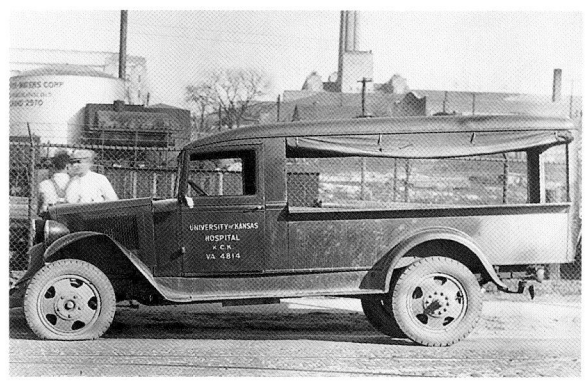

A hospital service truck after a minor accident, ca. 1933.

In 1937, the so-called corridor was built between the B Building and the Clinic Building. The term, "so-called," is used advisedly since it proved to be an unfortunate designation as well as an inadequate term, for it was more than a mere corridor—it housed the x-ray department on the second floor, the storeroom and postmortem room of the department of pathology on the first floor. When the building request involving $100,000 for the construction of a corridor was made, there were outcries against the extravagance of spending so much money for a corridor. However, when the matter was thoroughly explained, the appropriation was approved without too great opposition.
—Ralph H. Major, M.D., *An Account of the University of Kansas School of Medicine*, 1968.

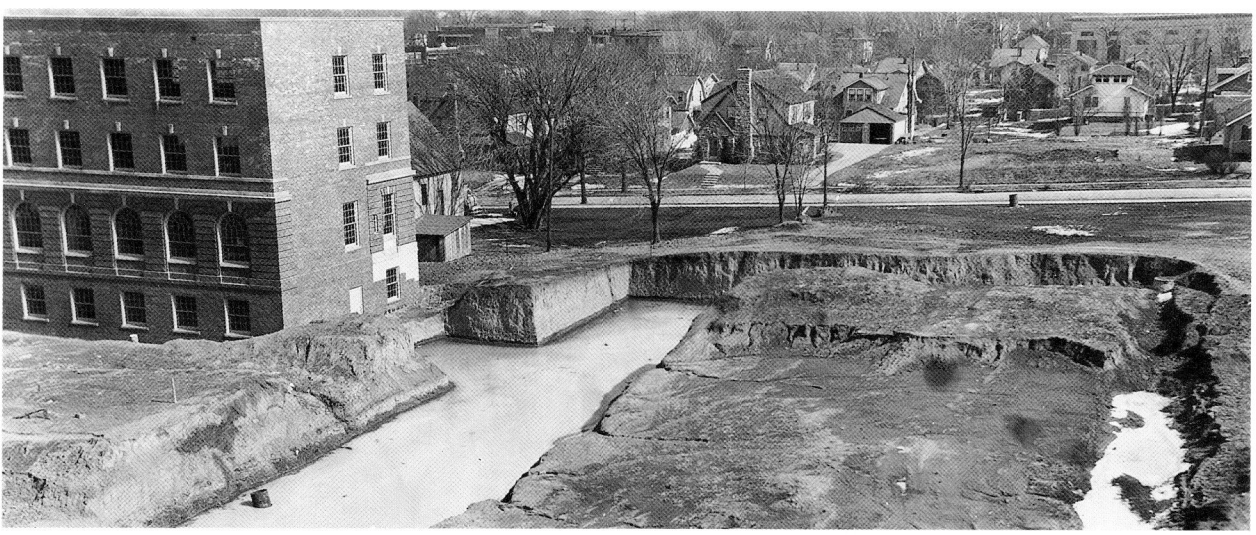

The excavation for the Connecting Corridor showing the south end of the Clinic Building, April 1, 1936.

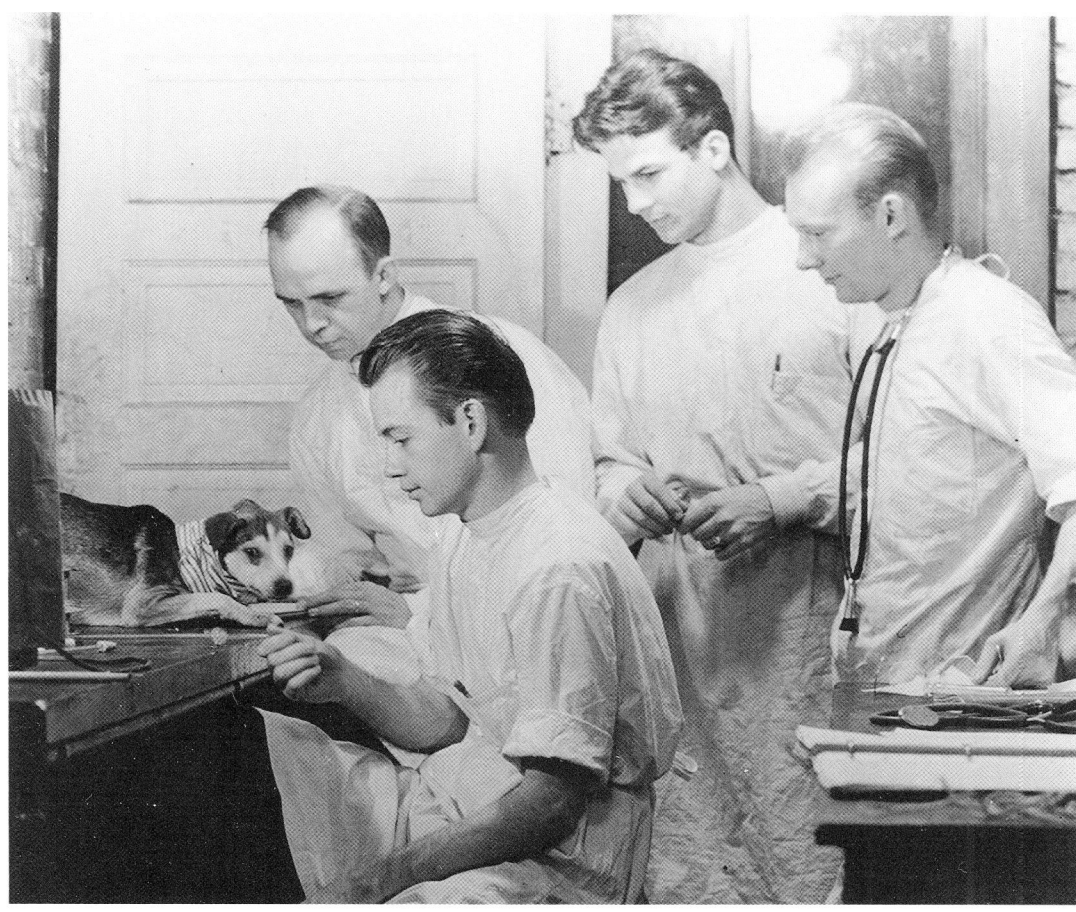

Students Ben Day, Philip Antrim, Dean Gough, and Vorris Reist
in the physiology lab, Lawrence campus, 1938.

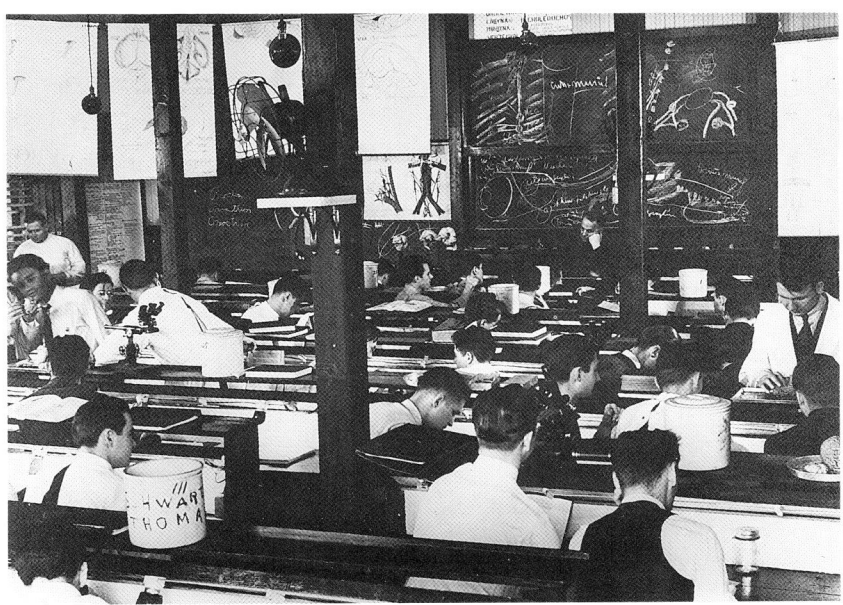

A 1930s anatomy class in Lawrence.

The number of students to whom an adequate medical education can be given by a college is related approximately to the laboratory and hospital facilities available and to the size and qualifications of the teaching staff. A close personal contact between students and members of the teaching staff results in an efficiency which is not possible in an institution where the number of students is excessive.
—William D. Cutter, M.D., to Harry R. Wahl, M.D., March 2, 1935.

I think one of the most important things to emphasize is that the state should do something more than it has in the past for medical education because of the fact that this is the only type of education, as far as I know, to which well qualified Kansas boys apply and are refused admission because of inadequate facilities. If a Kansas boy wants to enter the Engineering School or the School of Education, or any other professional school of the University, I do not believe he has any difficulty getting in because of the lack of facilities which the state provides.
—H. R. Wahl, M.D., dean, to R. A. McIlhenny, M.D., representative, February 5, 1929.

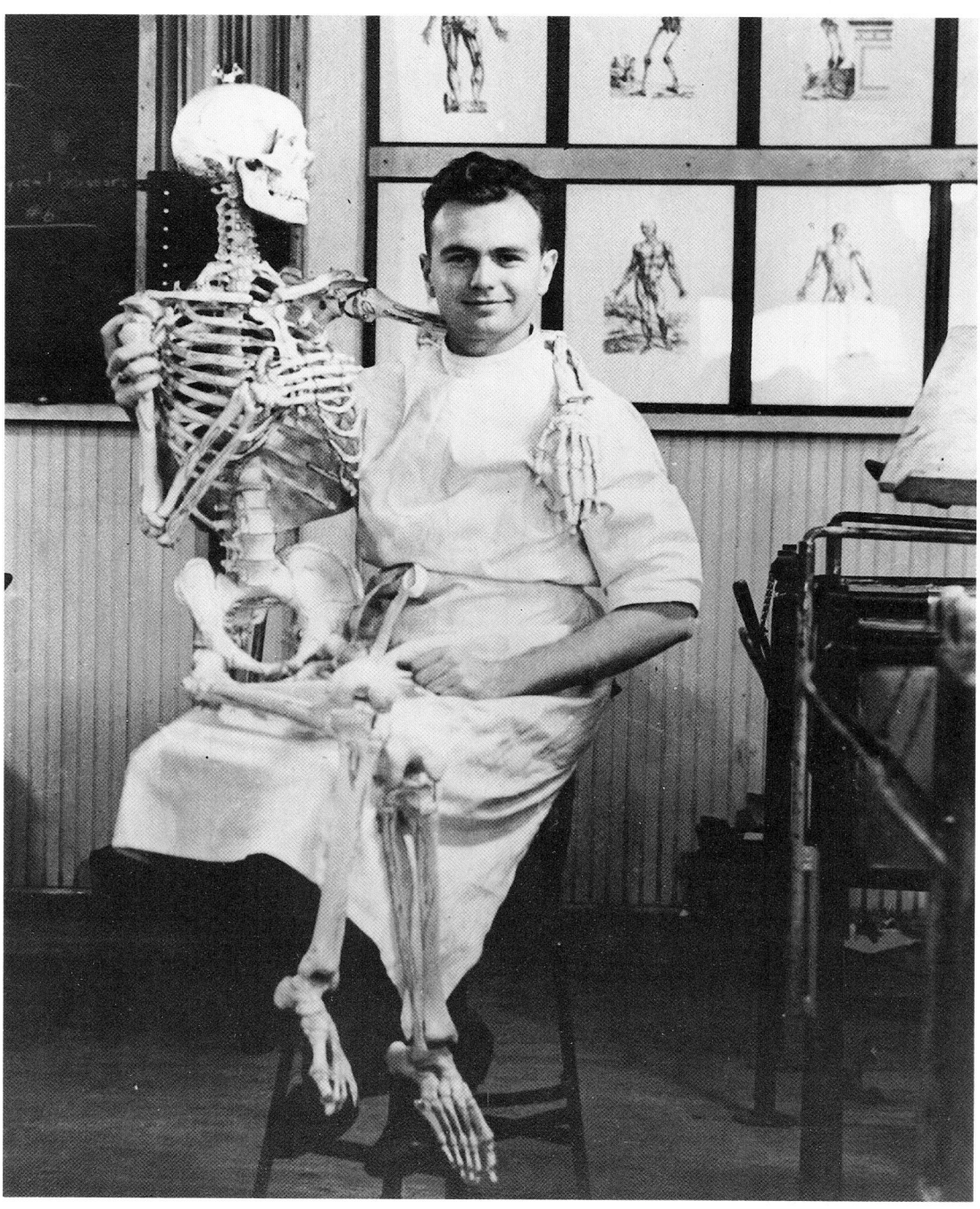

Medical student Philip H. Hostetter with a friend, 1938.

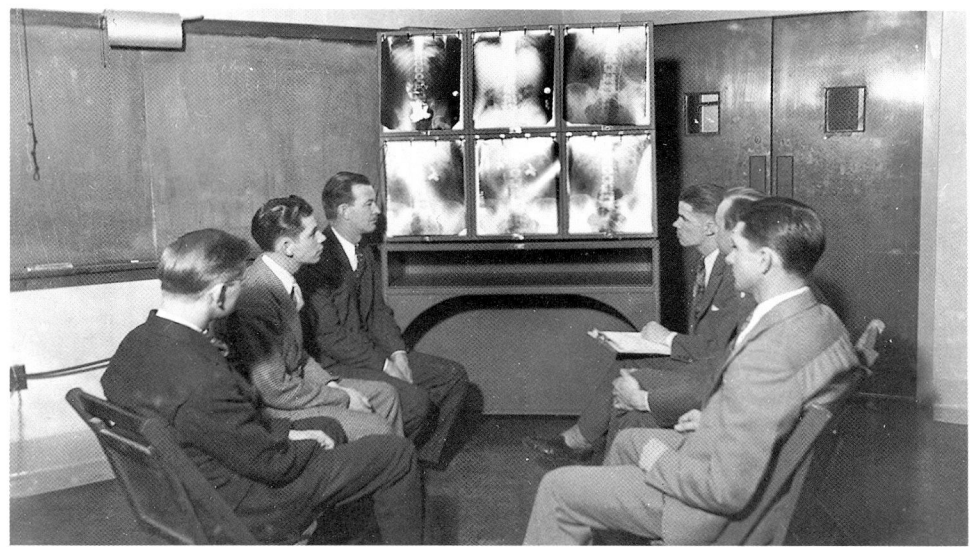

The University of Kansas has a good opportunity in medical education. It need not try to rival Johns Hopkins and Harvard Universities all at once. It needs time. It needs boosting instead of knocking, harmony instead of jealousy, co-operation instead of petty criticism. I believe the time is ripe for a big forward movement.
—E. P. Lyon, M.D., in *Graduate Magazine*, vol. XXIII, no. 1, October 1924.

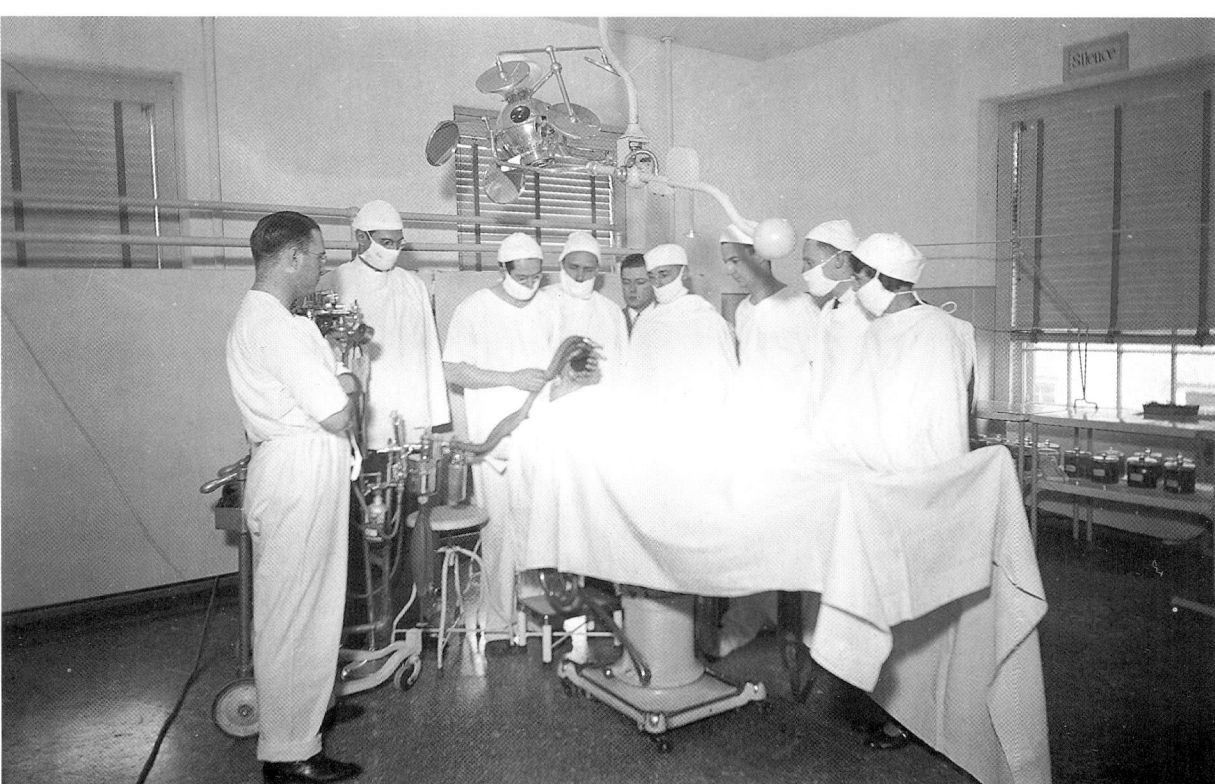

An anesthesiology demonstration, 1930s.

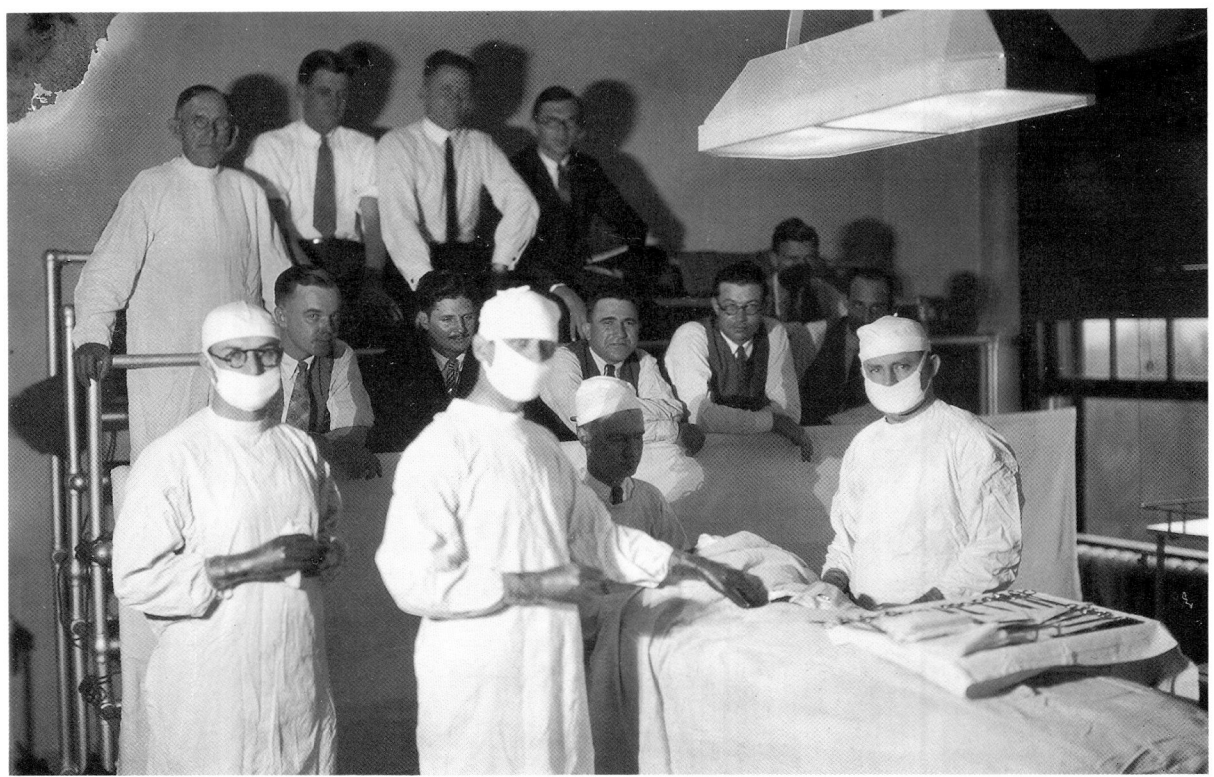

The operating theater, September 30, 1926.

The medical school has made considerable progress during the past six years and this year must determine whether we are going to continue progressing or turn back. We are asking this year, along with the rest of the university, for an increase in maintenance and for one new building. This new building is by no means a luxury, but a very great necessity. If completed, it will permit us for the first time to have adequate class rooms and teaching laboratories adjoining the hospital. At the present time, you may recall, most of the laboratories and class rooms are in the old building which is more than one mile away.—Howard E. Marchbanks, M.D., to Asa Messenger, February 26, 1929.

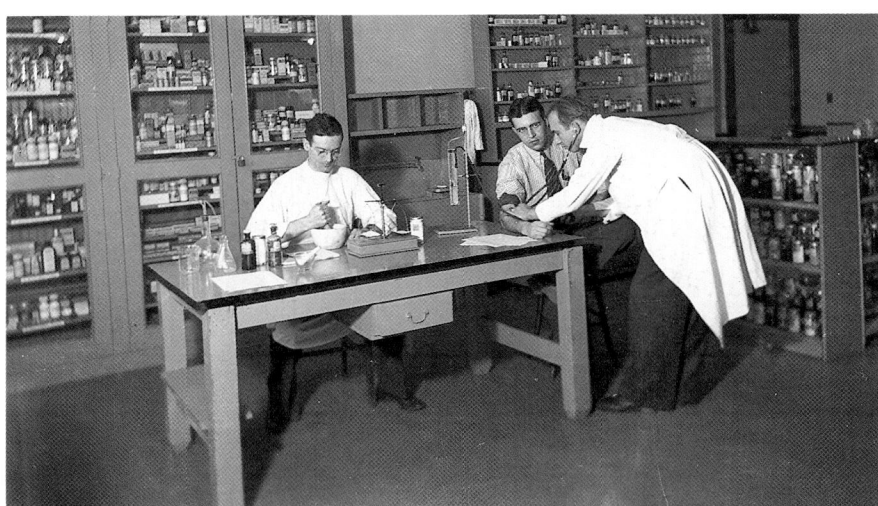

Students in pharmacology class, 1938.

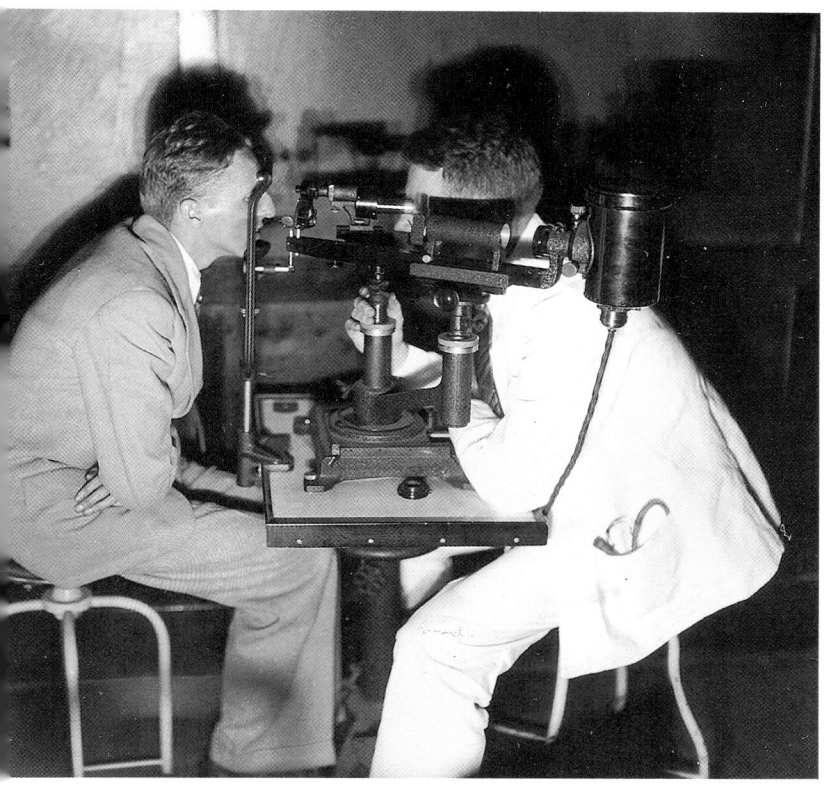

Patient receiving ophthalmology examination, September 29, 1926.

To the south of the B building is the new Children's Pavilion, recently erected through a gift of $60,000 by a loyal Kansas woman, and a PWA Grant of $57,270, the total cost being $117,270. Lack of funds has made it impossible to complete and equip this unit, and consequently has delayed its occupancy. The basement floor, however, is in active use. The building has a swimming pool, open air porches, and other facilities for children.
—Ralph H. Major, M.D., Report, 1938.

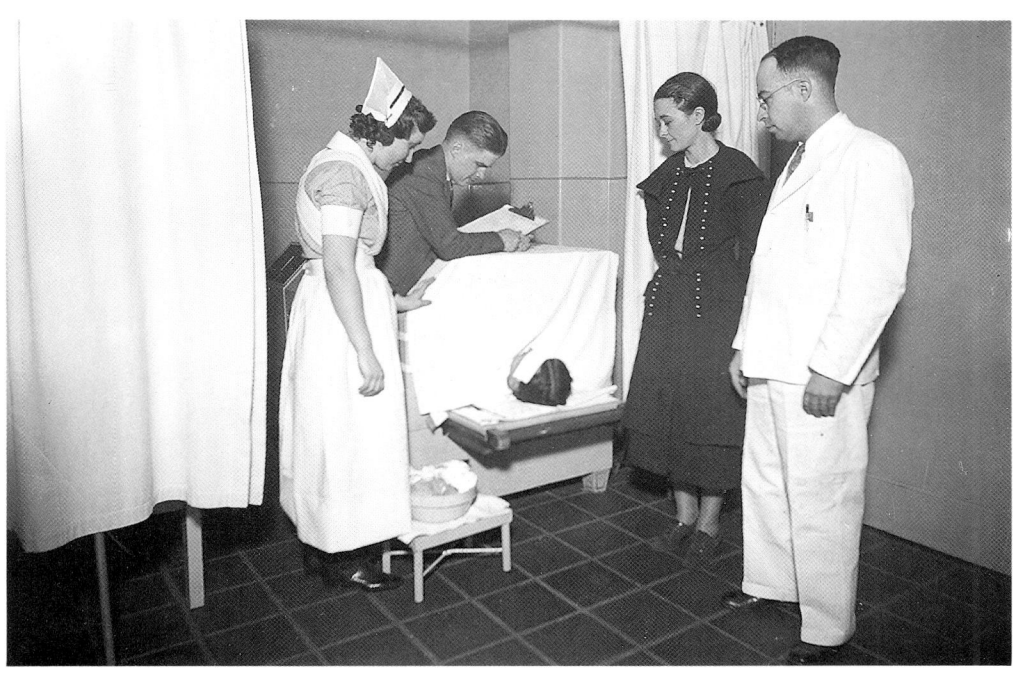

A patient undergoing fever therapy, late 1930s.

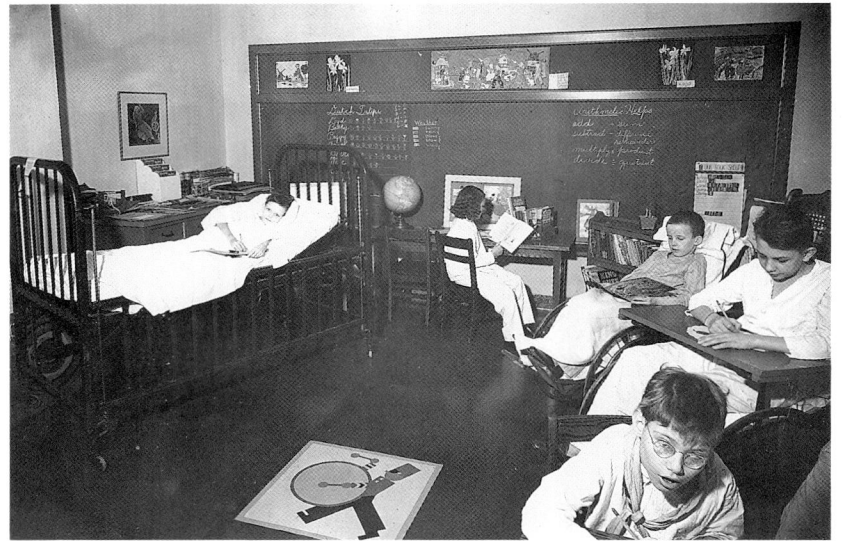

Interior of the Children's Pavilion, 1937.

When an order for breast milk is given by the doctor for one of the infants in the hospital, the parents, relatives, or guardians should pay for this in advance at the rate of 15¢ an ounce. This money should be turned over to the Supervisor of the children's ward, who shall make financial arrangements with the wet nurses employed, and is responsible for their payment. With the exception of extreme emergency such milk is not to be given to the child unless its payment has been provided for.
—House Order #5, Harry R. Wahl, M.D., 1925.

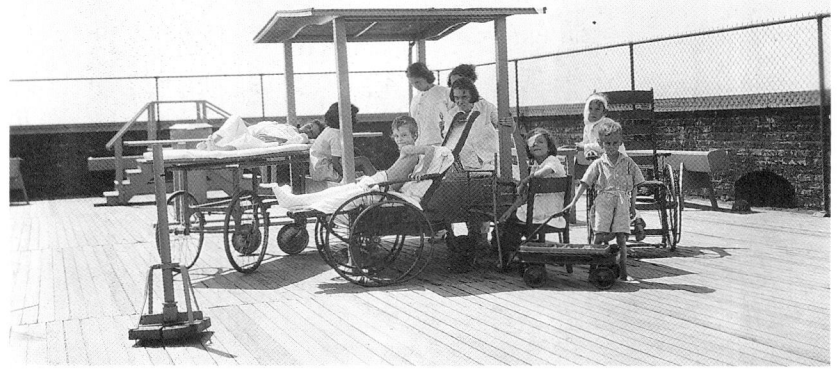

Patients on the roof of the Children's Pavilion, 1938.

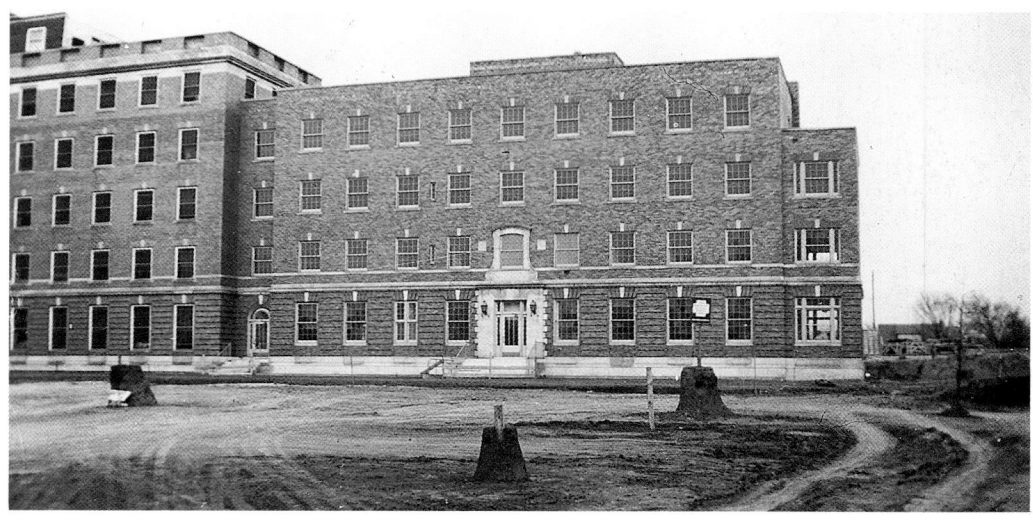

The new Children's Pavilion, April 1937.

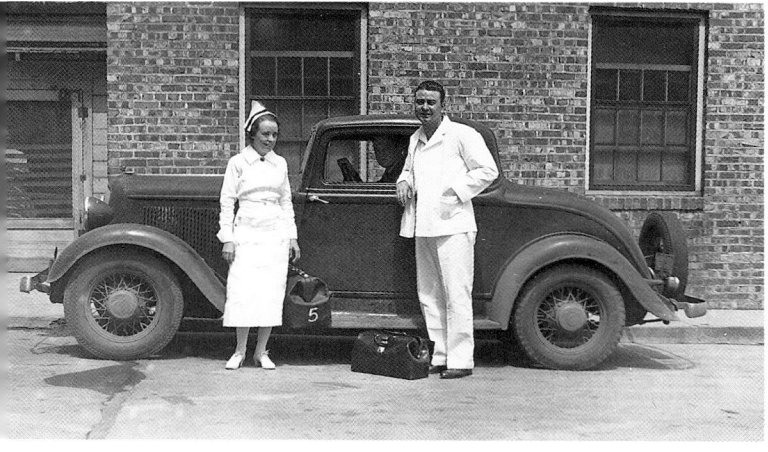

The past few years of stress have created an increasing demand for medical service. A few years ago the Out Patient Department averaged 150 visits daily. At the present time there are more than three times as many patients seen each day. The hospital, during the past year cared for 5,719 patients. The majority of the patients were sent in by various counties of the State who pay the hospital expenses. Provision is also made in the hospital for patients who can pay part or all of their expenses.
—Ralph H. Major, M.D., Report, 1938.

Entrance to the dispensary clinic, 1938.

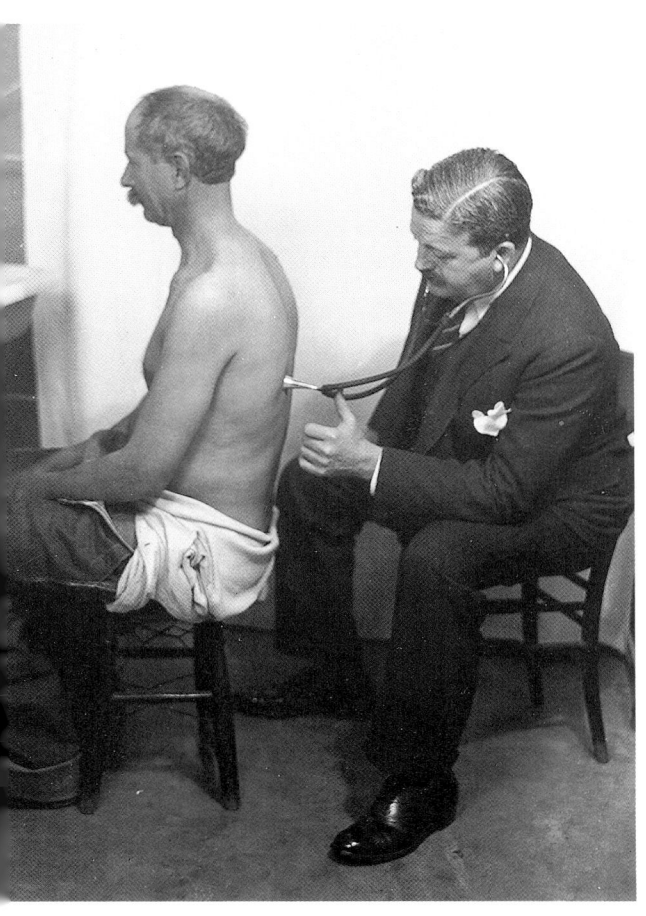

Dr. Logan Clendening examining a patient, late 1930s.

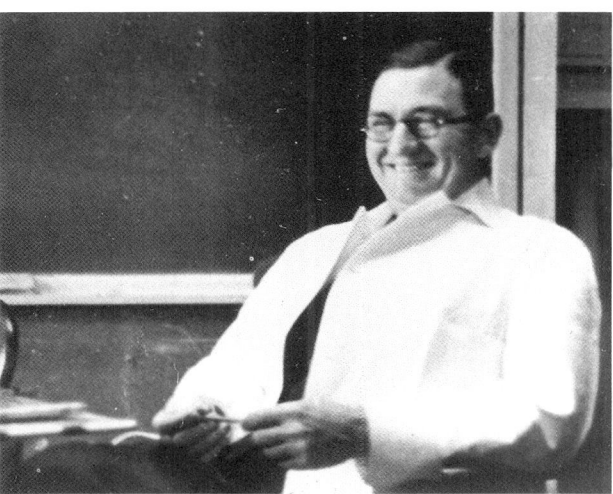

Thomas G. Orr, M.D., professor and chairman of surgery, 1938.

Dr. Orr was colorful when he was philosophic. At one time in 1931, while speaking to a group of medical students, he portrayed the lives of great men in medical history by accenting their little-known peculiarities, to make history come alive. He urged students to pick a hero, and added that "to study medicine without your medical hero is to pocket the nut without investigating the kernel." In his published thoughts concerning "Faith in Medicine," he urged young physicians to honor past medical discoveries and to apply the knowledge of their predecessors to the future.
—Stanley R. Friesen, M.D., "Thomas Grover Orr and Clinical Investigation," *American Journal of Surgery*, vol. 116, November 1968.

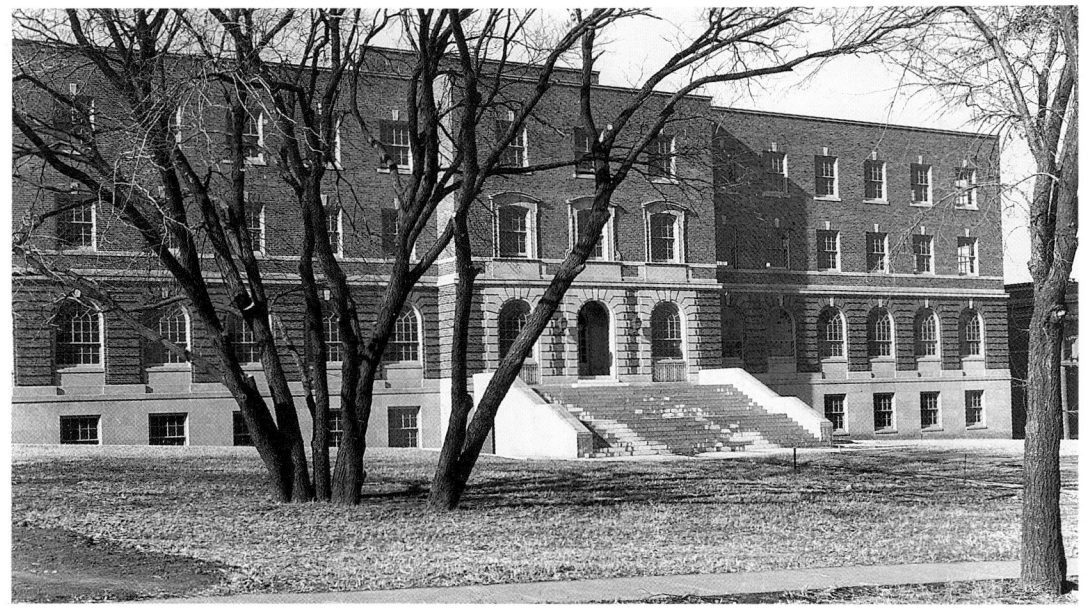

The Clinic Building, late 1930s.

This clinic building, erected on the order of the Board of Regents from funds not voted by the legislature, temporarily was under fire from a governor and some legislators, who insisted that, since the legislature did not authorize its construction, they were not obligated to appropriate money for its support. The flimsy old "cardboard" building, or the barracks, was abandoned and outpatients began to pour into the new building, which, to both patients and staff seemed like a palace when compared to the old dispensary. It was a beautiful, roomy, clean, airy, well-lighted, and cheerful building, efficient and well-designed.
—Ralph H. Major, M.D., *An Account of the University of Kansas School of Medicine*, 1968.

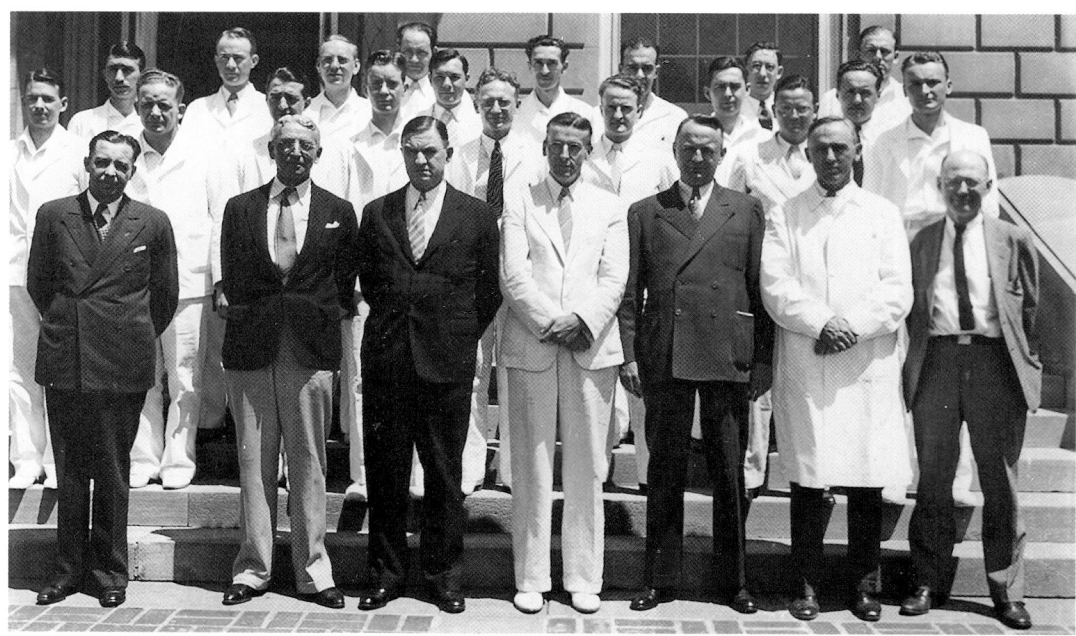

Medical school faculty, 1936

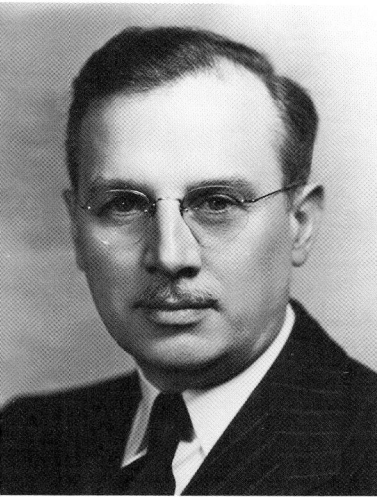

Don Carlos Peete, M.D., Department of Medicine.

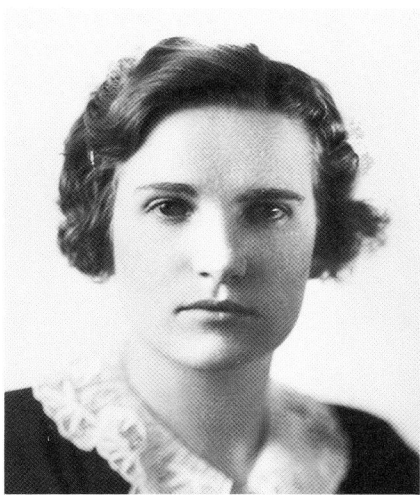

Nellie Walker, M.D., who eventually became the Kansas City, Kansas, health director.

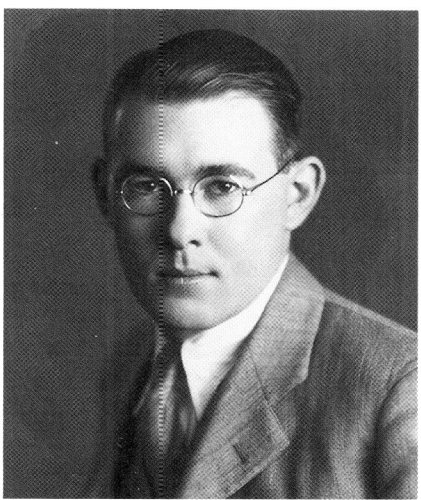

Richard L. Sutton, Jr., M.D., professor of dermatology.

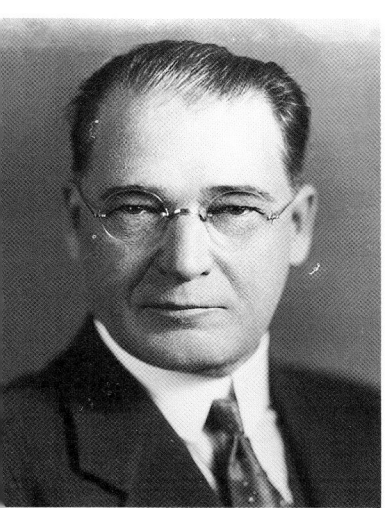

E. J. Curran, M.D., founder of the Department of Ophthalmology.

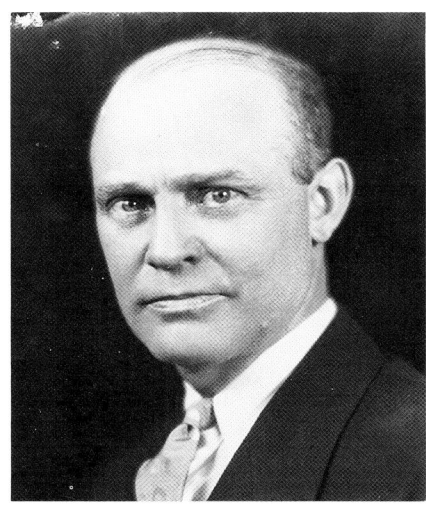

Albert N. Lemoine, Sr., M.D., associate professor in ophthalmology.

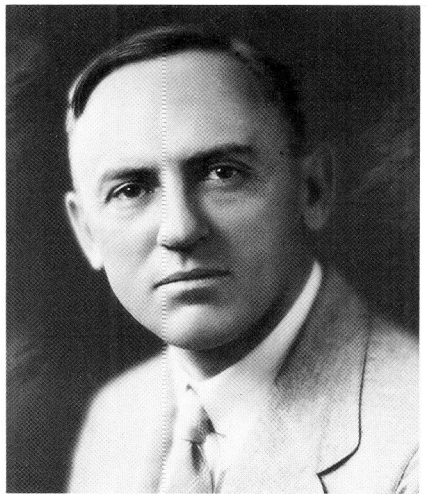

Ralph H. Major, M.D., chairman of the Department of Internal Medicine.

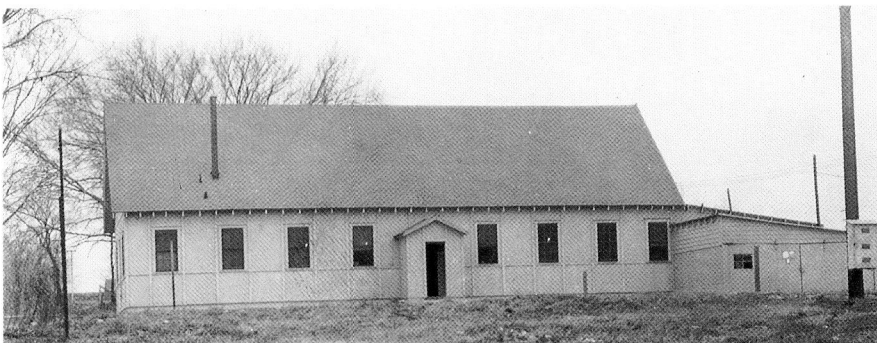

The experimental laboratory in 1934. This structure had originally been built to serve as a gymnasium.

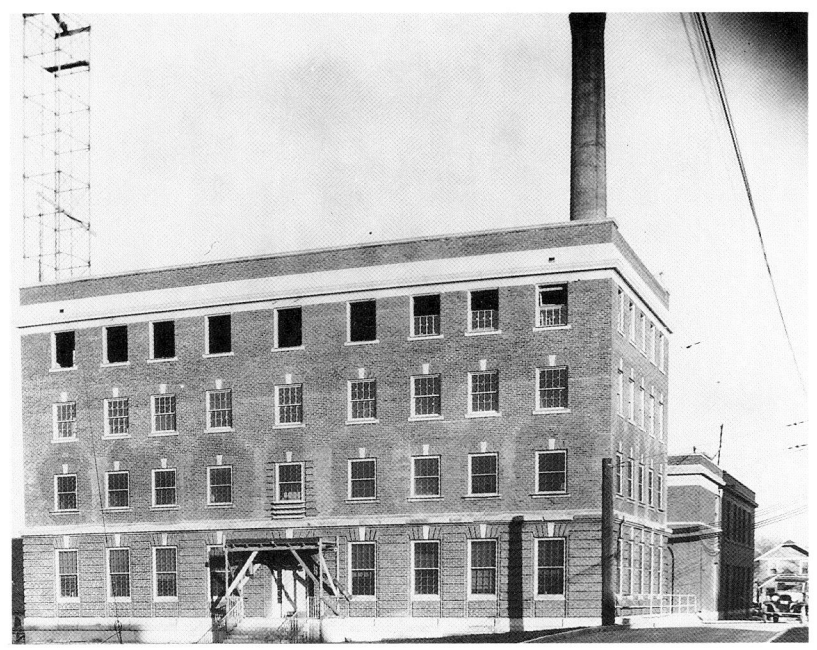

To the west of the Power Plant is the new Hixon Laboratory for Medical Research, now being completed. This unit was obtained through a private gift of $70,000, a PWA Grant of $56,088, and hospital earnings of $13,858, making a total cost of $139,944. This building houses the research activities of the entire hospital staff and medical school faculty. Many contributions are emanating within its walls. This research building is for the encouragement of all scientific and medical research.
—Ralph H. Major, M.D., Report, 1938.

The Hixon Laboratory, first occupied in 1936, was not finally completed until 1938.

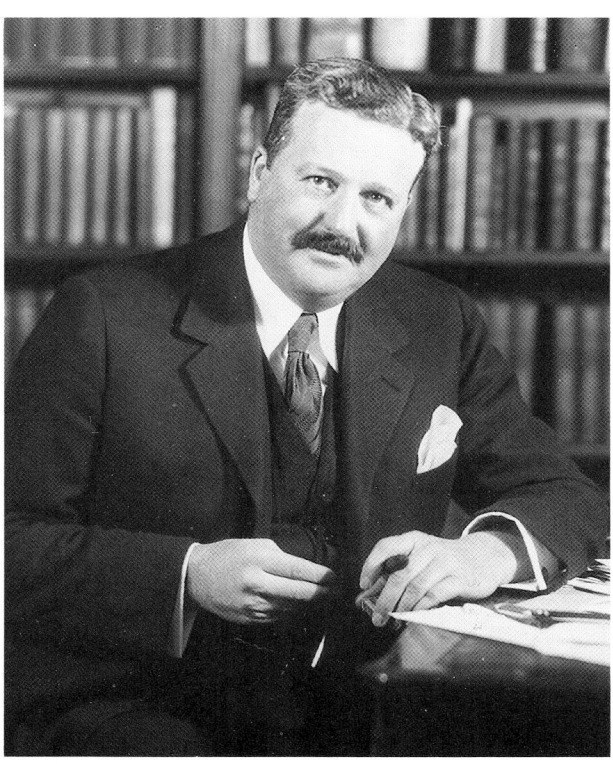

Logan Clendening, M.D., in his office, ca. 1935.

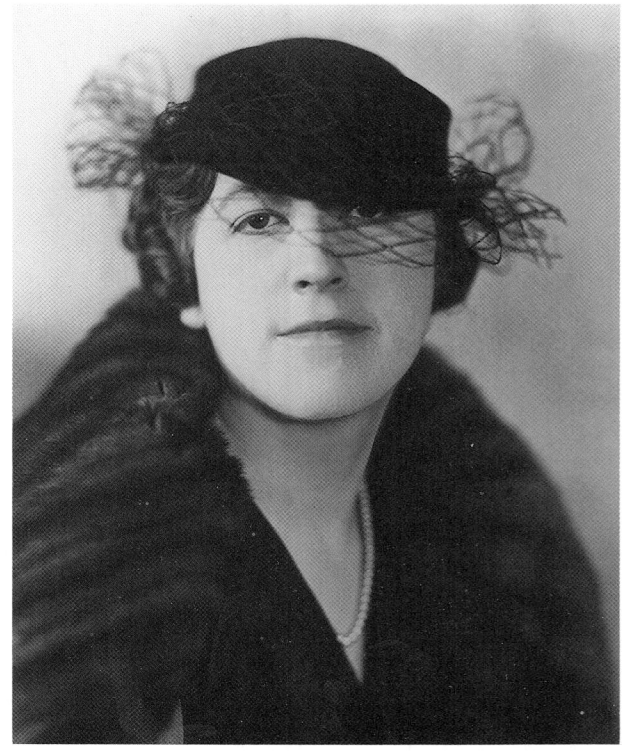

Dorothy Hixon Clendening, ca. 1935.

The present physical equipment is such that there is little opportunity for growth. The doctors are constantly complaining because there are not enough patients for demonstration to the students. County authorities are writing in to send patients into the hospital, and we have to refuse admission because of lack of beds. We ought to have more beds for maternity cases, orthopedic, and pediatric cases. The record room is crowded. We have hardly any place to put our files. The X-ray room is inadequate in that there is no proper ventilation, and to install such ventilation would be extremely expensive.—"The Work of the Hospital," in *University of Kansas School of Medicine Biennial Report*, 1926.

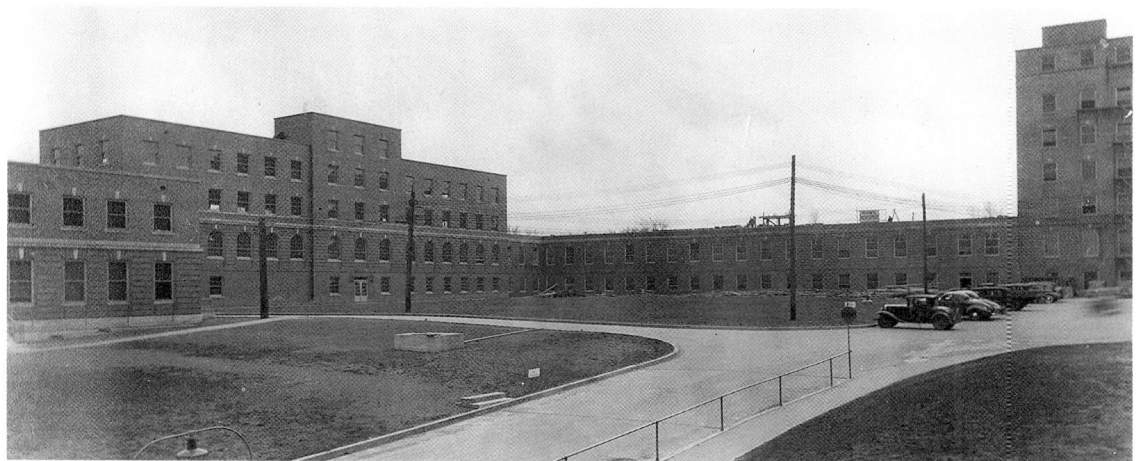

The Hixon Laboratory, Clinic Building, Connecting Corridor, and Ward Building from the 39th Street entrance, ca. 1937.

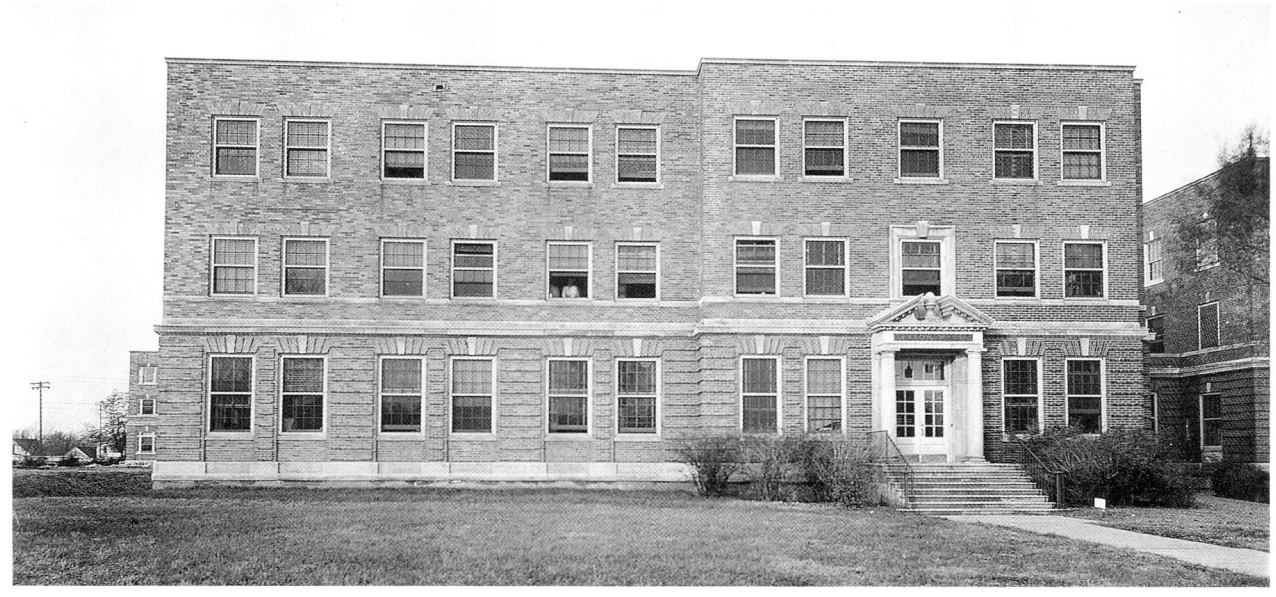

The Eaton Ward, 1940.

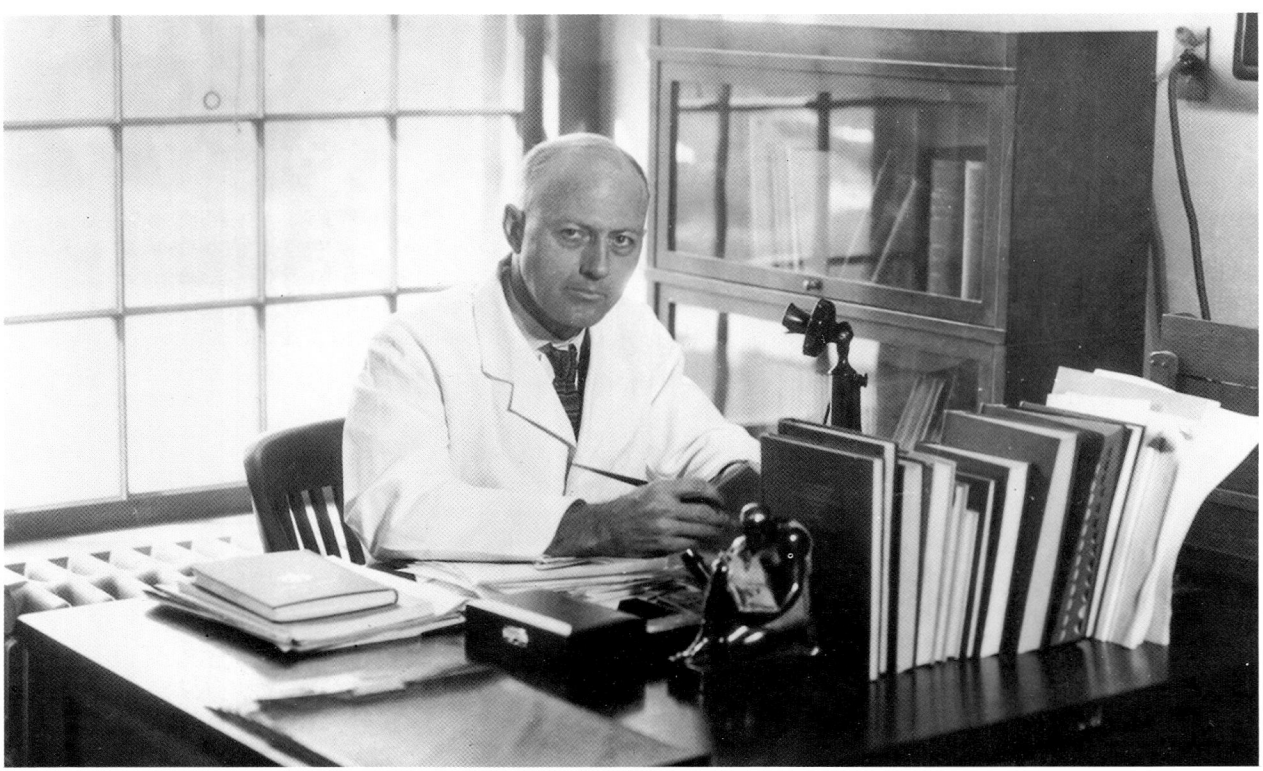

Dr. Wahl in his office, ca. 1940.

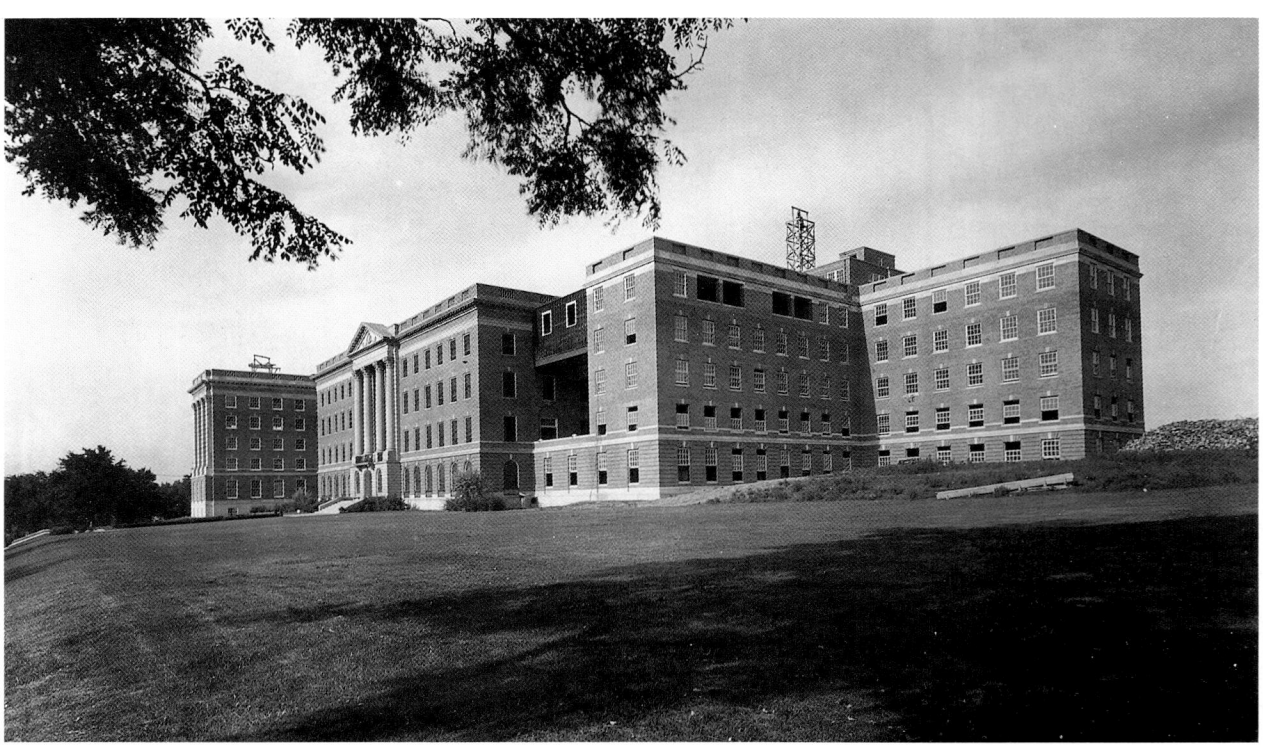

The University of Kansas Medical School campus, late 1930s.

Since my return to Kansas City I have heard from time to time a rather persistent rumor about moving the medical school to Lawrence. If there is any truth back of these rumors or any negotiations under way to bring about such a change, I would like to emphasize the fact that as an Alumnus, I think it would be the most grave and disasterous undertaking the forlorned and orphaned medical school has ever had to withstand in its years of struggle against the ravages of insufficient appropriation. In fact, as I recall from my experience . . . , I think such a change would be almost ludicrous.
—Ellis W. Willhelmy, M.D., to H. R. Wahl, M.D., February 16, 1926.

I am pretty familiar with the development of the Medical School down here adjoining Kansas City and I recently went over the request they are making for some improvements and additions at this time and I hope very much that the Legislature is able to grant them.

As a matter of fact we have no large medical school in Kansas City and I believe that there is a splendid opportunity for the growth of this medical school to serve quite a large area, located in Kansas City, Kansas, as it is, accessible by railroad to all parts of the state, and it is also available to clinical material so necessary for a good medical school.
—J. C. Nichols to Representative Joe Kramer, February 8, 1929.

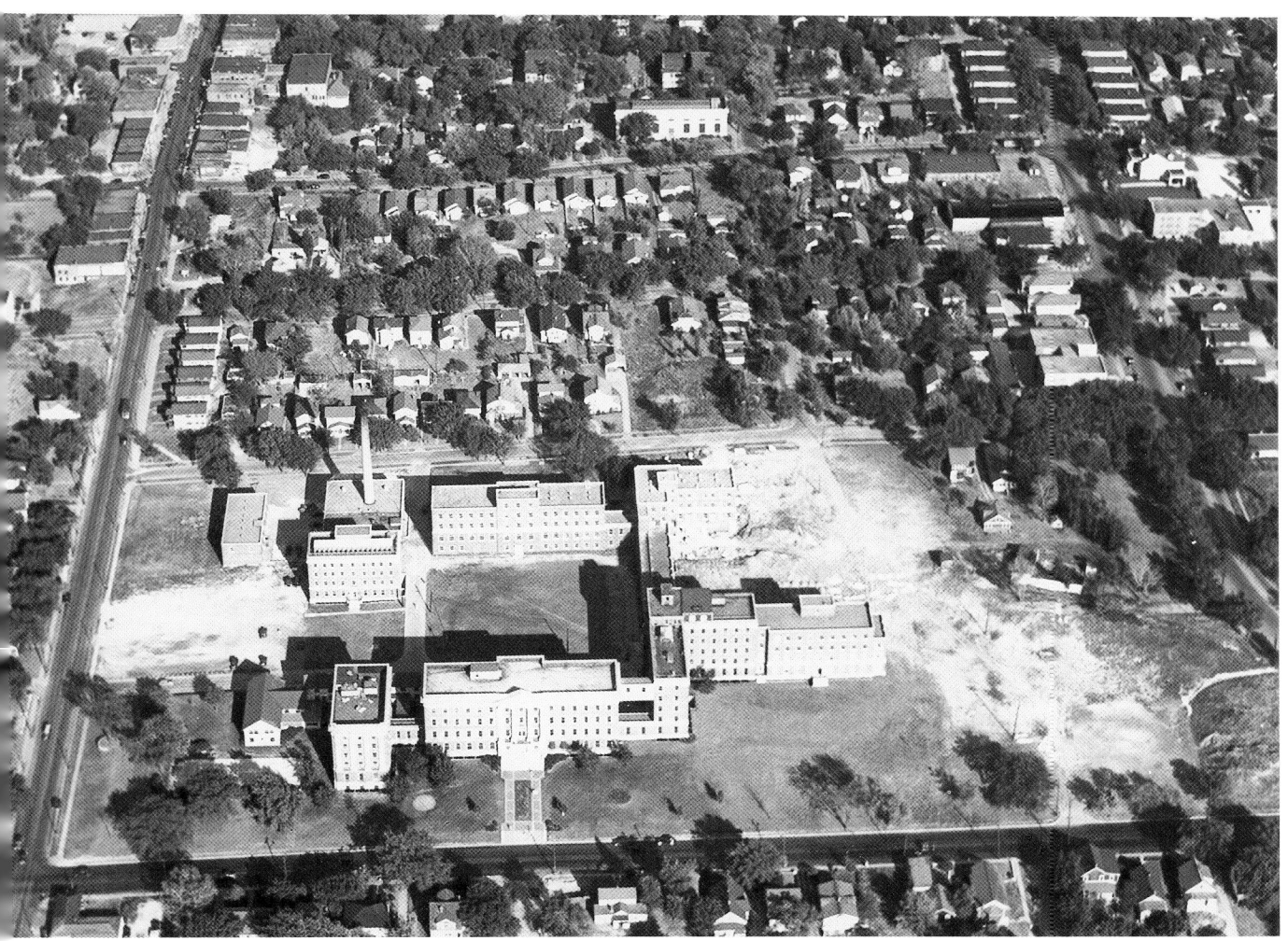

Aerial view of the hospital and medical school, 1939.

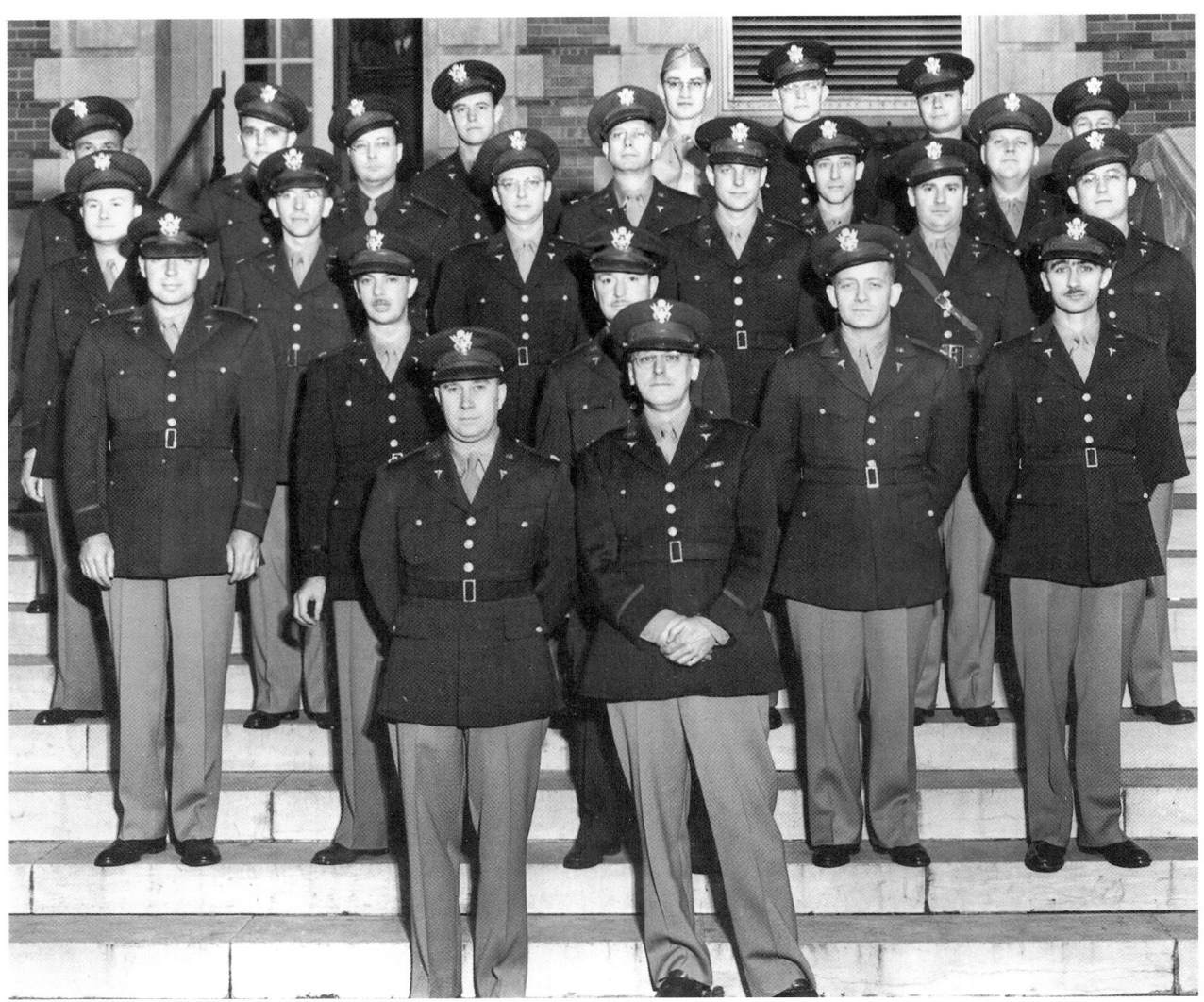

Medical officers of the 77th Evacuation Hospital Unit on the front steps of Bell Memorial Hospital, 1942.

4

Then Came the War

The advent of World War II checked any immediate hopes of notable progress at the University of Kansas School of Medicine. Although the state's financial position drastically improved with the rising price of agricultural products and the building of war plants, austerity remained the rule at 39th and Rainbow. The physical plant looked much the same as at the end of the New Deal. What passed for a major change was converting areas in the new Hixon Laboratory into a day-care center capable of accommodating twenty-five to thirty children. Although day-care facilities were needed, this worthy project occupied needed research space in a building designed specifically for that function. A research library housing Logan Clendening's history of medicine collection was also located in the Hixon Laboratory building. Throughout the war, then, meaningful medical research at the School of Medicine virtually ceased. Many faculty members went off to war, and those who remained behind undertook accelerated teaching responsibilities. As a result, in 1944 the school graduated two medical classes.

By the 1940s, the University of Kansas School of Medicine had gained a reputation as an institution that produced competent physicians and nurses who displayed a thorough knowledge of medicine and clinical duties, but were not especially research oriented. Since the budget for research in the mid-1940s was only $6,000 annually, the administration found it necessary to settle for a studied mediocrity—to consider institutional survival the primary objective rather than setting new goals designed to advance and modernize the school. With the onset of World War II, however, energies turned to coping with chronic shortages in supplies, equipment, and most importantly, staff.

The bright star of the medical school during the war years was the 77th Evacuation Hospital Unit. In the summer of 1940, the medical school accepted a proposal by the surgeon general of the United States Army to establish an affiliated military evacuation hospital. A paper organization grew up in the ensuing months that included physicians from the teaching staff and nurses, mostly from metropolitan Kansas City and surrounding areas. The leadership of this unit came from the medical school. Edward H. Hashinger, M.D., served as the temporary director and as head of the medical section. James B. Weaver, M.D., directed the surgical section. Young professors, including Mahlon Delp, M.D., and Max S. Allen, M.D., enlisted in the organization. The activation of the 77th occurred within six months after Pearl Harbor, in May of 1942.

Following basic training at Fort Leonard Wood in the Missouri Ozarks, the 77th traveled overseas to the United Kingdom in time to participate in the November 1942 invasion of North Africa and the ensuing Tunisian campaign. After providing medical support in the successful 1943 invasion of Sicily, the 77th returned to the United Kingdom. In the aftermath of D-Day, the 77th landed in Europe and participated in the great battles of liberation, from St. Lo to Paris to the Ardennes to the Remagen Rhine crossing, and on into Germany proper. In 1944 alone, the 77th admitted over 35,000 patients to a 750-bed hospital with an authorized strength of over 300 physicians and nurses, most of whom were from the original unit formed at the University of Kansas Medical School. The members of the 77th who returned to Kansas resumed their prewar positions, viewing with modest pride the service time that took them beyond usual medical concerns. Nevertheless, their shared experiences forged a permanent bond; the personnel of the 77th have continued to hold reunions through 1990. Moreover, the significant and gallant service of the medical unit impressed the people of Kansas, gaining additional support and recognition for the medical school.

During the war years as throughout its short history, the University of Kansas School of Medicine desperately needed financial support. Neither the school's survival nor its Kansas City location remained burning issues, but two decades of statutory neglect had helped to sap the vitality of the institution. Dean Wahl, in demonstrating the medical school's willingness and ability to survive on short rations during difficult times, gained credibility with the legislature by avoiding demands that might rekindle the regional problems and animosities that long vexed public medical education in the Sunflower State. So, the school struggled on. With many of its vibrant young people away at war, the institution remained much the same as in the 1930s—not necessarily out of step with the reforms initiated in response to Flexner's criticisms, but slow to advance beyond basic requirements.

While Wahl tended to stay in the background—he claimed to be a poor public speaker—popular syndicated medical columnist Logan Clendening, M.D., remained a visible spokesperson for the school. After Clendening's death in 1945, his wife, Dorothy Hixon Clendening Clark, provided support for the continued development of the school's history of medicine library. In addition, Clendening's friends raised money that resulted in the construction of a memorial fountain, still the centerpiece of the Medical Center. Besides Clendening, other prominent physicians supported the school through trying times—Clarence B. Francisco, M.D., in orthopaedic surgery for children; Thomas G. Orr, M.D., in general surgery; Ralph H. Major, M.D., in medicine; Frank Neff, M.D., in pediatrics; and Leroy A. Calkins, M.D., in obstetrics and gynecology.

As the photographic images demonstrate, the facilities were still meager and outdated. Even the relatively new red brick buildings at 39th and Rainbow look dull and institutional, and the inpatient and outpatient areas seem outmoded. The clothing worn by the medical and nursing personnel appears old fashioned and often reflects prewar styles. During the war, as in previous years, the school and hospital were performing many of the functions of a charitable institution for poor and indigent patients. As throughout the history of the school, the faculty continued to teach and perform their clinical duties. Many of the medical faculty who maintained outside practices, however, referred their paying patients to other hospitals. Their often voluntary medical school responsibilities frequently conflicted with maintaining successful private practices.

Wahl, beset by the usual funding woes, realized that he had stayed dean too long. Over twenty-four years, through depression, war, and inflation, his annual state budget had only increased from $140,000 to $625,000. In real dollars the budget had declined. During 1948, Wahl left his twin posts as dean and director of the hospital, but continued to teach and conduct research until his death in 1955. His successor was Franklin D. Murphy, M.D., recommended to Chancellor Deane W. Malott of the University of Kansas by Wahl and other senior faculty members. Murphy exhibited the strong public relations and organizational talents that would be needed to bring the school into the mid-twentieth century.

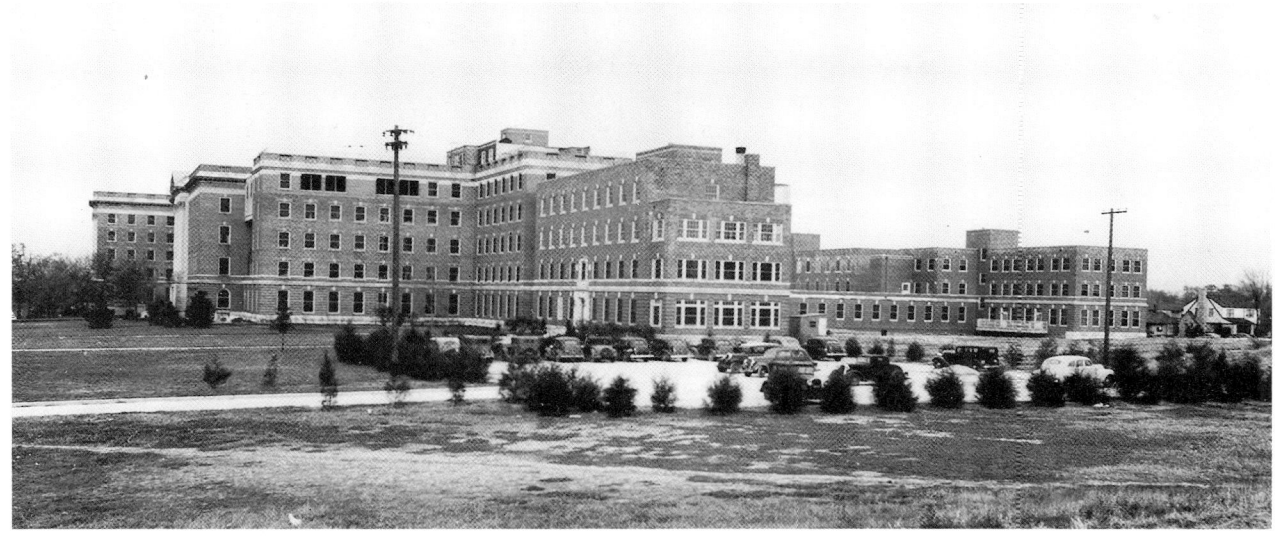

The Medical School from Olathe Boulevard, 1940s.

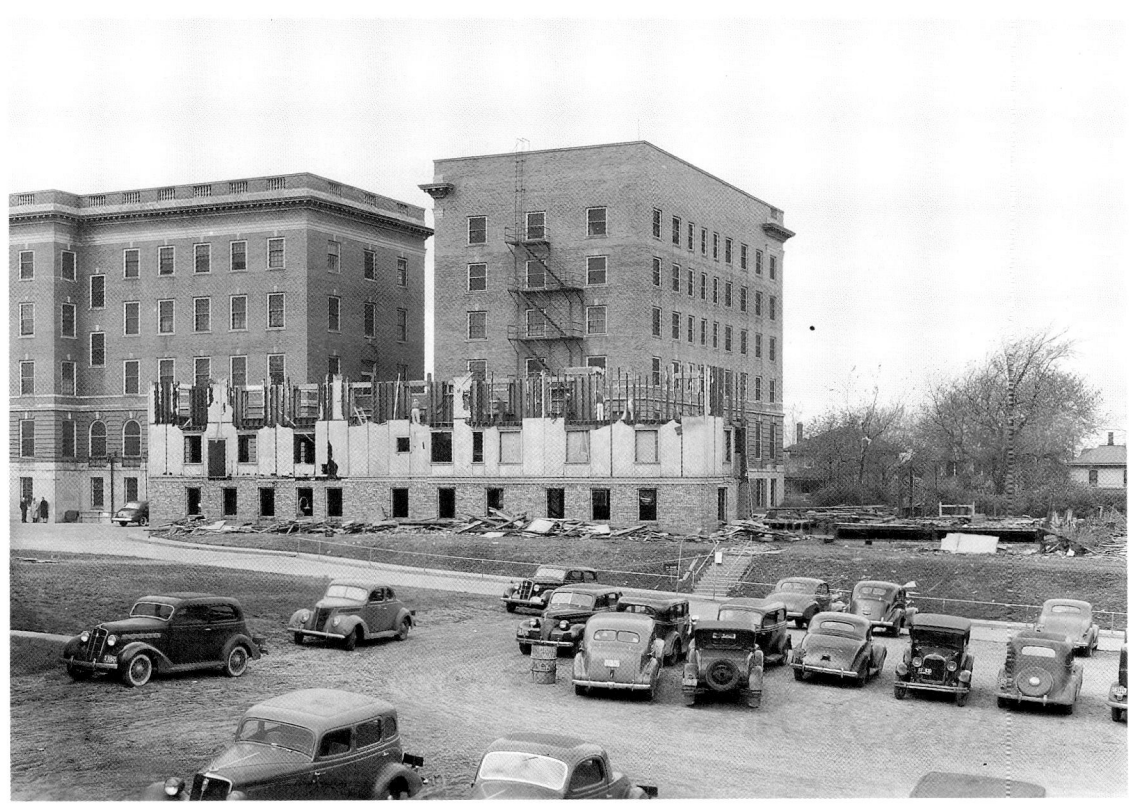

Demolition of the barracks, October 23, 1940.

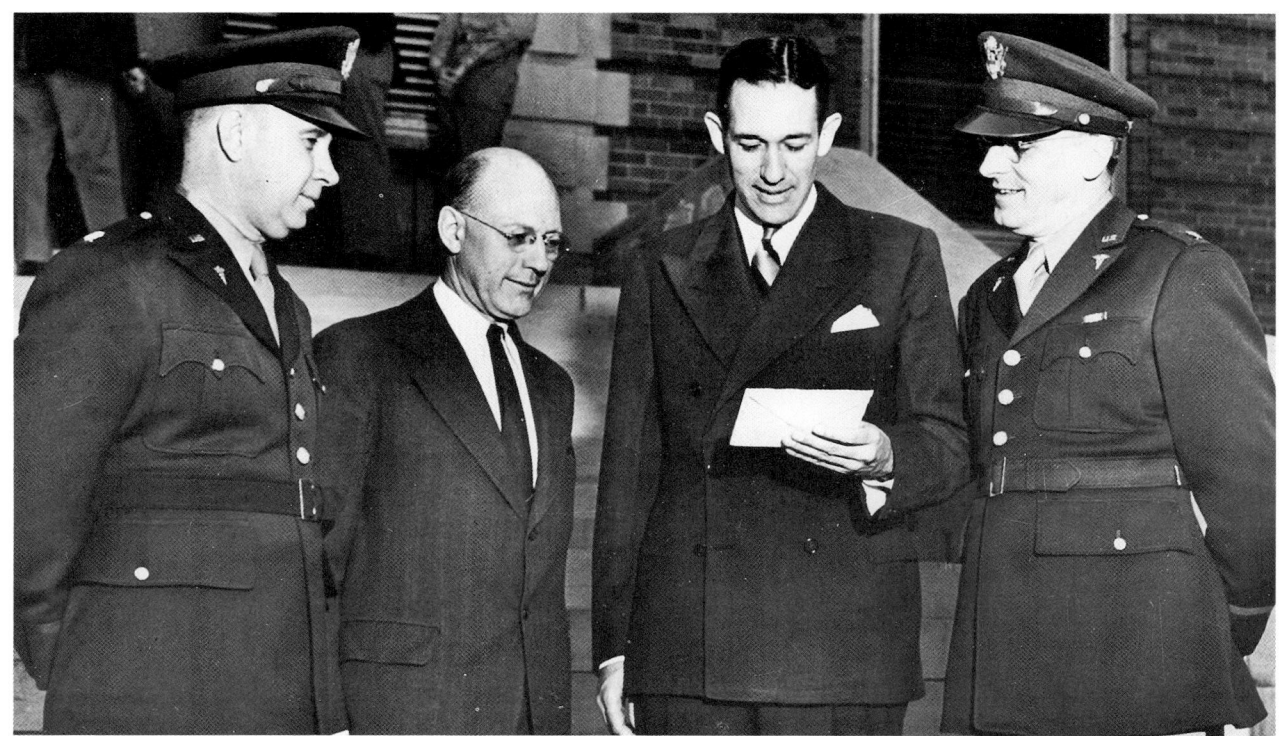

Dr. James Weaver, Dean Harry R. Wahl, Chancellor Deane Malott, and Dr. Edward Hashinger at the official activation of the 77th Evacuation Hospital Unit, May 16, 1942.

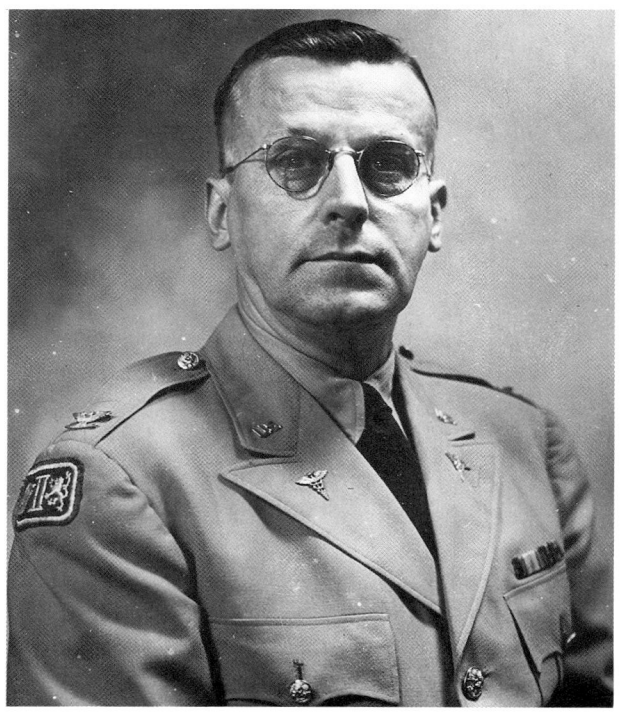

Colonel Edward H. Hashinger, M.D., organizer and commanding officer of the 77th.

In the summer of 1940, following a request from the Surgeon-General, an evacuation hospital unit was formed. With Pearl Harbor on December 7, 1941, this paper organization became a living, throbbing thing under the command of Dr. Hashinger, and recruits literally began to pour in, both officers and men. In addition to members of the hospital staff, a number of physicians and dentists practicing in Kansas City, as well as alumni of the Medical School, joined. On May 22, 1942, a farewell banquet and party were given in honor of the 77th Evacuation Hospital, and the following day 35 officers reported at Ft. Leonard Wood. We were all proud of them as our representatives on the field of battle and quite expected the magnificent account they gave of themselves.

—Ralph H. Major, M.D., *An Account of the University of Kansas School of Medicine*, 1968.

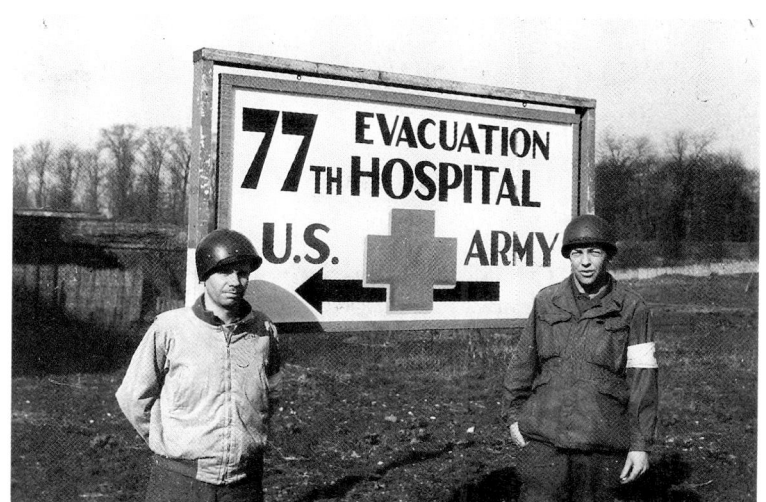

The 77th in Europe.

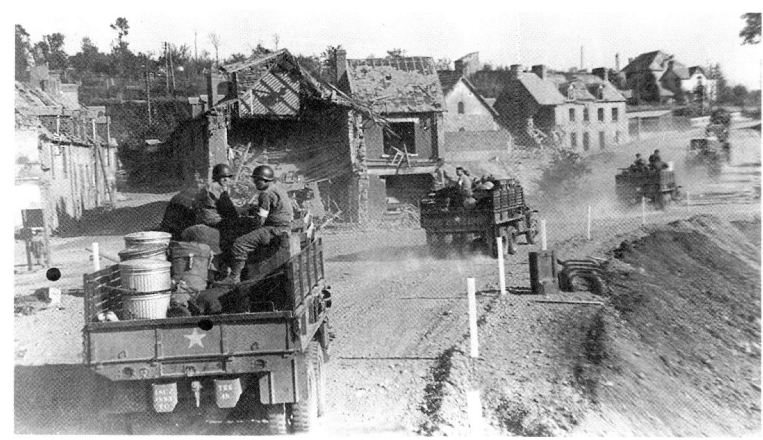

The 77th Evacuation Hospital Unit moves through a bombed-out St. Lo, France, in August 1944.

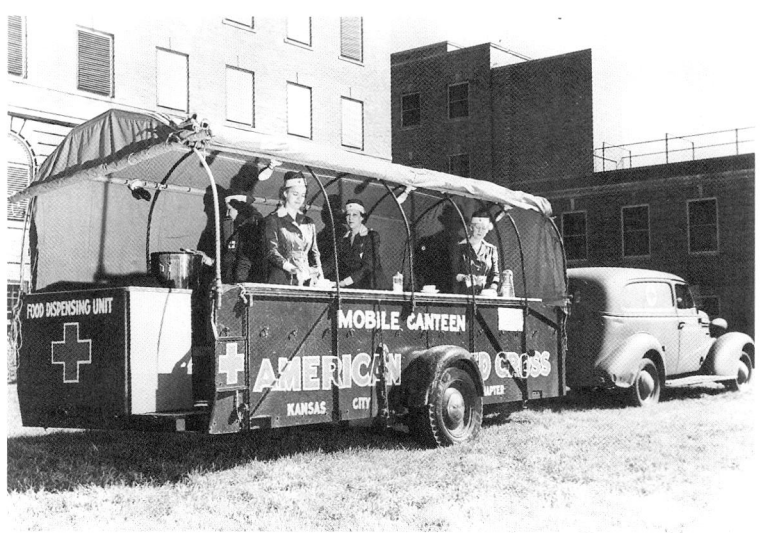

An American Red Cross mobile canteen visits the campus on October 10, 1942.

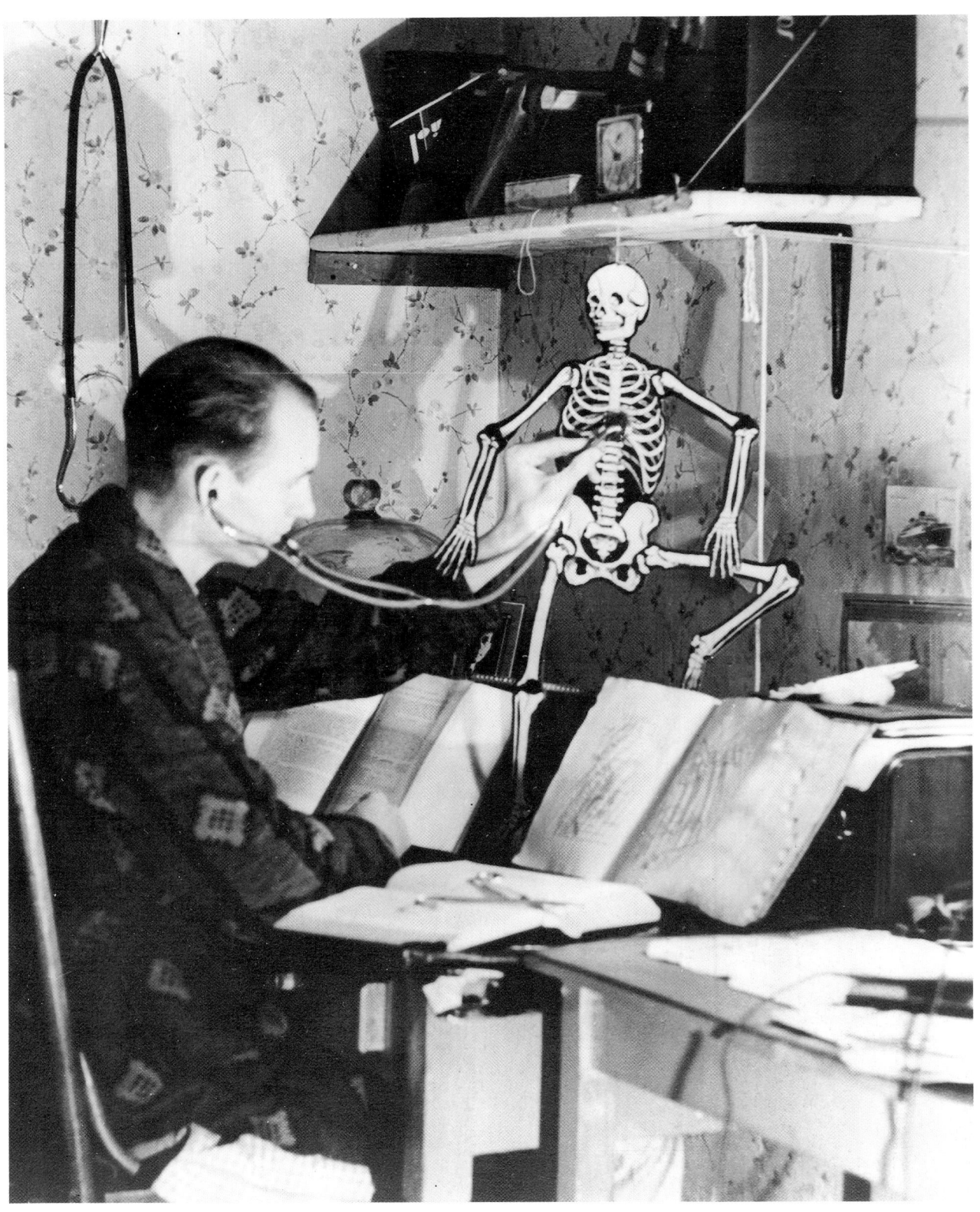

Auscultation by student Hal McLean, 1940.

One of the first hospital units to be activated was the 77th Evacuation Unit, composed of members of the faculty and nursing staffs of the KU Hospitals. With a characteristic esprit de corps under the effective direction of Drs. Hashinger and Weaver, the unit rapidly gained renown.

They have participated in invasions on three fronts. In with the shock troops at Oran, they handled 25,000 patients before moving to Sicily. Recognizing their efficiency, General Bradley requested that they be returned to England to be on hand for D-Day. Request granted, they are following the First Army into Germany.—*Jayhawker MD*, 1944.

One of the new-fangled theories of progressive medical education, which was developed at the University of Kansas and which is slowly being accepted among medical students in the East, is that it takes more than a student body to build an educational institution—it also requires the presence of a faculty. The original hypothesis as incorporated into the policy of this University stated that if a group of learned men could be torn away from the humdrum of a medical practice, their accumulated experience could be applied towards aiding a small full-time staff in taking rolls, curbing cribbing, and providing the student body with conversational material. Such a system, we are proud to state, has proved successful at KU, and it is hoped that other schools will benefit from the results obtained.—*Jayhawker MD*, 1944.

The work of the first year and a half is given at Lawrence. It consists of fundamental scientific branches, anatomy, biochemistry, bacteriology, and physiology. The instruction is given by men who devote themselves entirely to teaching and research. The medical students have all the advantages of the University laboratories, libraries, museums and lectures.

The work of the last half of the second year and of the third and fourth year is given at Kansas City, Kan. It is intended largely to familiarize the students with the various manifestations of diseases and their treatment. Much of the work is done by the bedside, and the student has an opportunity to observe all the processes of making a diagnosis and prescribing the treatment.—*Bulletin of the University of Kansas*, Catalogue of the School of Medicine for 1940–1941 and 1941–1942.

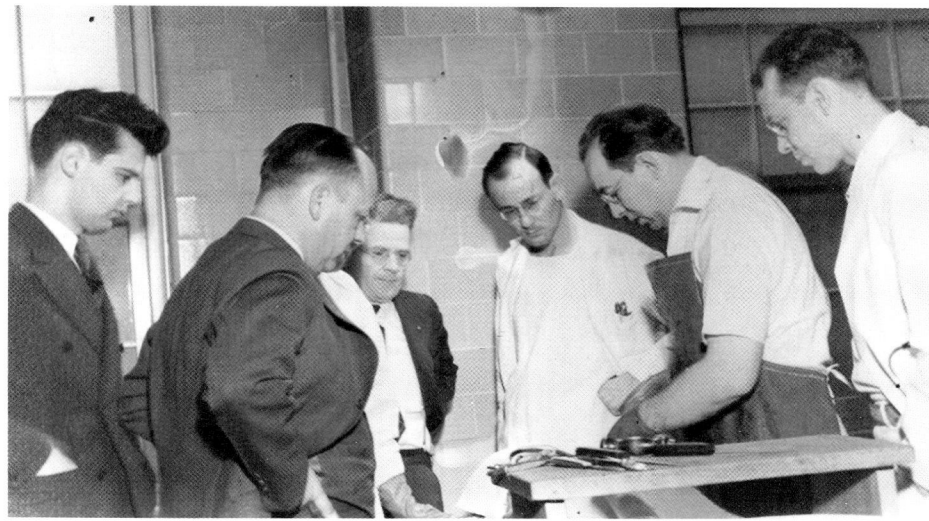

A teaching session with Graham Asher, M.D., ca. 1940.

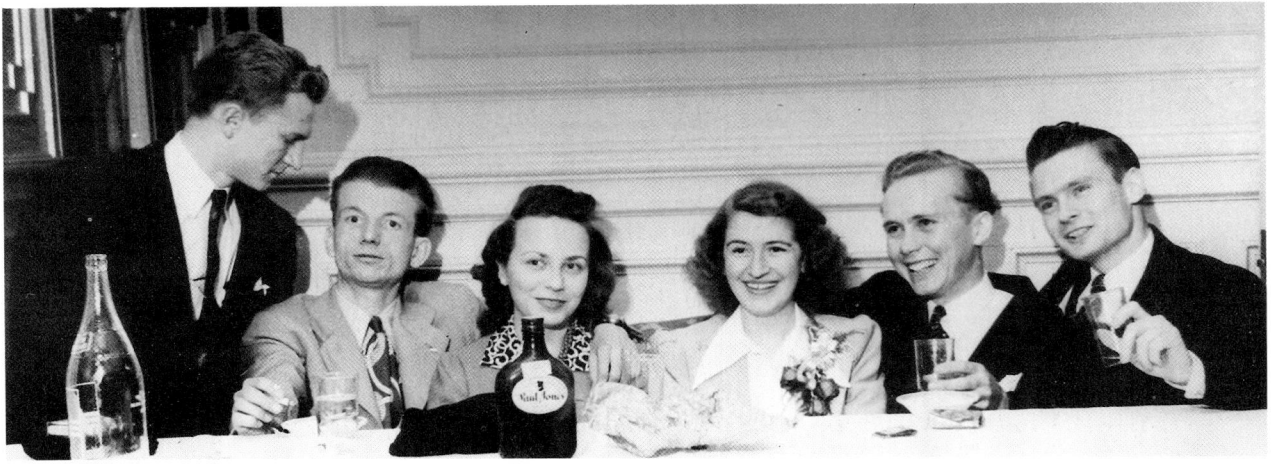

A medical student party, 1940.

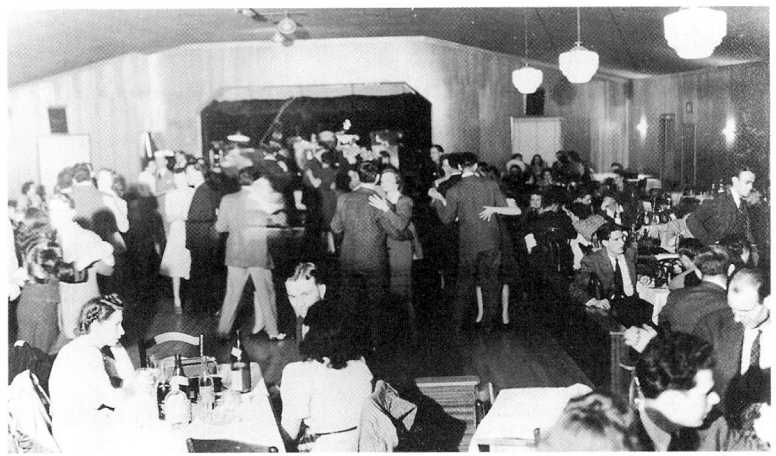

Students dancing at a 1941 social event.

Medical Dames was what I enjoyed most. This was an organization of the medical students wives. We met monthly and some of the meetings were on campus. I enjoyed the activities which were in the homes of the faculty. Ones which made a lasting impression on me were in the homes of Mrs. Don Carlos Peete and Kay Wahl. They were gracious hostesses. They were interested in all the Medical Dames and eager to help in any way they could. From their wealth of experience they were helpful when one of the young women had a problem she wanted to talk about. They were like mothers to us.
—Correspondence: Helen Hostetter to Nancy Hulston, February 13, 1989.

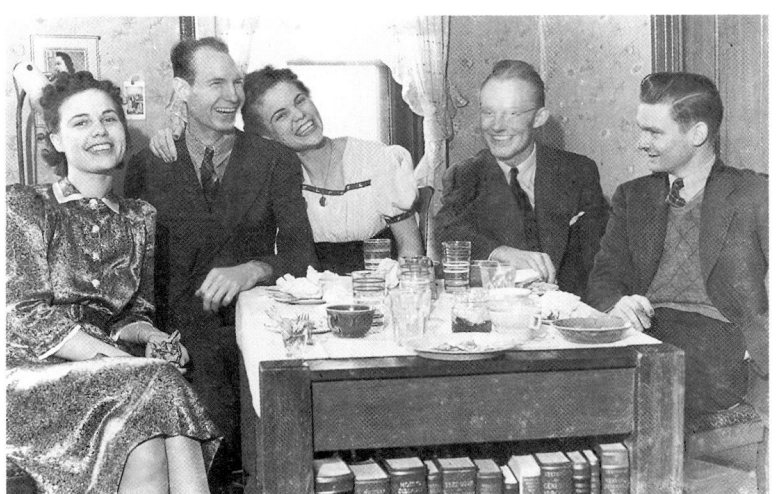

Helen Whitman (Hostetter), Hal McLean, Dorothy Whitman, Vorris Reist, and Morton Brownell, 1940.

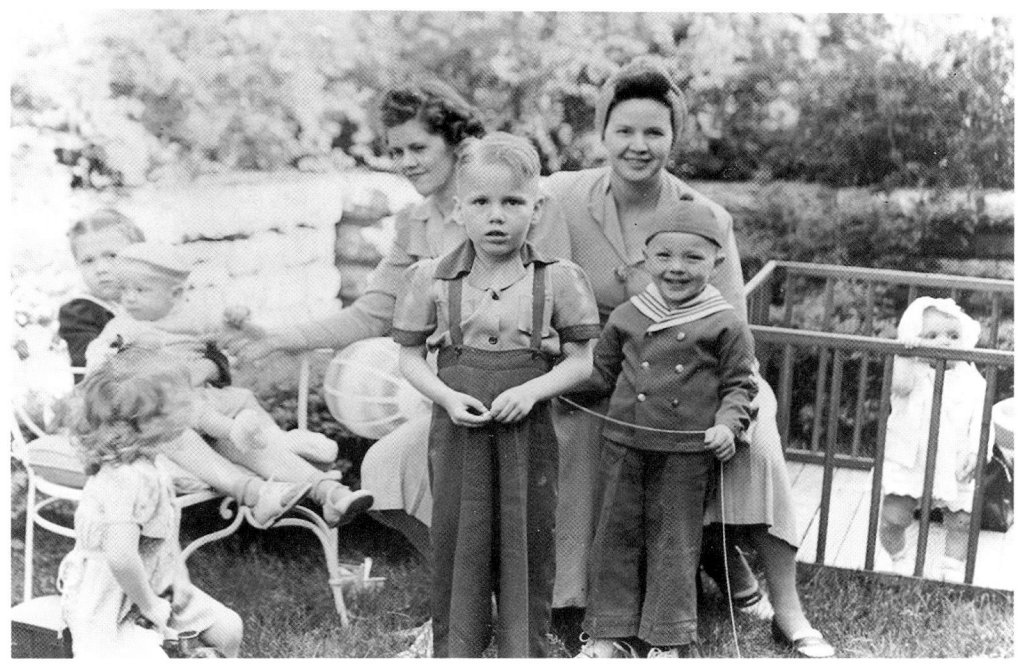

Medical students' families, 1942.

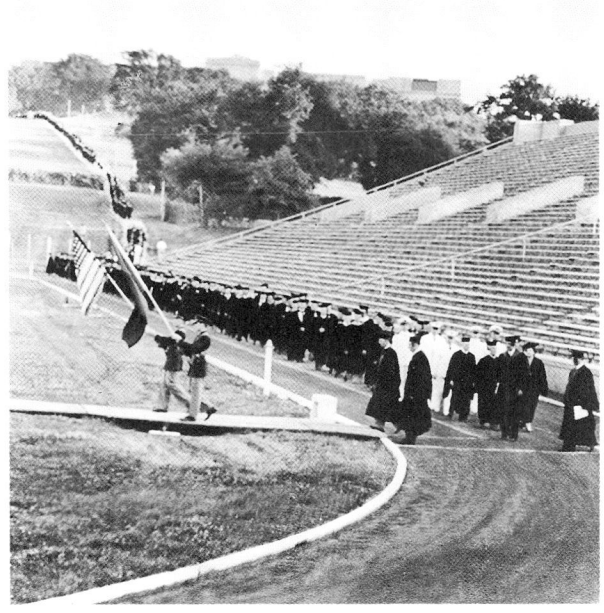

Class of 1942 graduation at Lawrence.

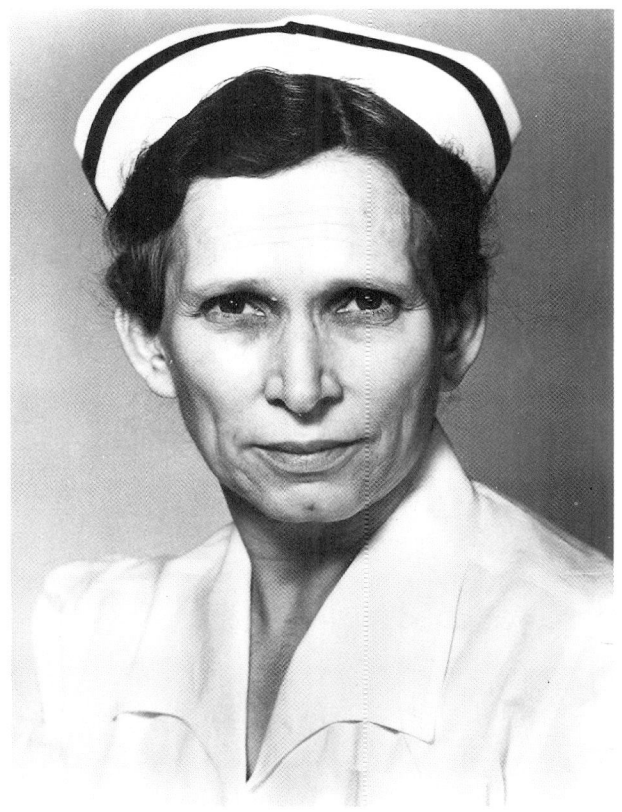

Sara A. Patterson, R.N., acting superintendent of nurses, 1941–1944.

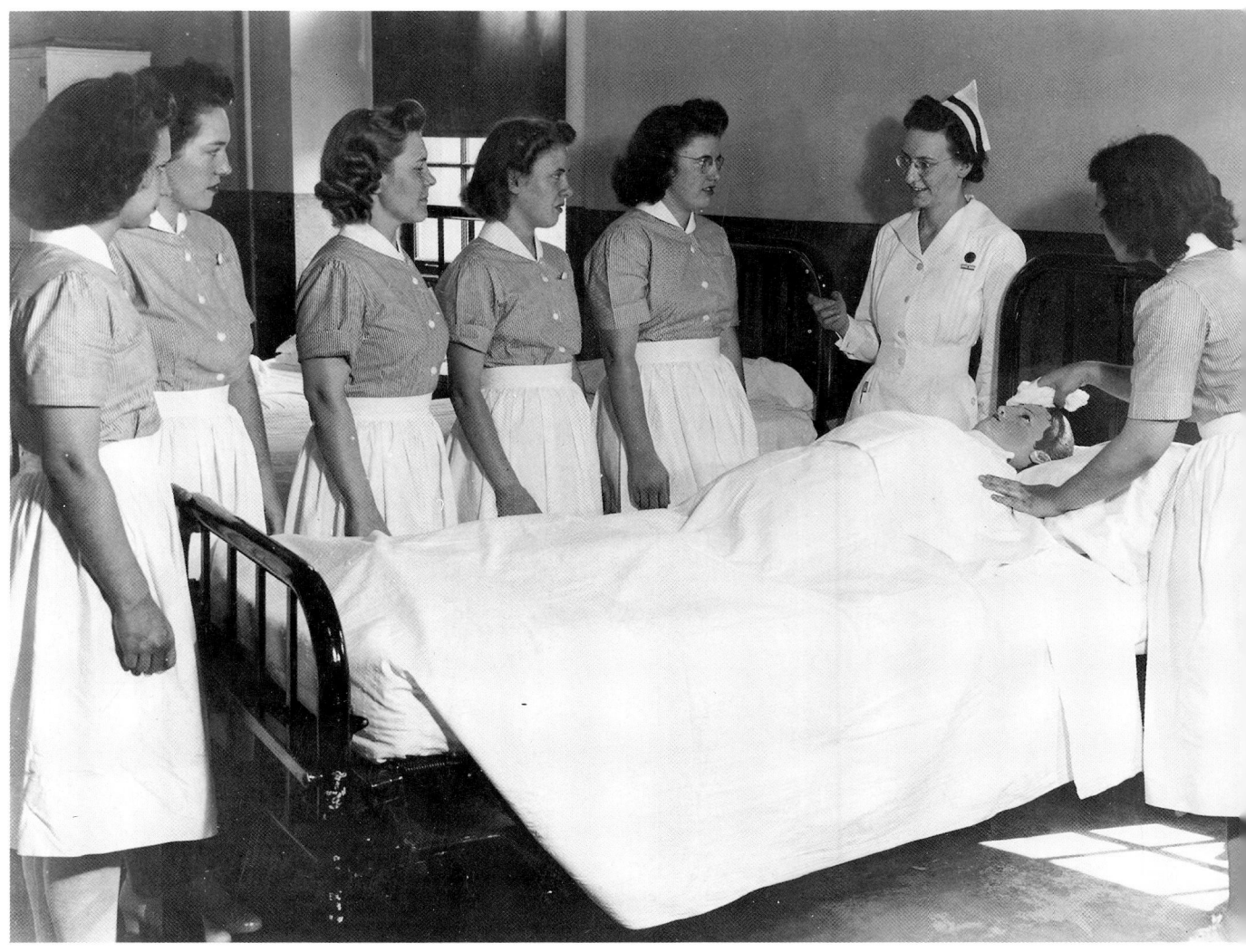

A demonstration with a mannikin for the student nurses, ca. 1940.

Then came the war. . . . During these three years the pressures were great. More nurses needed, programs accelerated, increased enrollment, three classes admitted each year, fewer and less well prepared faculty, and graduate nurses volunteering for military services leaving more of the nursing service to the students. The amount of service given by students had always been in excess of educational needs but now more was expected of them. These students all deserved service medals for their contribution to the war effort because service was often given at the sacrifice of their education. Housing for students had to be found in the community as Hinch Hall could not accommodate the increased enrollment.—Sara A. Patterson, R.N., "Out of Our Past," 1966.

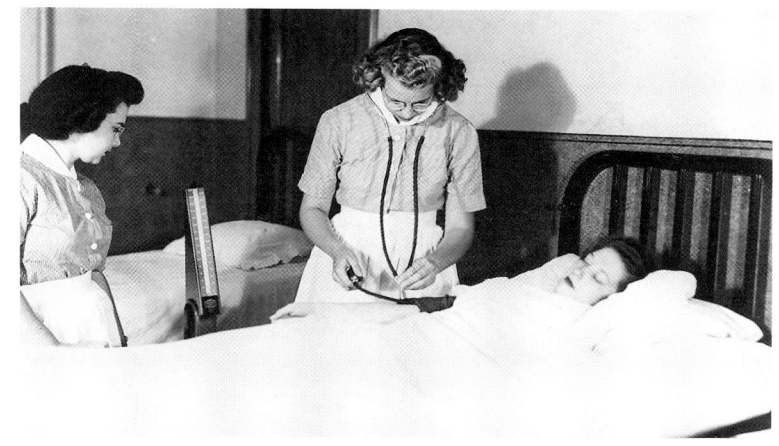

Student nurse Karleen King taking a patient's blood pressure, early 1942.

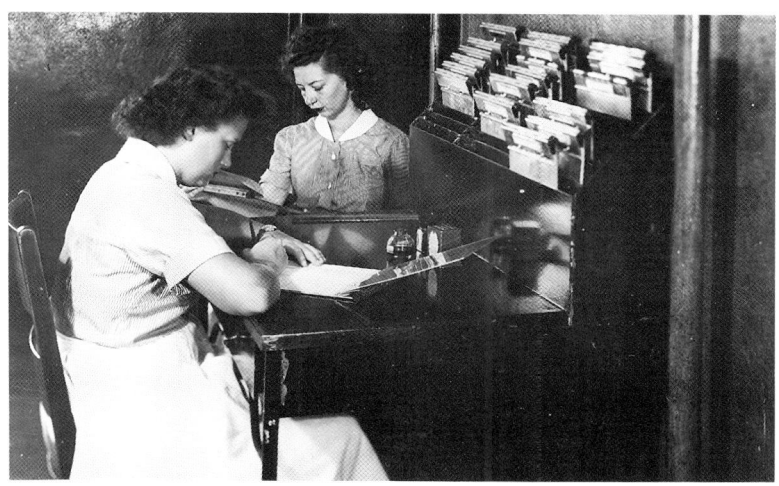

Working with patients' charts, early 1940s.

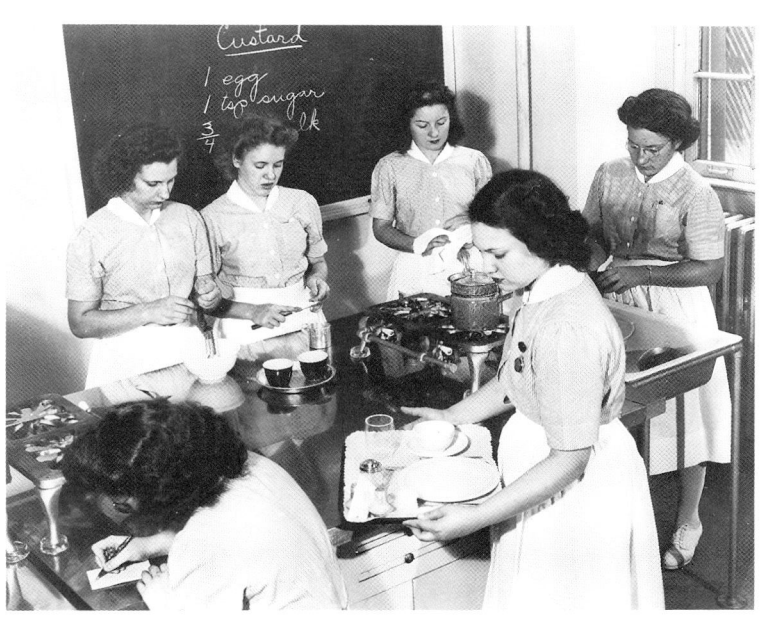

Student nurses in nutrition class, 1942.

April 18, 1941, is an important date because of a change in a policy concerning students. On this date the Nursing Committee met and discussed, "Should the students be allowed to marry?" As anyone who was a student here prior to that date knows, out of every class that graduated at least one member was "secretly" married. The Dean moved that "hereafter the marital status of an applicant to the school of nursing is not to play any part in the future admission or continuance in school." Motion carried. The reason a decision had to be made at this time was that a student had married and had gone to her minister to discuss the possibility of her dismissal from the school. The minister called the administration. It was a timely decision as this would have been a real problem during World War II. Allowing students to marry brought criticism from various sources. One doctor objected saying that it would "take something away from nursing to allow students to marry." He didn't explain this statement.
—Sara A. Patterson, R.N., "Out of Our Past," 1966.

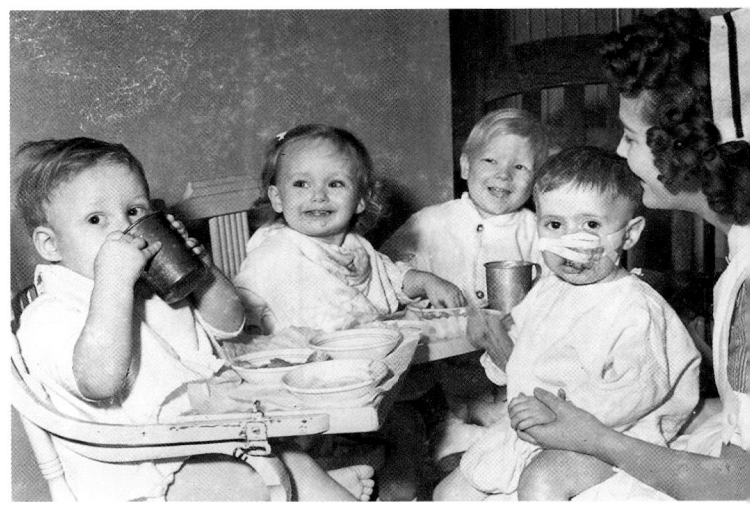

A student nurse feeding pediatric patients, 1941.

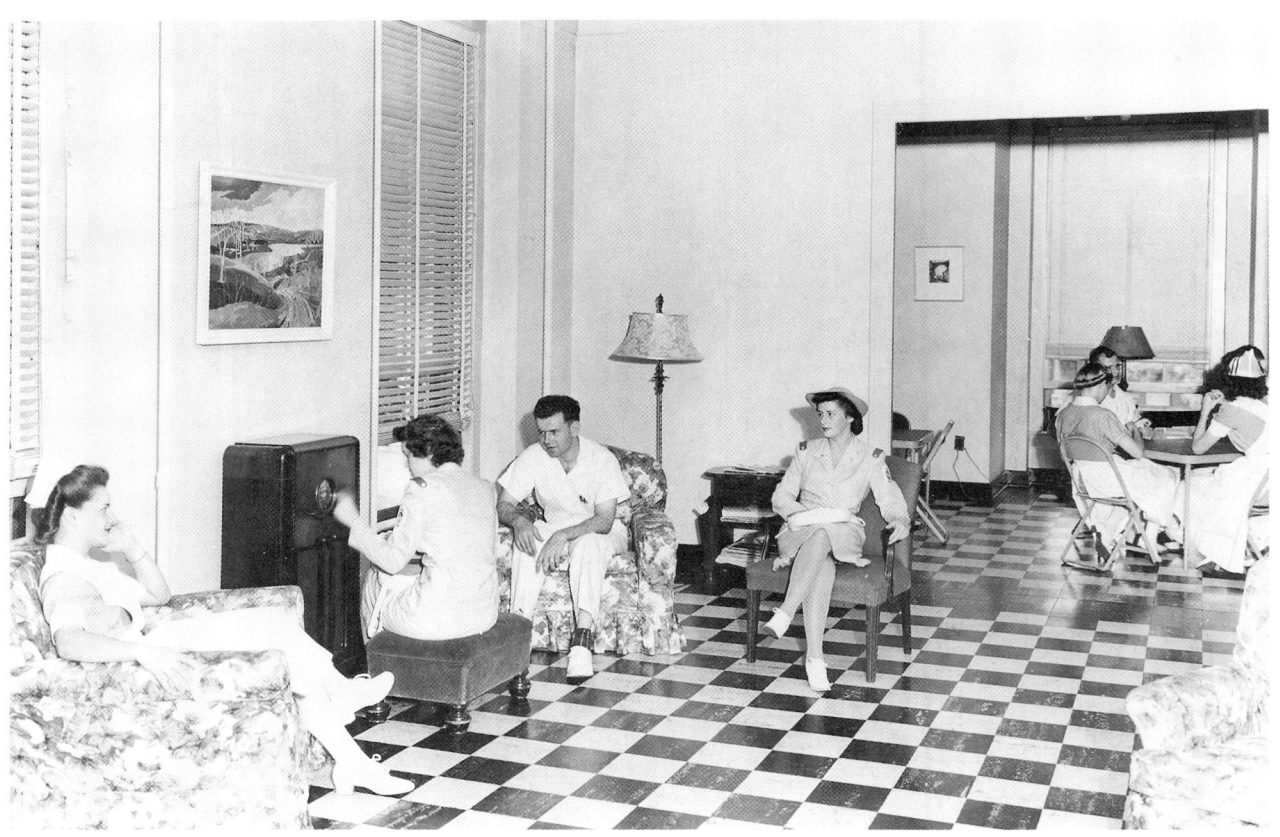

The recreation room in the nurses' residence during World War II.

On February 23, 1944, the class lost a true friend in Dr. C. B. Francisco. Any expression of the significance of his passing is of necessity wholly inadequate, for it is impossible to measure in words the profound effect which he had upon all those with whom he came in contact. To us, his students, he will remain as one of the great personalities in our medical careers. While his lectures did not show the polish or style of a philologist, they were not long and dry, but were steeped with common sense and good medicine.

Many of us recall his simple and sound method of evaluating every case. "First, is it something or nothing? Second, if it is something, is it a mechanical condition or what disease is it?" He never lectured to us without subtly reminding us of the evils of incompetence. The recollection of his admonition, "It is forever too late," constantly reminds us of the fact that if we are not well trained, we are forever a failure. But again, he would fortify our misgivings by telling us, "Try to be a good doctor, and don't worry if you are not a great doctor."
—*Jayhawker MD,* 1944.

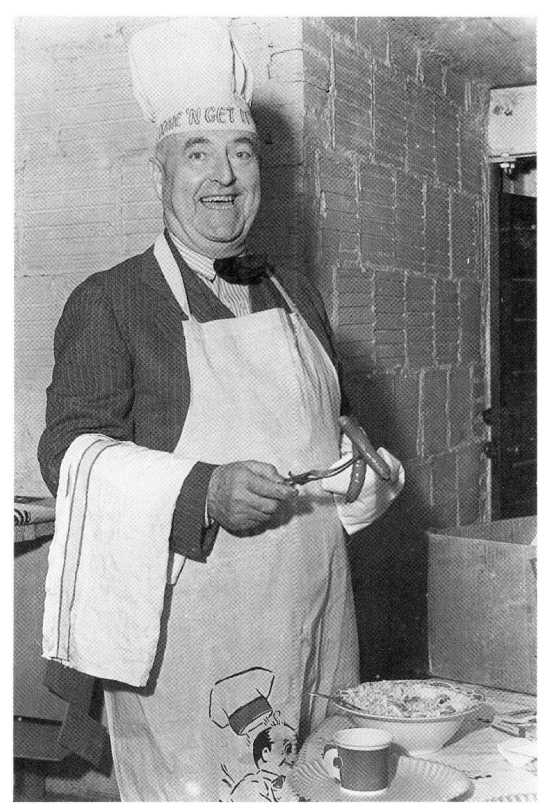

C. B. Francisco, M.D., serving hotdogs at his annual picnic for medical students, ca. 1940.

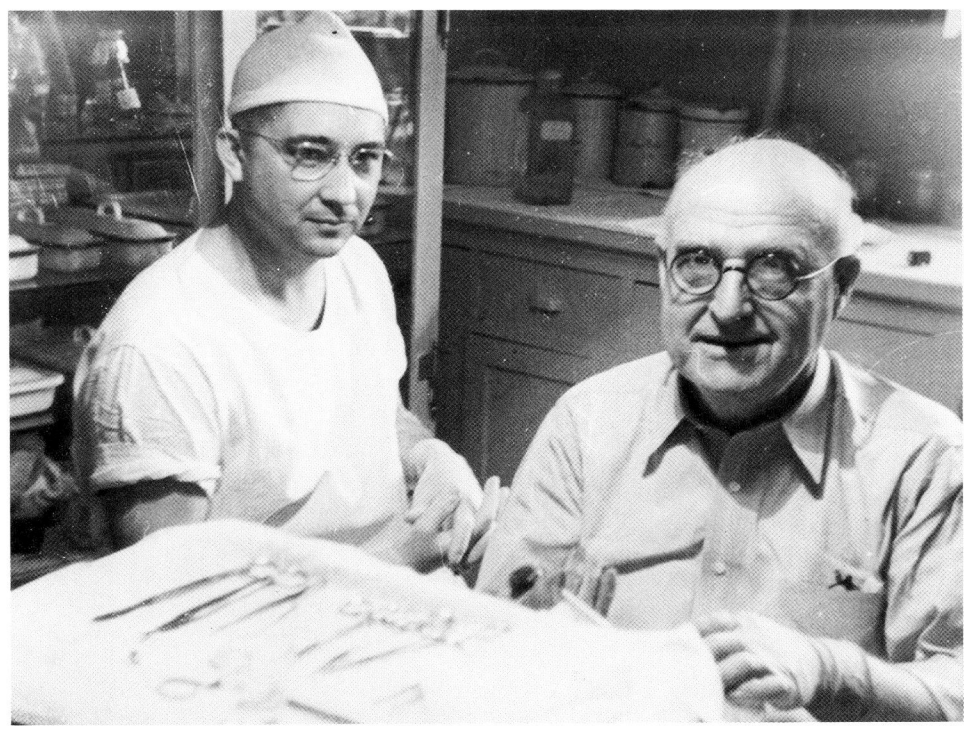

Dr. Francisco, professor of orthopaedic surgery, with a student, 1941.

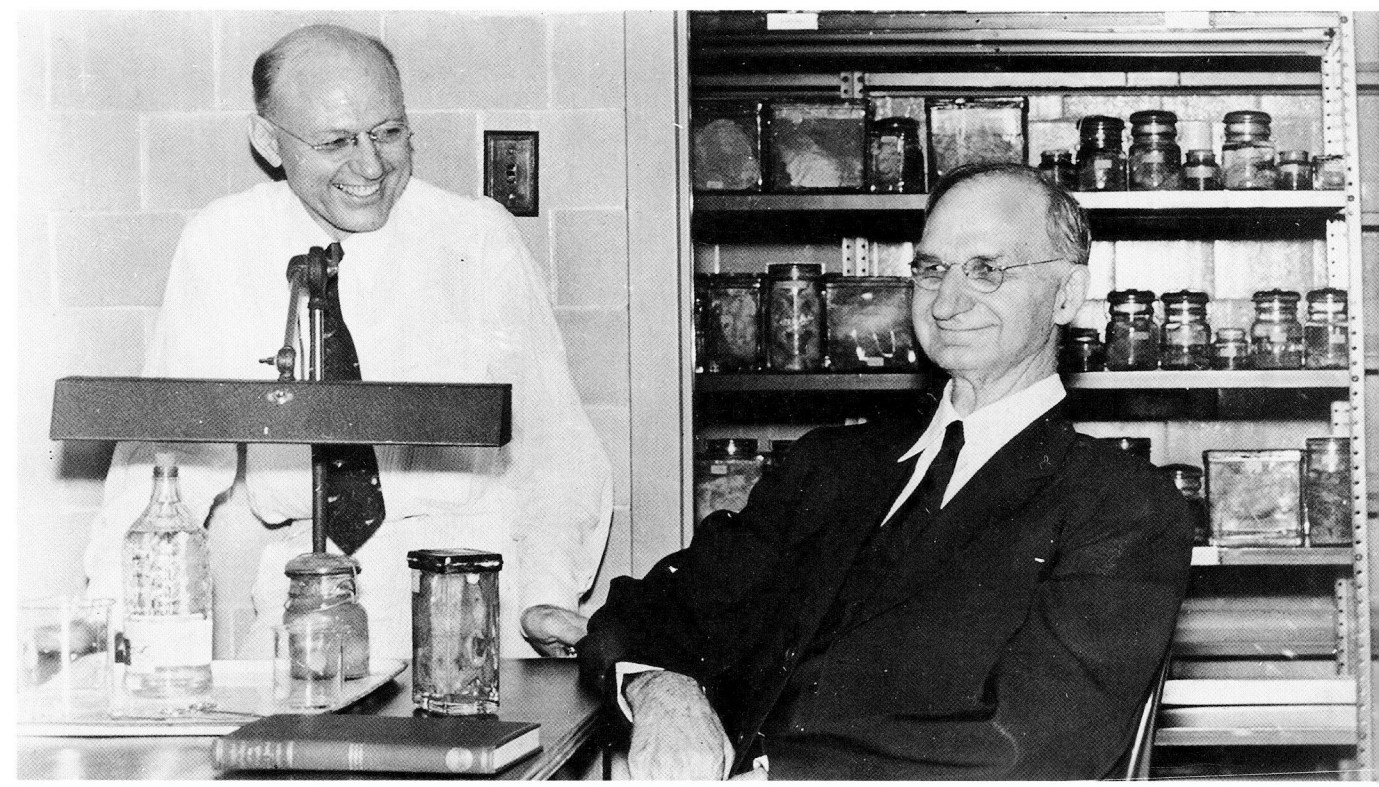

Drs. Harry R. Wahl and Arthur E. Hertzler in the pathology
museum located in the Hixon Laboratory, 1942.

While many other doctors were buying faster horses for their buggies, Hertzler
bought books and collected tumors. He started a book about tumors and lugged
many of them to St. Louis by train, in the smoking car because the odor from the
not-too-well-sealed buckets made him unwelcome elsewhere.
—Newspaper account, April 13, 1959.

"I am positively convinced that the most effective clinic is one where the teacher
spends at least half of his time quizzing the students. The students not only like
it, but they realize it is the only way they can learn; and, what is more important,
it breaks the monotony and makes it very much easier on the teacher."
—Peter T. Bohan, M.D., in *The Man Who Became a Tradition*,
compiled and edited by Helen Sims, 1974.

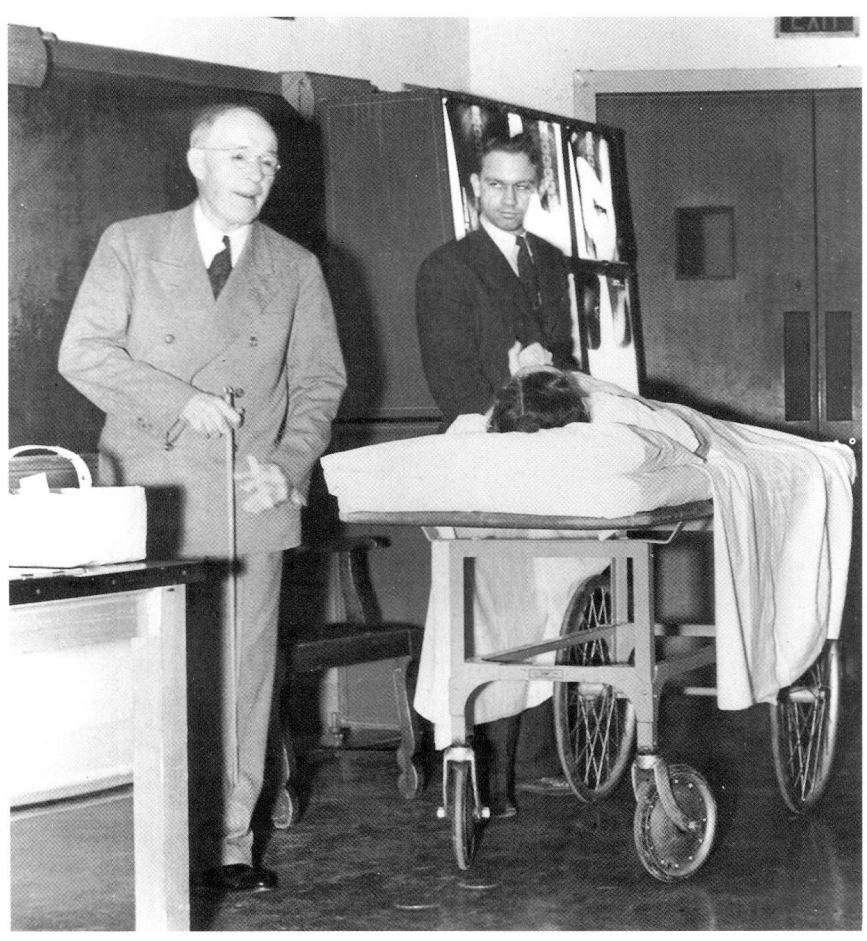

Peter T. Bohan, M.D., professor
of medicine, with student
Lewis L. Coriell, 1940

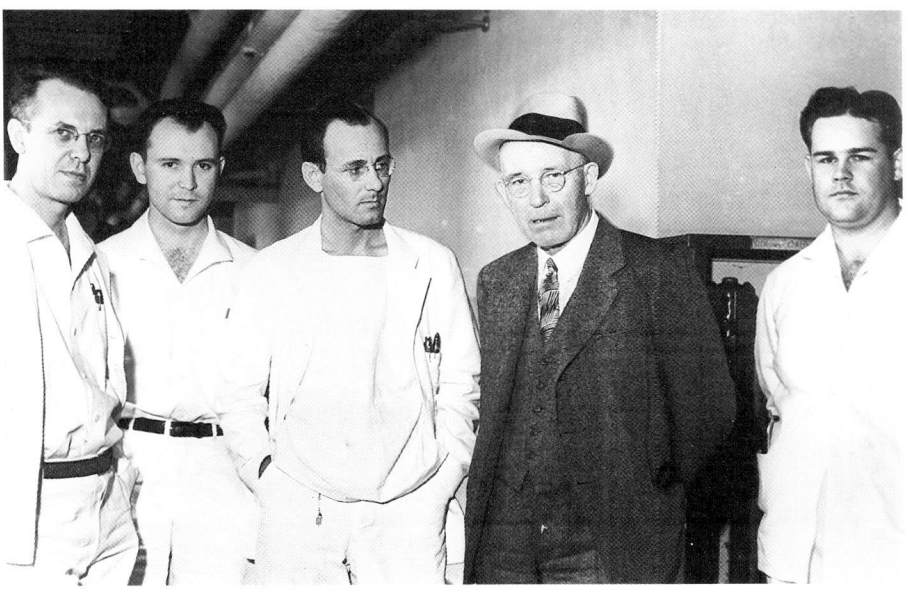

By 1942, Dr. Bohan was internationally known in the field of
hematology and internal medicine.

Another problem is that of permitting our staff to practice in the Hospital. At the present time, the policy is to allow only the heads of departments to practice here in order that they should concentrate their activities and interests on this one place. It is understood that such practice is limited to consultation work or such work that will not interfere with one's duties as a teacher and head of the department. While theoretically this may lead to abnormal profits, it is balanced by the fact that the department head has only a limited number of private beds available, no department head having available more than three private rooms at any one time. It does enable the institution to secure outstanding men for a relatively low salary because they can increase their income by means of these private patients.

—University of Kansas School of Medicine Biennial Report, 1944–1946.

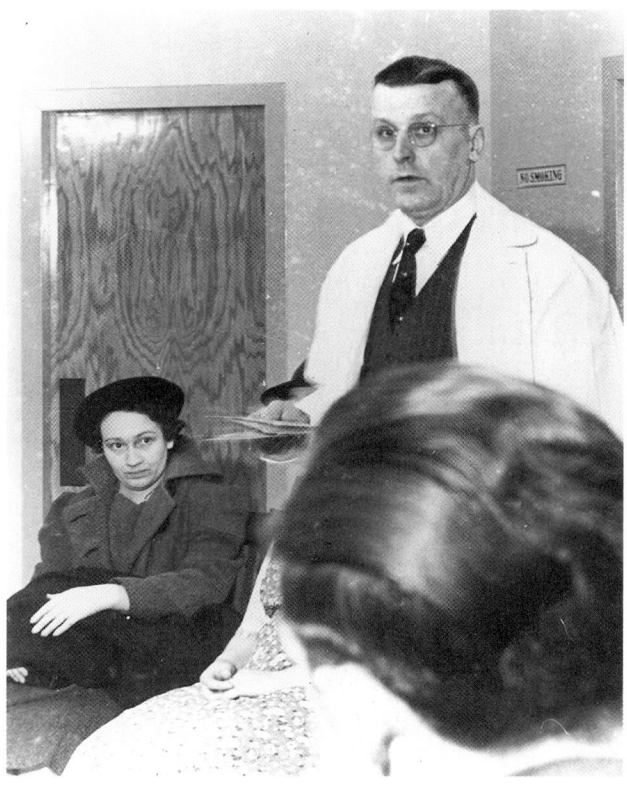

Edward Hashinger, M.D., director of the
Outpatient Department.

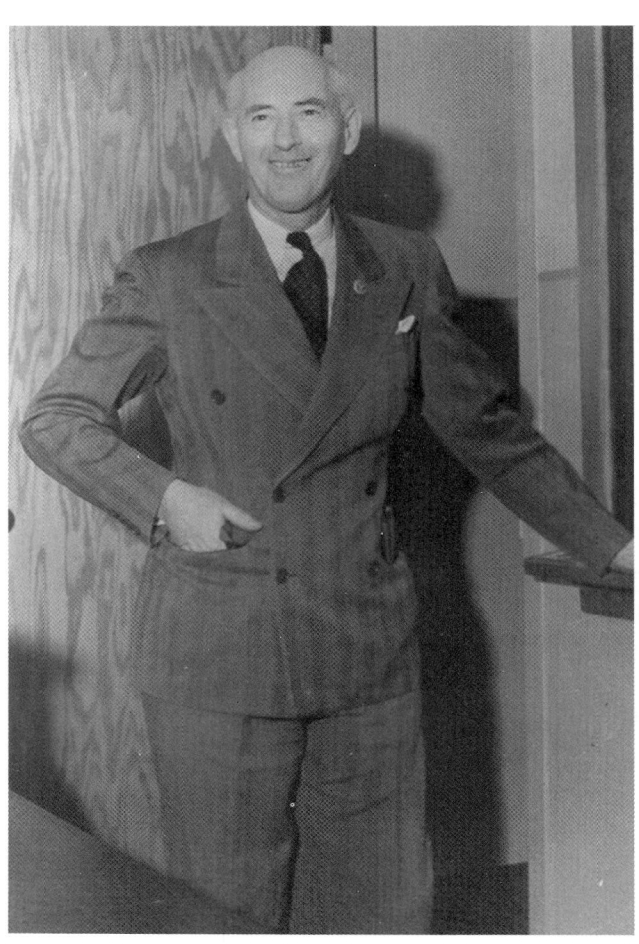

Don Carlos Guffey, M.D., chairman of the Department
of Obstetrics and Gynecology.

The financing of the hospital activities of the Medical School has indeed been difficult over the past two years. Cost of hospital maintenance has risen sharply and in spite of the fact that the hospital charges have also been raised, it has not been possible to keep pace with the dizzy spiral of rising costs. . . . It should be remembered in the field of hospital costs that the cost of this institution to care for a patient per day is somewhat over $12.00, and that fees obtained from county patients are in the neighborhood of $5.00. The same holds for the children being supported by the Crippled Childrens Commission. In essence, this means that the Medical School is paying a greater share of the costs of the county and crippled children patients than are the various agencies who send these patients to the Hospital.
—University of Kansas Medical Center Biennial Report, 1946–1948.

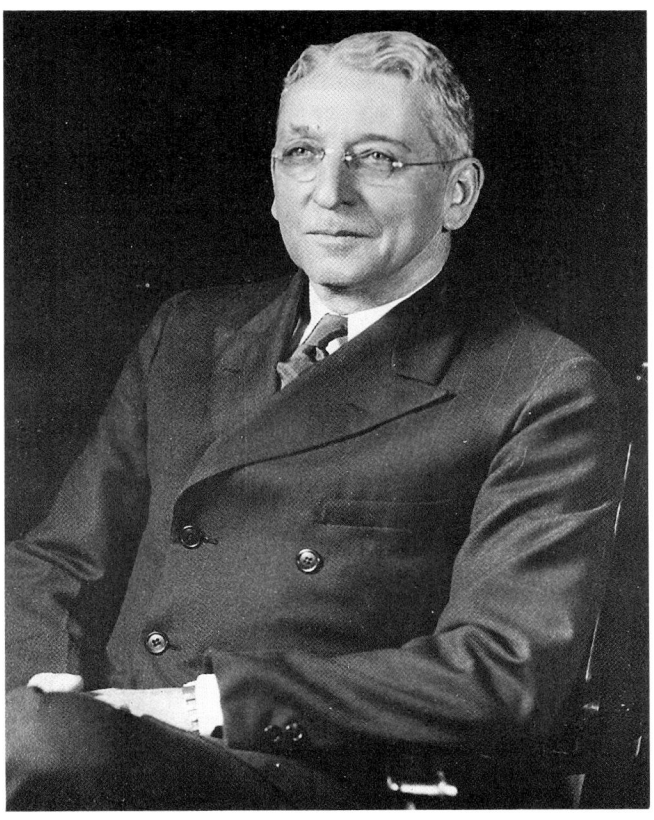

Frank C. Neff, M.D., emeritus professor of pediatrics until his death in 1947.

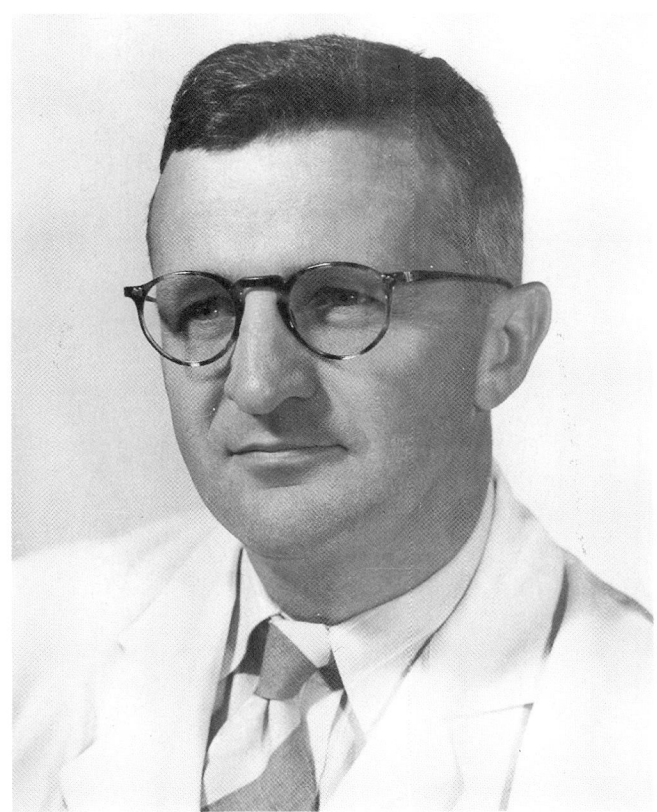

Herbert C. Miller, M.D., was appointed chair and professor of pediatrics in 1945.

As the only medical educational institution in Kansas, it is clearly the obligation of the Medical School to guarantee the people of Kansas the best continuing type of medical care through postgraduate instruction of their doctors. The Medical School administration is working in the closest relationship with the Kansas State Medical Society and the State Board of Health in the field of postgraduate medical education, and it is becoming increasingly apparent that in the years to come the postgraduate instruction directed by the Medical School will be of as great significance as is the undergraduate education.—University of Kansas Medical Center Biennial Report, 1946–1948.

A request was made by the interns that they not be called to the phone during meal time except on necessary occasions. Many calls are not of immediate importance, and can be held until after meal time. A complaint was also made that the tennis courts are used by the public to such an extent that they are not available for the nurses and employees. It was requested by Dr. Wahl that a deputy be appointed in the Engineer's Department, and that the tennis courts be watched for these intruders.—University of Kansas Hospitals Department Head Meeting Minutes, April 1939.

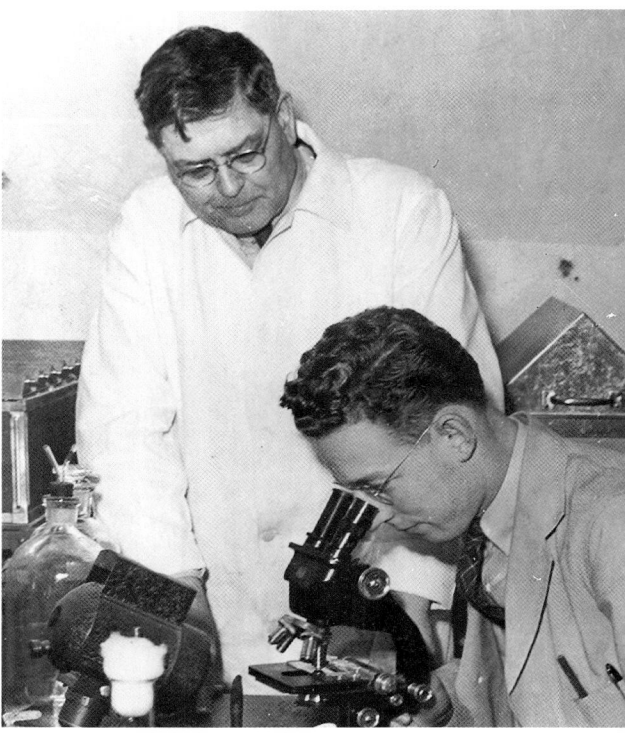

Noble P. Sherwood, M.D., professor of bacteriology, with a student, early 1940s.

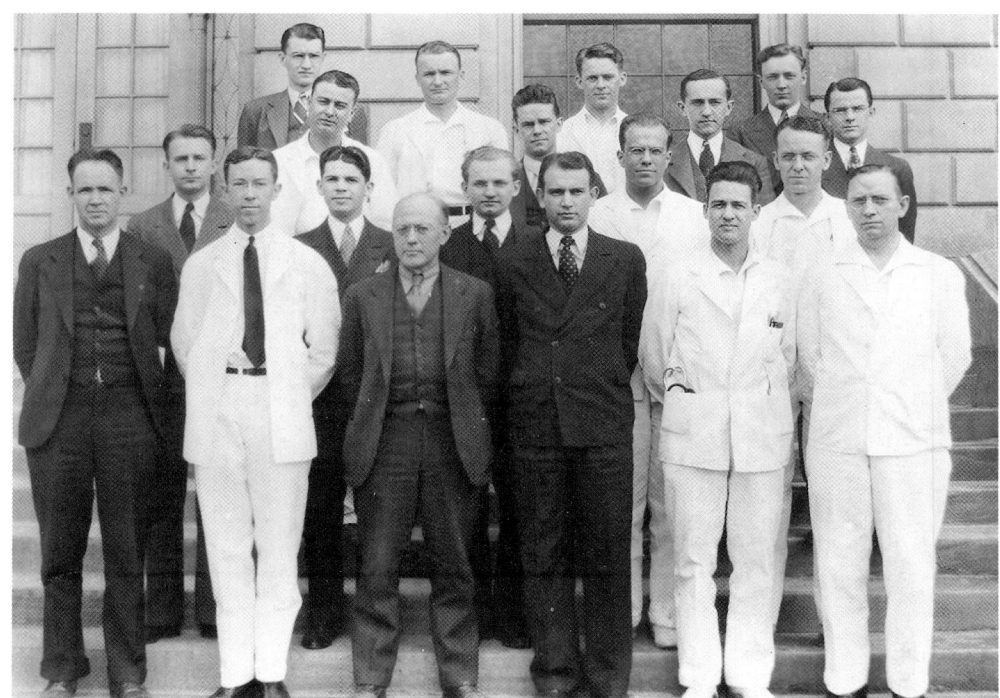

Alpha Omega Alpha Honorary Society, early 1940s.

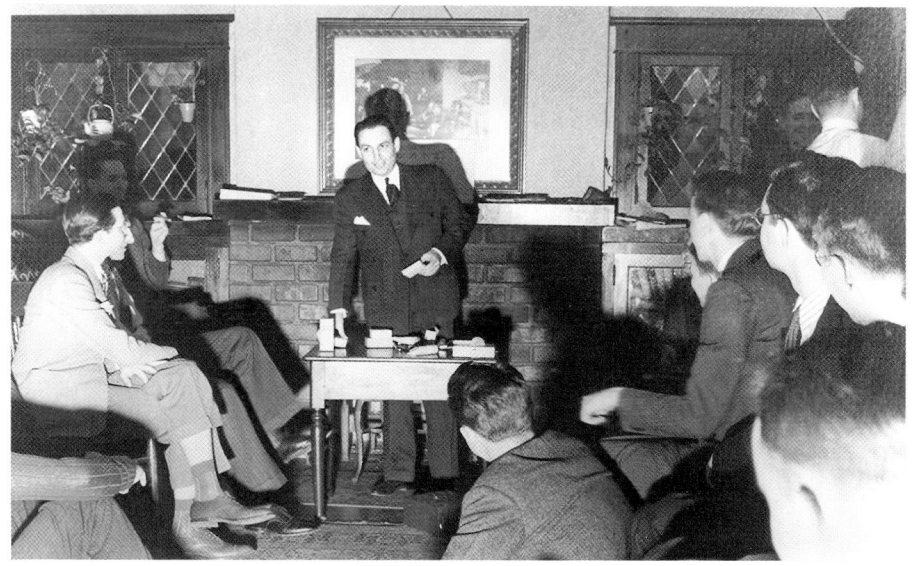

The Phi Beta Pi medical fraternity in 1940.

My fraternity Phi Beta Pi maintained a house but I seldom attended meetings. I was indeed a struggling student and not "in" socially. Most of us had virtually no social life.
—Philip H. Hostetter, M.D., to Nancy Hulston, February 13, 1989.

The first building on the new site, designated on the architect's plans as the Administration Building and now known as the A Building, was officially called the Bell Memorial Hospital. . . . Later, when the new buildings were added, it was deemed advisable to call the entire plant the University of Kansas Hospitals, this name appearing first in the catalogue of 1936–37. With the growth of the institution and the development of other departments with instruction in physical therapy, occupational therapy, dietetics, speech and hearing, laboratory technique, and the stress laid on postgraduate instruction, it seemed proper to employ the designation popular elsewhere, so, in 1947, the name, "University of Kansas Medical Center" was officially adopted.—Ralph H. Major, M.D., *An Account of the University of Kansas School of Medicine*, 1968.

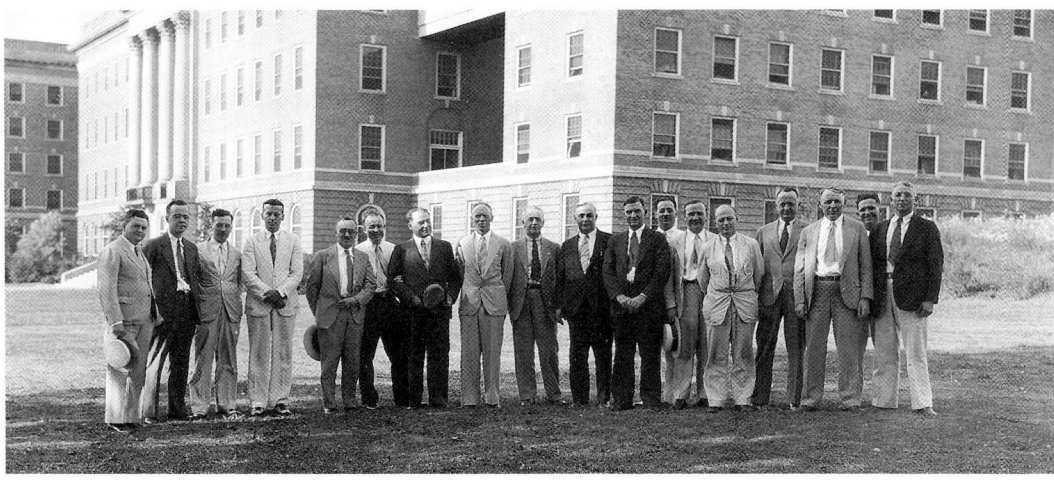

A group shot of faculty members in front of the Bell Memorial Hospital and B Building, 1940s.

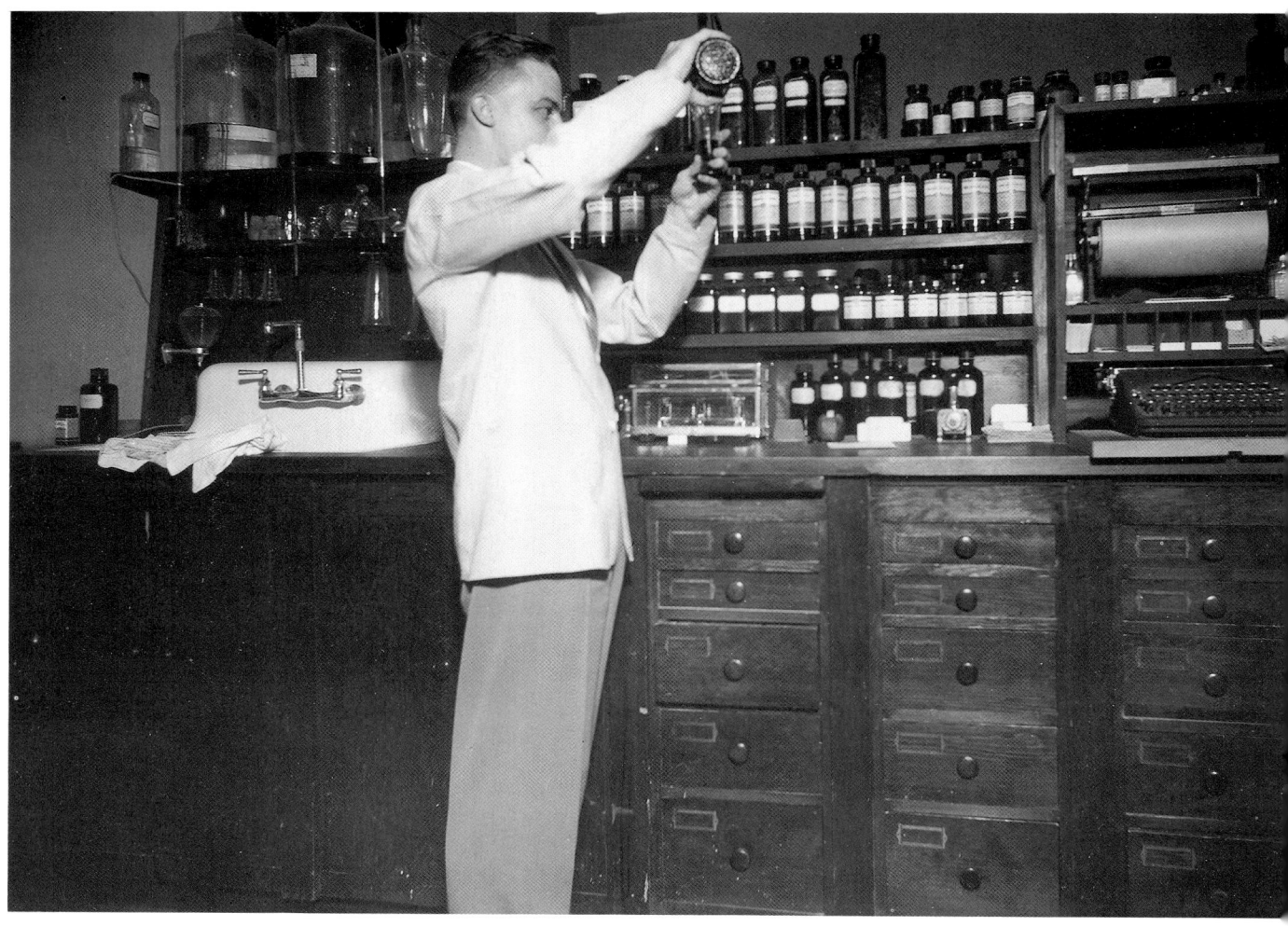

Pharmaceutical room, March 1942.

An evaluation of the needs and plans of the Medical School can be made only in the light of the health needs of the State of Kansas. There is a general recognition of the fact that there is a country-wide shortage of medical personnel in all categories, i.e., doctors, nurses, technicians, etc. This shortage is more acute in rural areas, and informal surveys carried out by the School of Medicine and the Kansas State Medical Society indicate that Kansas reflects the national situation and, being essentially a rural state, reflects it more acutely than some of the more urbanized states. The office of the Kansas Medical Society in Topeka as well as this office are constantly in receipt of letters of inquiry from Kansas towns concerning the desperate need for physicians. We in the School of Medicine, therefore, are confronted with the continually frustrating situation of finding, at one end of the spectrum, many fully qualified young men and women who are Kansans and who desire to study medicine in Kansas and practice medicine in Kansas. At the other end of the spectrum we find a crying need for doctors, nurses and technicians in Kansas. The bottleneck, the reason why this raw material cannot be converted into the finished medical product, is the physical plant of the Medical School. . . . It must be made clear to the people of Kansas, then, that if they wish to have more doctors and more medical personnel of all types and, in addition, if they wish to guarantee their doctors continued training, they must provide the physical facilities.
—University of Kansas Medical Center Biennial Report, 1946–1948.

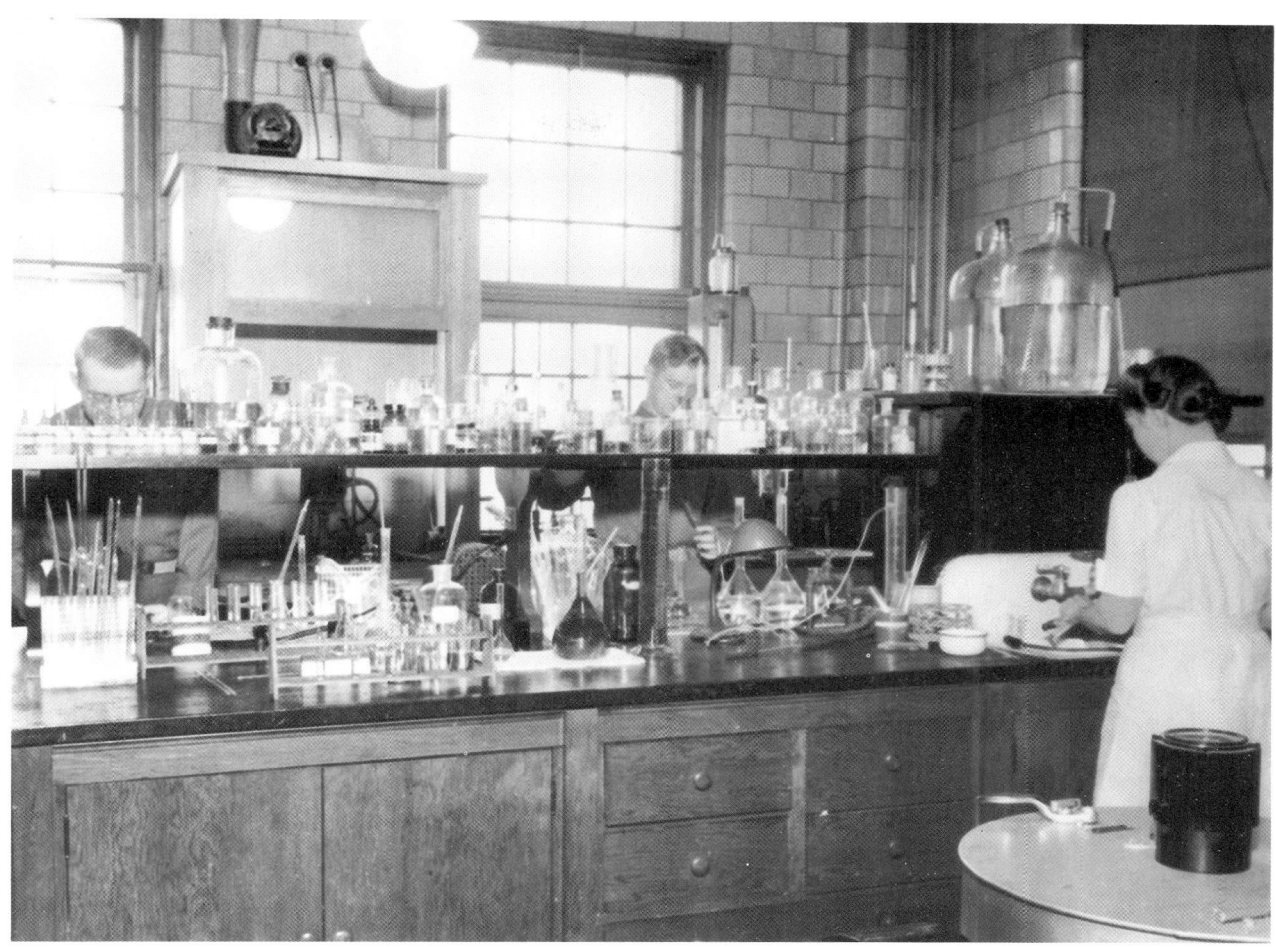

The biochemistry laboratory, 1940s.

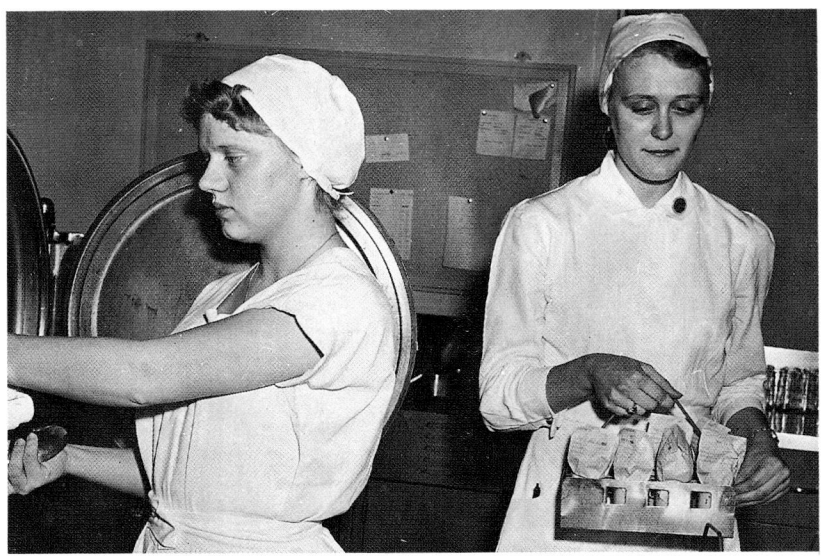

Dietetics and Nutrition students preparing infant formula.

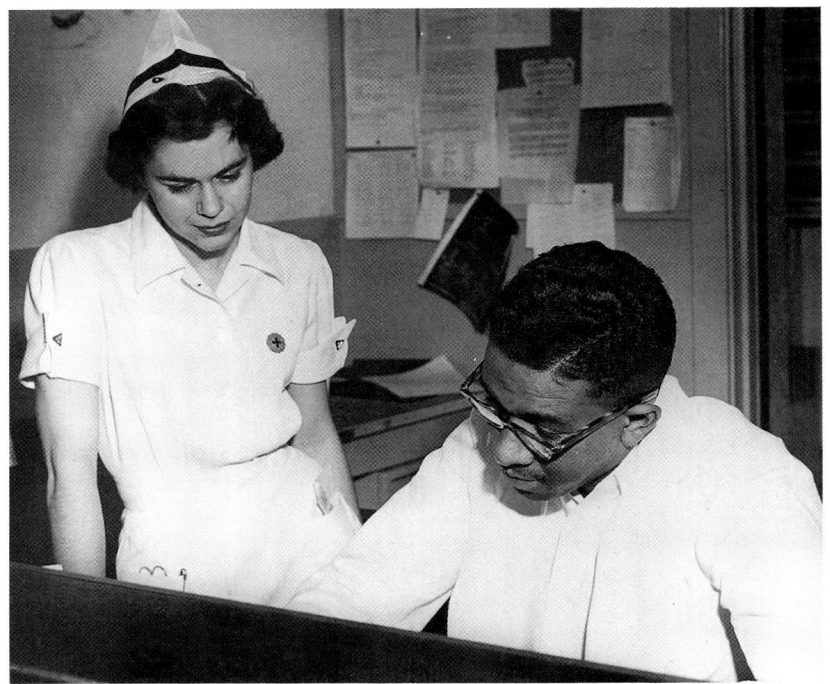

Medical student Lewis Napier Bass, Jr., with Marlene Frohn, R.N., 1945.

The problems of personnel are becoming of more importance than the physical needs of the institution. The current labor shortage, the increasing salary scales in all branches of employment resulting from the war, the increased cost of living, the competition of large local defense industries with their exorbitant salaries, and the accumulation of elderly instructors on the faculty make the personnel factor of paramount importance in the coming biennium, and of necessity the salary budget must be considerably increased if the efficiency of the school and hospital is to be maintained.
—University of Kansas School of Medicine and University of Kansas Hospitals Biennial Report, 1942–1943, 1943–1944.

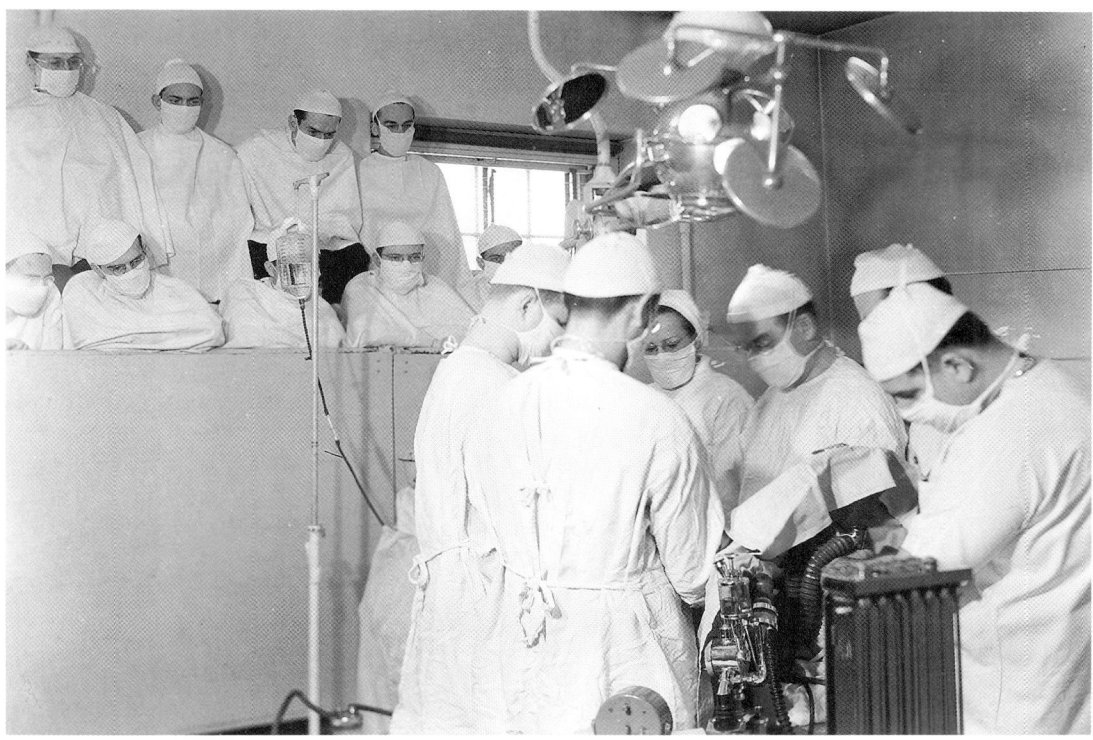

Surgery in progress, March 29, 1944.

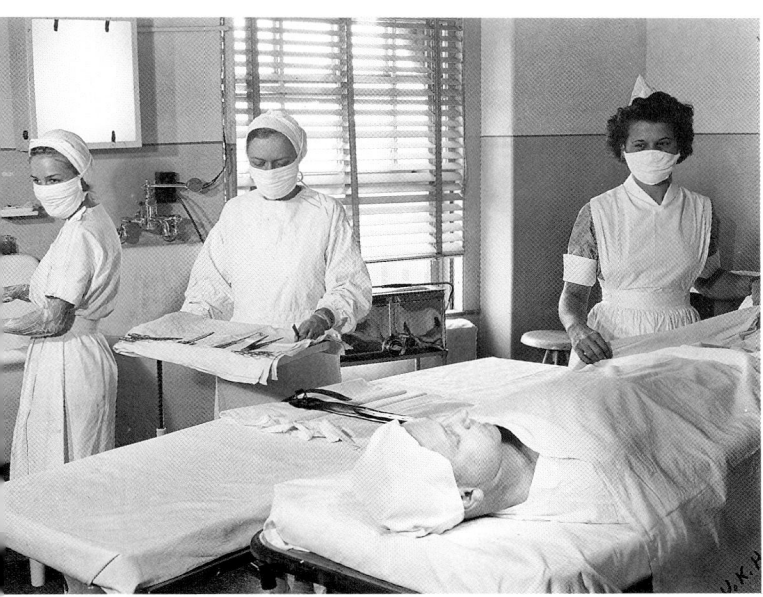

Nurses in surgery, ca. 1942. Student nurse
Aileen Brooks is on the far right.

The Medical School is the nucleus of the University of Kansas Medical Center—an institution that supervises directly or indirectly all activities that contribute to the health of every citizen of Kansas. The School is just emerging from the educational and service stage of its development, when it struggled to obtain the bare physical facilities to provide space and equipment for a laboratory for the instruction of doctors and nurses. Now, it is entering into a period where it will also actively contribute to medical science. New investigations in the Hixon Laboratory for Medical Research, in the fields of infectious diseases, cardiac disorders, and cancer, should soon make the School a Medical Center of which every graduate may well be proud. Especially will this be true if the School will aid in a program of restoring every physically handicapped individual back to his home as an independent, productive member of society.
—Message from Dean H. R. Wahl, *Jayhawker MD*, 1948.

Recent personnel problems threaten the efficient development and management of the Medical School and Hospitals almost as much as the physical plant needs. These difficulties have been increased by the war and have made the operation of the four major divisions—the Medical School proper, the Nursing Department, the Out-Patient Clinic, and the Hospital—correspondingly difficult. Low salaries, inadequate help, defective housing and recreational facilities for both employees and students, limited budgets faced with rising costs of all supplies, personnel losses from military demands, the competition of labor with numerous defense plants, and the limitation of many supplies because of priorities has complicated the efficient management of these divisions. Especially is this true with the fact that almost one-third of our medical staff has been called into military service.
—University of Kansas School of Medicine and University of Kansas Hospitals Biennial Report, 1940–1941, 1941–1942.

One of the most serious problems affecting this School and Hospital is the lack of clinical facilities, little relief having been obtained even though funds were available for additional construction. The general building restrictions, incidental to the war, and the material and labor shortages have prevented the use of these funds. The result has been a desperately acute shortage of beds. Even with additional buildings constructed, there is some question, under the present conditions, as to whether, with the shortage of technical and personnel help, we could keep the beds filled. Certainly there is no doubt that we could fill three or four times as many beds if nurses could be obtained for floor duty.—University of Kansas School of Medicine Biennial Report, 1944–1946.

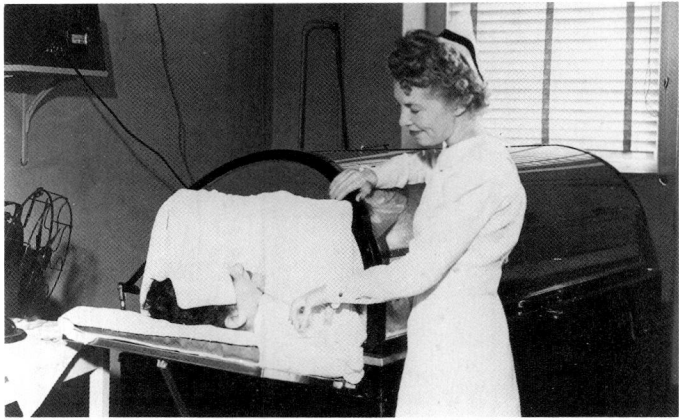
Artificial fever treatment in the Physical Therapy Department, July 1946.

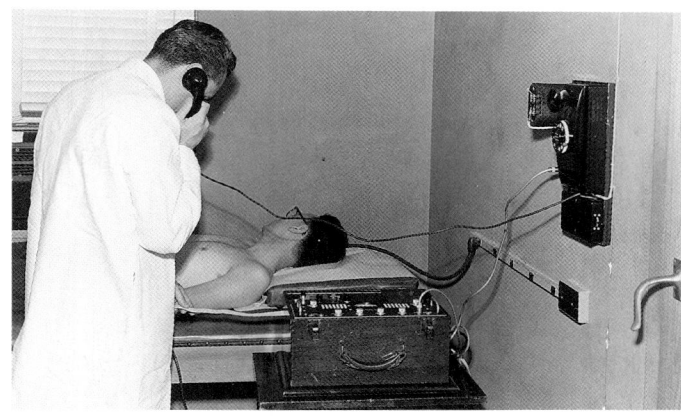
A cardiovascular researcher performing an experimental electrocardiogram transmission, late 1940s.

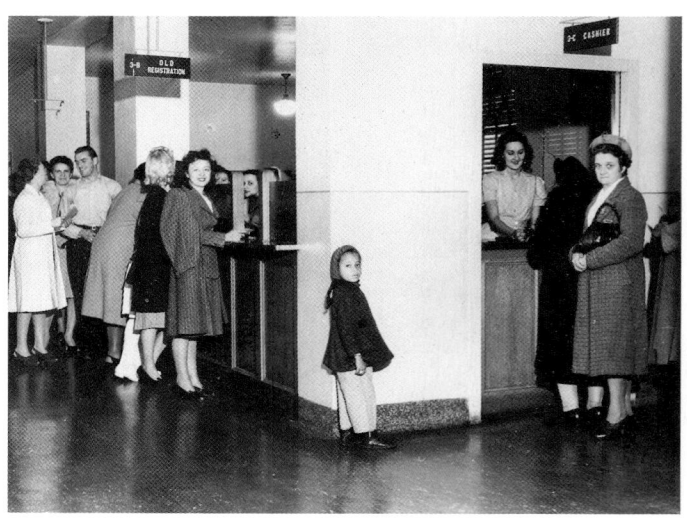
The registration desk and cashier's office, late 1940s.

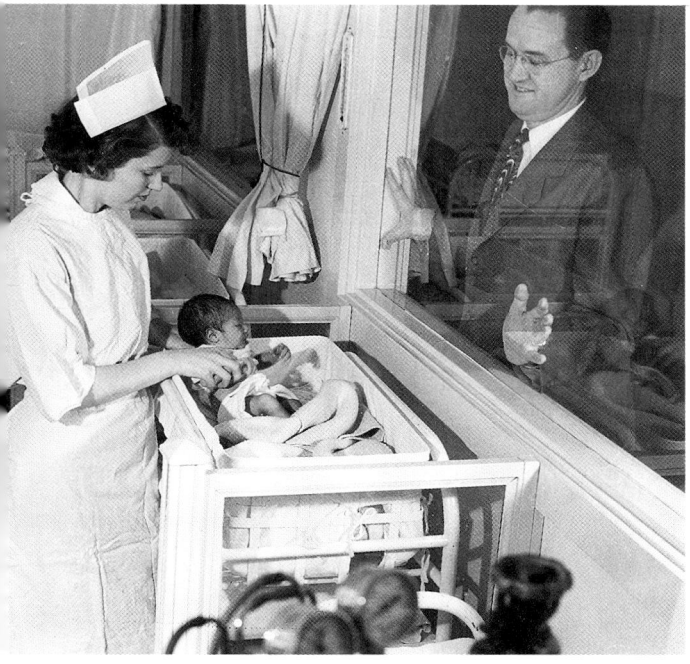

A proud father viewing a newborn infant, 1940s.

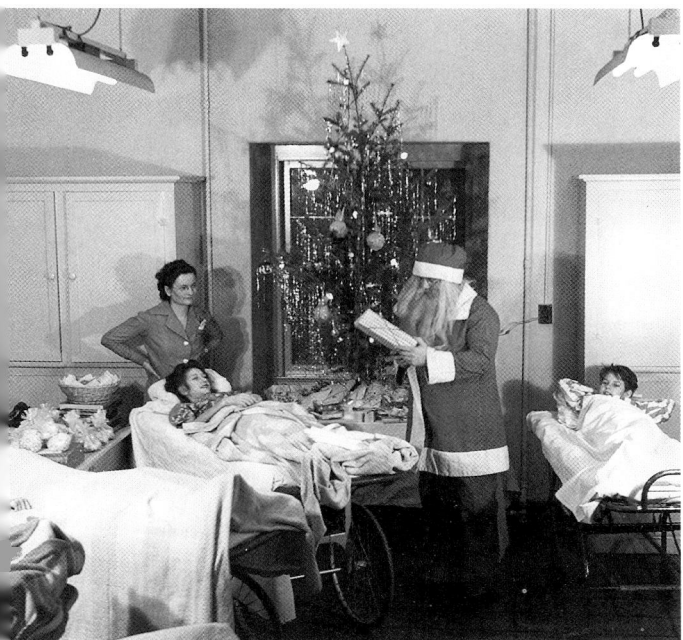

Santa visits the pediatrics unit, December 8, 1941.

Last summer the University of Kansas Hospitals and Medical School applied for a defense grant for additions to the connecting corridor, clinic building and the children's ward to provide accommodations for defense workers in the Kansas City, Kansas area. . . .

Inasmuch as several defense projects are being constructed in Johnson County, especially at the new airport at Gardner, and since Johnson County has no hospital facilities we are the logical place to which the defense workers and their families would look for medical service, especially if they are unable to provide for their own hospital and medical treatment. Last year our hospital took care of 90 indigent patients from Johnson County alone and this does not include the patients who come to the out-patient department. Our hospital is quite crowded at present, and with the influx of new patients from Johnson County and the adjacent areas, we would be faced with demands for care of these patients without having available beds. If this grant were requested defense workers and their families would be given priority in this addition.
—Harry R. Wahl, M.D., dean, to D. R. Kennicott, regional director, Federal Works Agency, March 6, 1942.

Mr. Applegate stated that the War Production Board had asked we have no outside Christmas lighting this year. After discussion it was decided the only inside Christmas trees and decorating would be in the Children's Ward, Nurses Home and Eleanor Taylor Hospital.—University of Kansas Hospital Department Head Minutes, December 1, 1942.

Dr. Jennett stated that the first official blackout would be Monday night, December 14, at 10:00 P.M. and would last twenty minutes. He stated that the only lights that would be left on would be the room call lights. Blackout sheets would be placed in every room and if it was necessary to use a light it should be a flashlight and should be pointed to the floor. No light would be on at the front entrance during the blackout. Mr. Applegate was asked to see that buckets of sand were available on the roof. Mr. Applegate stated that the Volunteer Air Raid crew would be on duty on each floor and our telephone operator would be officially notified of the blackout and it would be announced over the auto-call system.
—University of Kansas Hospital Department Head Minutes, December 1, 1942.

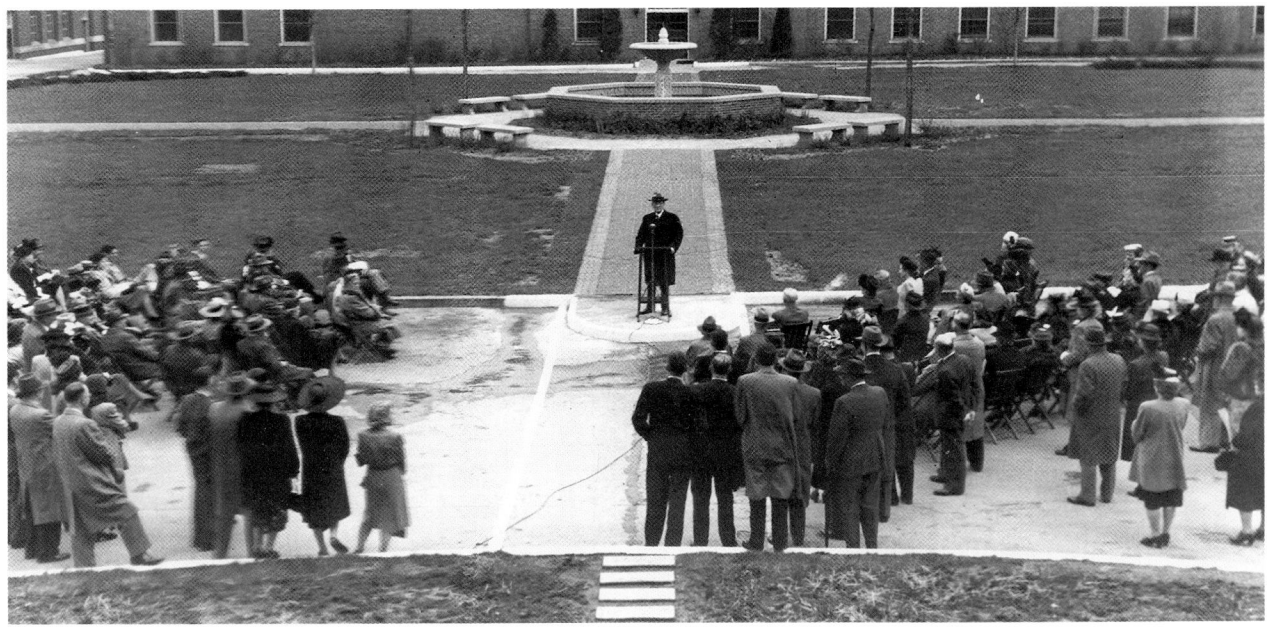

Guests at the dedication of the Clendening Memorial Fountain, April 17, 1947.

It is appropriate that the memorial to Logan Clendening should take the form of a fountain. A fountain is no inert thing. It is full of life and interest, the movement of water suggests sparkle and animation—the qualities that were so conspicuous a part of Logan's endowment.

The setting is appropriate. Any memorial to Dr. Clendening belongs in this great medical center which so absorbed his interest and to which he devoted so large a part of his life. Here for more than thirty years he taught. In the fine Hixon Research Laboratory, testimonial to Mrs. Clendening's concern in her husband's work, he developed the superb medical history library that has become such a valuable adjunct to the institution.

For most of his life Logan Clendening heard the pipes of pan and responded to them with an infectious gayety that spread to all with whom he came in contact through either the spoken or the written word. . . . And we hear again the pipes that Logan heard as we listen to the splash of the water in the fountain set up in memory of our friend.
—Henry J. Haskell, *Kansas City Times*, April 21, 1947.

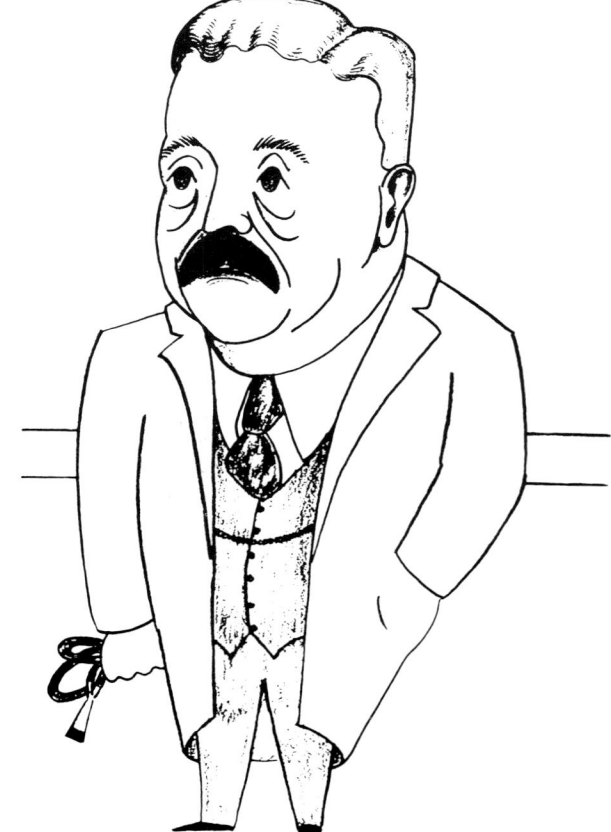

Dr. Logan Clendening, by
Hubert Floersch, M.D.

The matter of installing a garbage disposal unit in our drains was brought up. Doctor Jennett suggested we investigate the possibility of securing one for our T.B. Hospital to eliminate the hauling of all garbage down to the Missouri River twice a week as now required by the Health Department.
—University of Kansas Hospital Department Head Minutes, May 5, 1943.

The elevators in both the "A" and "B" Buildings should be either replaced with new equipment or, if satisfactory, overhauled and modernized. The laundry equipment in the institution is woefully inadequate and overtaxed. It is hoped that some new equipment can be obtained during the next fiscal year, but it is very doubtful that the operating budget will allow sufficient funds to obtain all that is needed. The four motor trucks, owned by the institution, are all in poor condition and have passed the time when they should be replaced.—University of Kansas School of Medicine Biennial Report, 1944–1946.

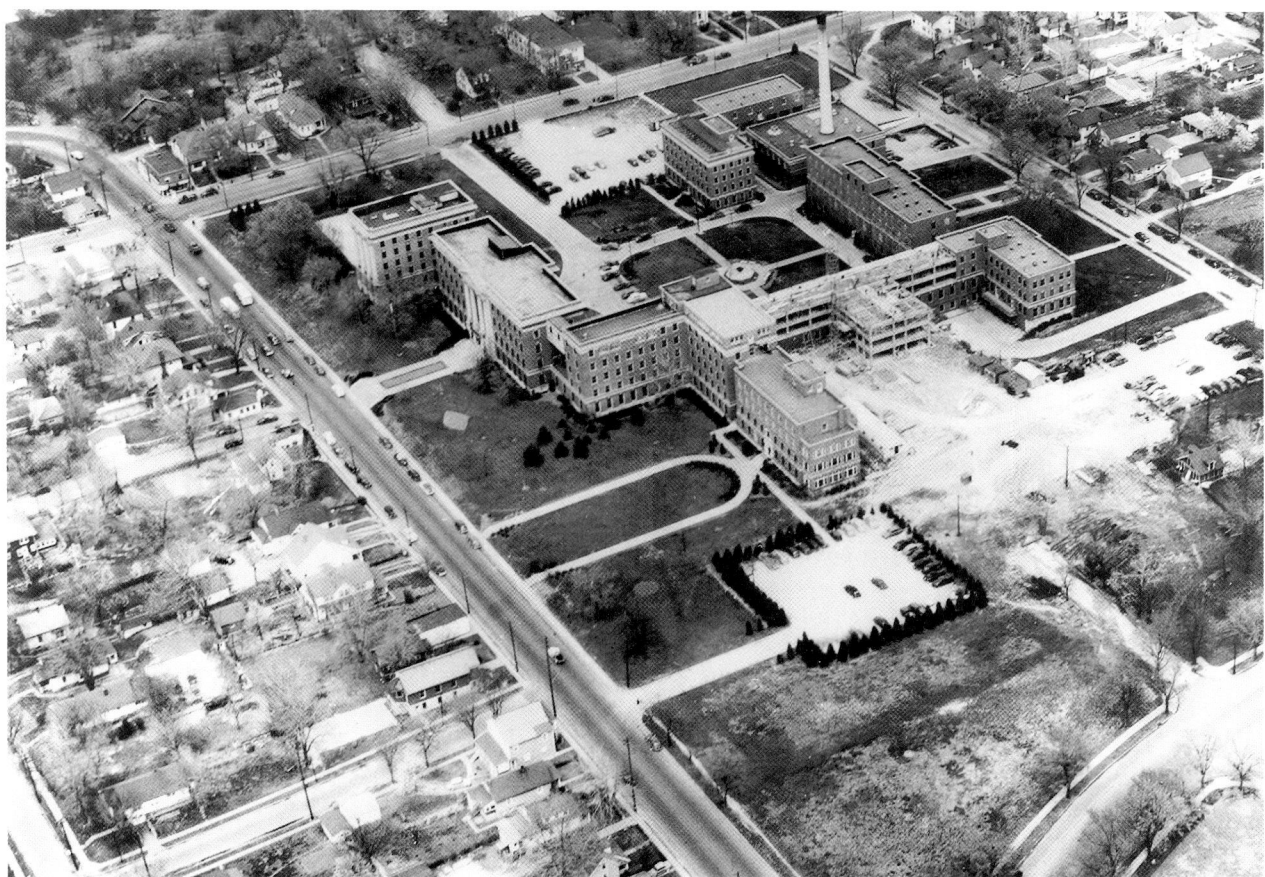

Aerial view, 1947.

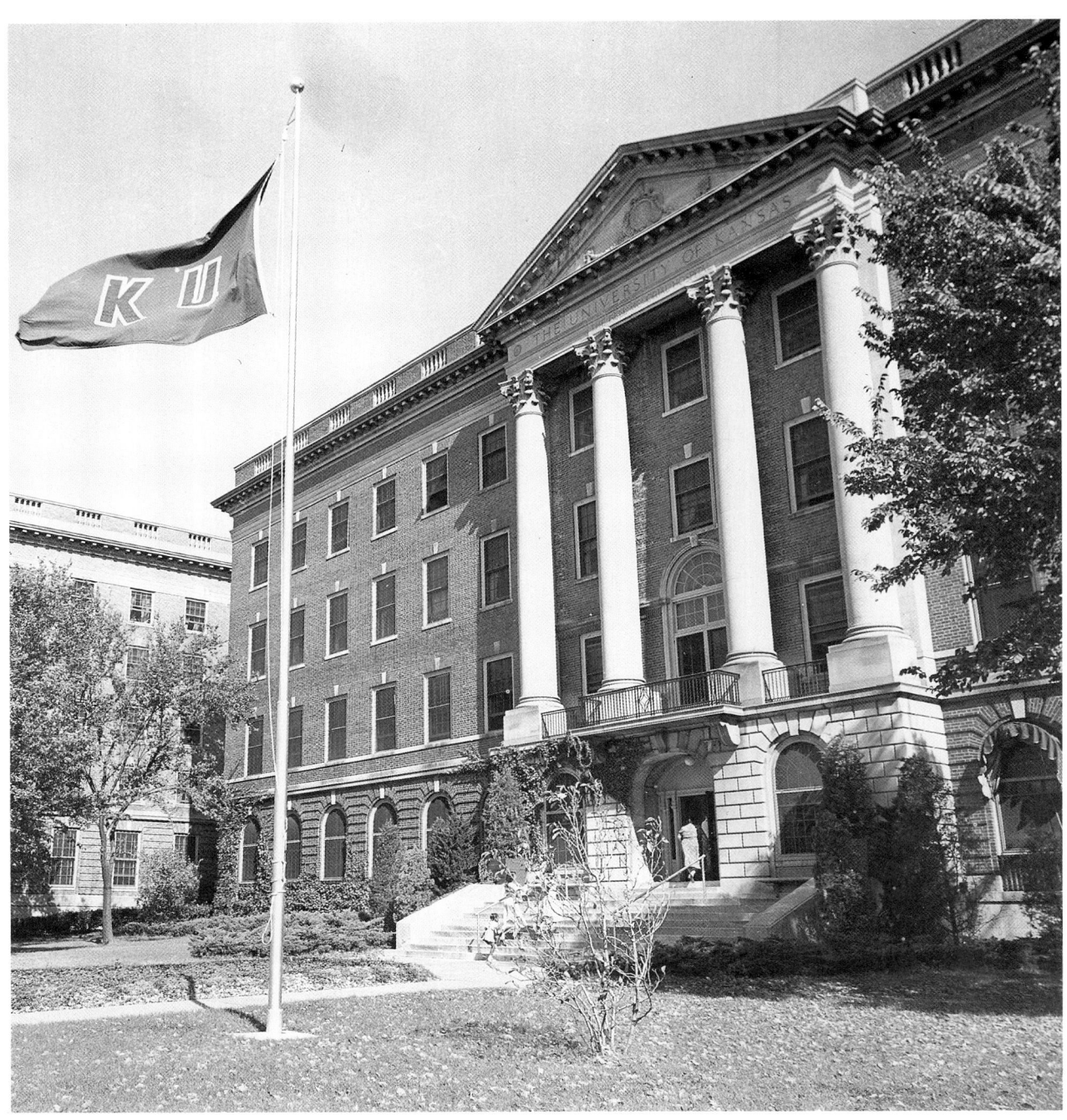

Entrance to the University of Kansas Medical Center.

5

Entering into a New Generation

In 1947, only months before Harry Roswell Wahl relinquished his administrative responsibilities, the University of Kansas School of Medicine was renamed the University of Kansas Medical Center. Officially, the change reflected the growing, multi-faceted educational functions of the institution. Unofficially, the new designation afforded an opportunity for a fresh start, a way of breaking with the political upheavals of the mid-1920s and the cautious stability that defined the "Wahl Years."

Wahl had been thirty-eight when he took charge; the new dean, Franklin D. Murphy, M.D., was even younger at age thirty-two. His father, Franklin E. Murphy, M.D., a founder of the medical school, had served Wahl in a number of advisory capacities. The younger Murphy, through his wartime work in the military as a pioneering penicillin researcher, appeared to have a promising medical career ahead. A graduate of the University of Pennsylvania School of Medicine, his shift from research to administration represented a significant change of direction in his life, a change that he regarded as only temporary. (This new direction would become permanent, however. In 1951 he would become chancellor of the University of Kansas, and in 1960 he would assume a similar position at the University of California at Los Angeles.) When he assumed the deanship of the Medical Center in 1948, Murphy already had achieved recognition as a man on the rise in the medical profession. Kansas was ready to support a medical school and Murphy was the man with the necessary leadership capabilities and political savvy to make that a reality.

The crowning achievement of the three-year Murphy deanship was the Kansas Rural Health Act of 1949, also called the "Kansas Plan" or the "Murphy Plan." The drain of physicians and registered nurses from rural Kansas to urban areas both in and out of the state reflected nationwide

problems. Urbanization trends and the concentration of hospitals and, hence, medical opportunities in large cities, had a tremendous impact on the health profession. The centralization of medical talent improved the quality of medicine in the country, encouraging specialization and creating opportunities for group research. Unfortunately, it also created a marked decline in the number of rural family practitioners—the kind of fabled country doctor immortalized by Arthur E. Hertzler, M.D., in his best-selling 1938 account of his experiences in rural Kansas, *The Horse and Buggy Doctor.* The fact that many of the old-time medical men had undistinguished credentials, usually from proprietary schools, was not the issue. Rather, the problem had become finding and training qualified medical personnel to serve much of the state.

The rural health plan became law because it gained widespread support throughout much of Kansas, especially from such powerful organizations as the Kansas Medical Society, the Kansas State Chamber of Commerce, the Kansas Farm Bureau, and the Kansas State Board of Agriculture. Republican Governor Frank Carlson and a bipartisan majority in the legislature favored the plan. Almost all of the newspapers in the state backed the proposal, contributing editorials and stories illustrating the poor quality of medical care in small Kansas towns. The need for action had been apparent for many years—the state medical society had established a committee to study rural health problems in 1947—but action only came after Murphy very effectively promoted the rural health concept through articles, speeches, and lobbying. As he later said, he discovered political skills of persuasion that he had not imagined he possessed. He found that for him, leadership meant the ability to provide a vision—in this case one already in place—and to persuade people to follow and implement it. The main elements of the plan were straightforward and, most importantly, easily understood.

Murphy's proposal involved combining various parts into a whole. This meant an expanded medical school to produce more physicians, nurses, and technicians; a large postgraduate medical education program; and a commitment by Kansas communities to provide offices and other facilities for young medical men and women. The cost, close to $5 million in state and matching monies, seemed astronomical, given the past parsimonious funding of the Medical Center. At first, the Kansas Plan worked well enough to become a model for the rest of the nation. However, further rural decline was an inevitable consequence of the urbanization of America. In the final analysis, the Kansas Plan proved a stopgap measure despite its initial successes. The claim made in the 1950s that all citizens of Kansas were within twenty minutes of medical help could no longer be made by the 1980s.

Some observers argued that the plan channeled resources of the University of Kansas Medical Center in the wrong direction, thereby undermining efforts to obtain research money by emphasizing continuing medical education courses around the state instead of medical research. Yet, the Rural Health Act of 1949 enhanced the Medical Center's role as a statewide institution. The school, under attack at one time for supposedly favoring a metropolitan Kansas City, rose in public esteem in Kansas by reasserting rural values.

In a radical departure from past practices, Murphy oversaw a restructuring of the relationship between physicians and the Medical Center. Groups of faculty physicians now practiced full-time rather than part-time on the premises. In exchange for space and other privileges, they paid a percentage of their annual income to the school and to a medical endowment fund. This concept effectively ended the old problem of physicians practicing in Missouri and sending patients to hospitals other than the Medical Center.

After Murphy moved to Lawrence, longtime faculty member Edward H. Hashinger, M.D., functioned as acting dean for eighteen months until the 1952 selection of W. Clarke Wescoe, M.D. At the time of his appointment, Wescoe was thirty-two, the same age Murphy had been when he took charge. But unlike Murphy, Wescoe had no strong ties to the school, having arrived at the Medical Center only the year before as a professor of pharmacology.

A native of Allentown, Pennsylvania, and a graduate of the Cornell University Medical College, Wescoe had shown promise as a researcher, working on drugs designed to relax muscles during surgery. Characterizing Wescoe as knowledgeable, articulate, and decisive, with demonstrated abilities in building an "interesting department," Murphy selected Wescoe to succeed him as dean. The two men became close associates and worked well together.

Wescoe proved especially good at turning ideas proposed by others into concrete plans, and he worked well and persuasively with faculty, legislative, and alumni committees. Like Murphy, Wescoe had a vision for the Medical Center. "He smiles as he talks of the expanding services of the medical center," a Kansas City Star reporter wrote about Wescoe on April 11, 1954. "It is pleasant to think along with him as he talks of the hopes and possibilities of a great medical plant which has its headquarters, appropriately, on a boulevard named Rainbow."

During the 1950s, the University of Kansas Medical Center underwent a tremendous expansion, almost unbelievable in light of its past history of dire financial straits, shoestring levels of operation, and hand-to-mouth funding. The Medical Center's state appropriation soared by 1957 to $3 million a year. With the addition of private donations, grants, and hospital operating profits, the school had become over a $7 million operation. The research budget alone totaled $750,000. The school moved closer towards consolidation when the second year medical class moved to the Rainbow campus for the 1951-1952 school year, leaving only the first year program in Lawrence. Several new buildings went up, including new science, psychiatry, library, and nursing facilities. The first section of the Student Union Building opened in 1954. The Kenneth Spencers donated Spencer House, an expansive English-style home on Mission Drive in Johnson County, Kansas, for use as an official residence.

Another change of tremendous significance occurred during this period: formal segregation of the clinics and hospital ended with the rejection, at long last, of the argument that paying white patients would accept neither the services of black medical personnel nor the close proximity of hospital beds occupied by blacks. In 1955, Lewis Napier Bass, Jr., M.D., became the first black resident to serve the Medical Center.

By the end of 1958, the seventeen-acre Rainbow

campus with fifteen major buildings—many quite new—had an upbeat appearance. Innovative programs of national importance accompanied the new look. Starting in 1949, the Medical Center pioneered the use of television in medical education. Just as significantly, in a typical year over five thousand health care professionals participated in continuing education courses offered by the school. The Kansas Plan, especially its preceptorship program (under which students spent from four to six weeks in the field working with practicing family physicians), received much favorable publicity. The student body in medicine, nursing, and allied health numbered over eight hundred, and fifteen departments offered a wide range of instructional opportunities. The Medical Center also had nearly two thousand employees, marking it as a significant Kansas City area employer.

Even the location had become a positive factor. By 1960, metropolitan Kansas City had a population of over one million, and the University of Kansas Medical Center actively served both Kansas Cities and the entire state of Kansas. For the first time, Kansas appeared on the road to having a top-ranking American medical school.

The tone of the photographs taken during this period reflects the changing conditions. In the medical buildings at 39th and Rainbow, the students and faculty, ensconced in modern facilities, appear confident and optimistic. From all quarters, a new spirit of progress characterized life at the Medical Center as it vaulted ahead during the Murphy-Wescoe period. In a time of tremendous change in medicine in general, the University of Kansas Medical Center was prepared to continue its rapid advance to prominence.

There is no such thing as a cheap medical education. As knowledge of medicine has expanded, so has the death rate fallen. There is no way to bring down costs and at the same time keep up this declining death rate.

It may come to a question of subsidies, but when you mention the word, you hear a cry of 'socialized medicine.' What is socialized medicine? Among other things, it is control of the individual by the government. You take what the government assigns you to. It's absurd to say that subsidies for medical education of students is government control of individuals.
—Franklin D. Murphy, Dean

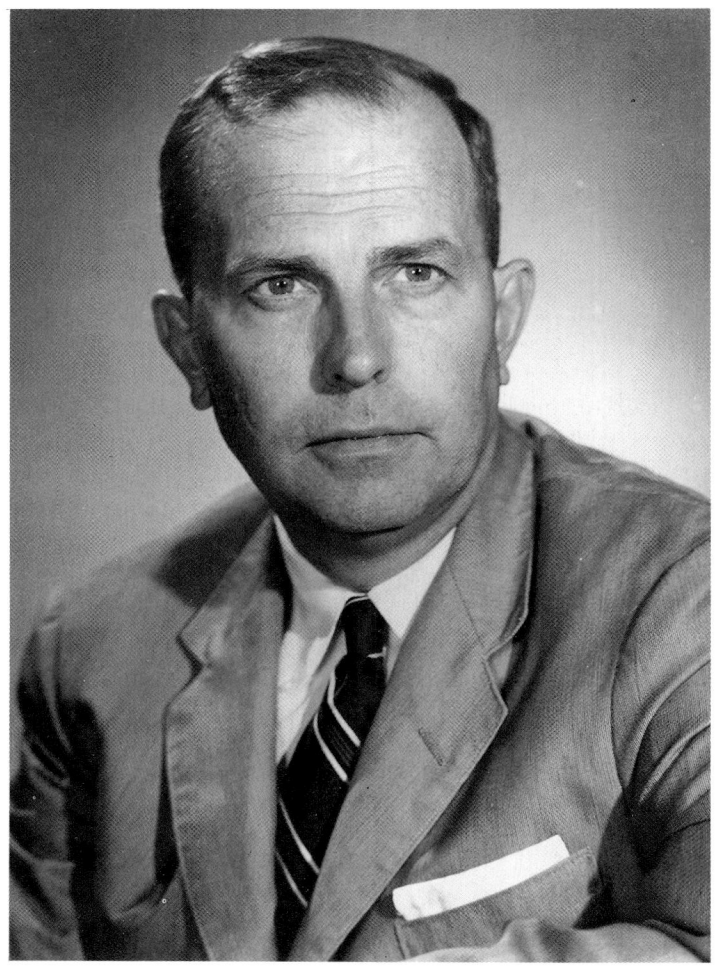

Franklin D. Murphy, M.D., dean of the School of Medicine and associate professor of medicine from 1948 to 1951.

When a young man is asked to peer into the future, he frequently does so without fully recognizing that the future in no small measure depends upon the past and the present. What is the foundation on which we can hope to build for the future?

In a sense it can be said that our medical school is entering into a new generation, for more than forty years have elapsed since the establishment of a four-year medical school at the University of Kansas. In retrospect, the accomplishments of that small band of founders seem truly prodigious in the light of the handicaps and struggles associated with their efforts. The handsome physical plant and, more importantly, the scores of graduates of the Kansas Medical School who have made outstanding names for themselves in the field of medicine stand as a tribute to the vision, vigor, enthusiasm, ability and unswerving determination of that group of men, who can truly be called fathers of the University of Kansas School of Medicine.

Those younger ones of us who have been handed the responsibility for carrying forward the torch of academic medicine in this medical school can continually take strength and courage from those men and certainly with all humility, we can say, "Well done."
—Franklin D. Murphy, M.D., *Jayhawker MD*, 1949.

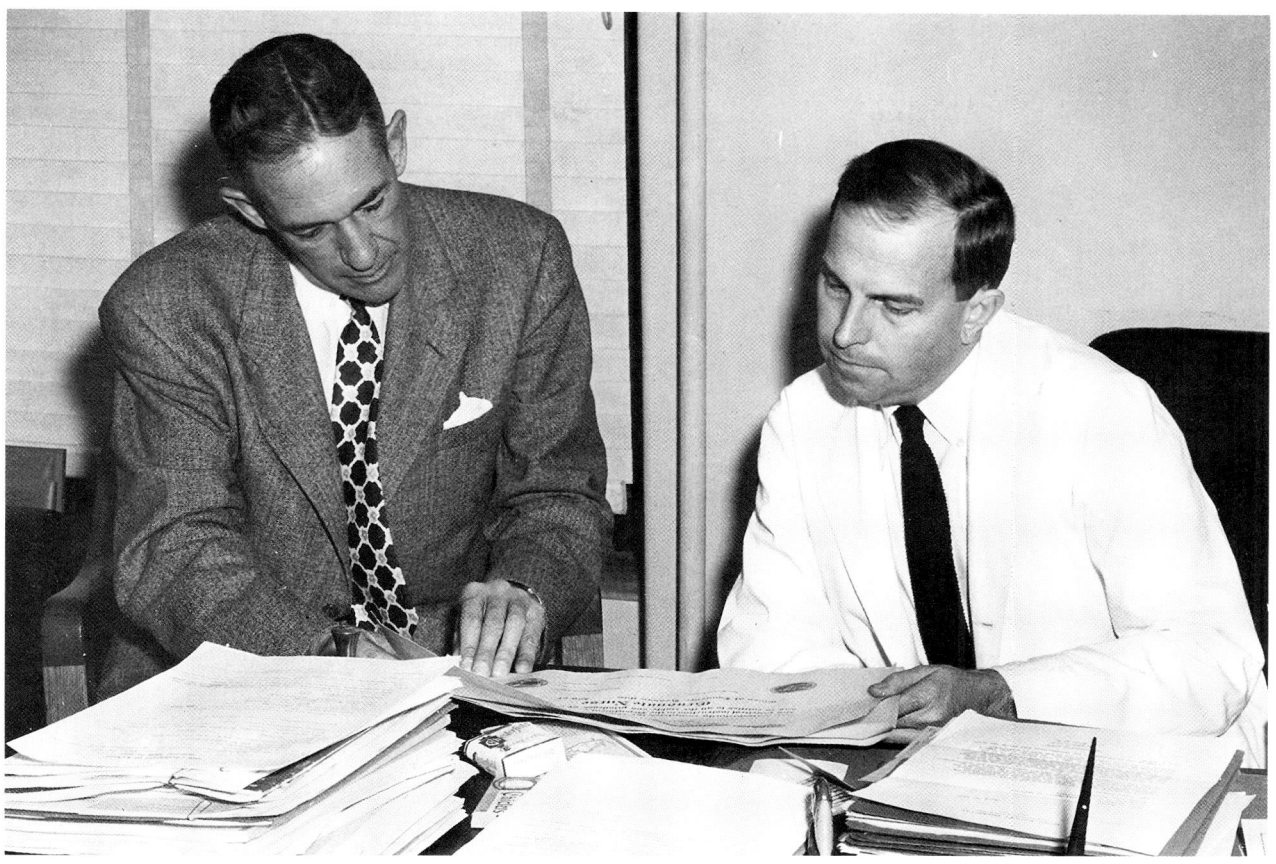

Dean Franklin D. Murphy and Chancellor Deane W. Malott signing diplomas, 1948.

Many of you graduating seniors saw service in what has been called World War II, and you had every reasonable right to assume that you had seen the last of the horrors and dislocation of war, at least in your generation. And yet these same ones of you face the prospect of additional military service.

It is difficult to explain to anyone's satisfaction why leadership here and abroad has not been able to make it possible for us to all live out our lives in a peaceful pattern of progress with our families and our profession. And yet we must constantly remind ourselves that all of the privileges to which this American Democracy entitles us carry with them responsibilities. Men and women fought and sacrificed so that we might enjoy the fruits of freedom. Many of these sacrifices in their way were more terrible than most which you and I will be asked to make. The system of state-supported medical education which provided for each one of you a medical education at far less than its actual cost represents one of the privileges of the American system. It would then appear that when our freedoms and opportunities are threatened, we have the obligation to rise up in their defense. In some respects no generation of Americans will be measured as firmly and realistically against the sacrifice of our forefathers as ours. We must, then, try to understand the annoyances and interferences with our hopes and plans, not in terms of discrimination, but rather in terms of the opportunity and responsibility of proving that we are indeed worthy of our forebears.
—Franklin D. Murphy, M.D., *Jayhawker MD*, 1951.

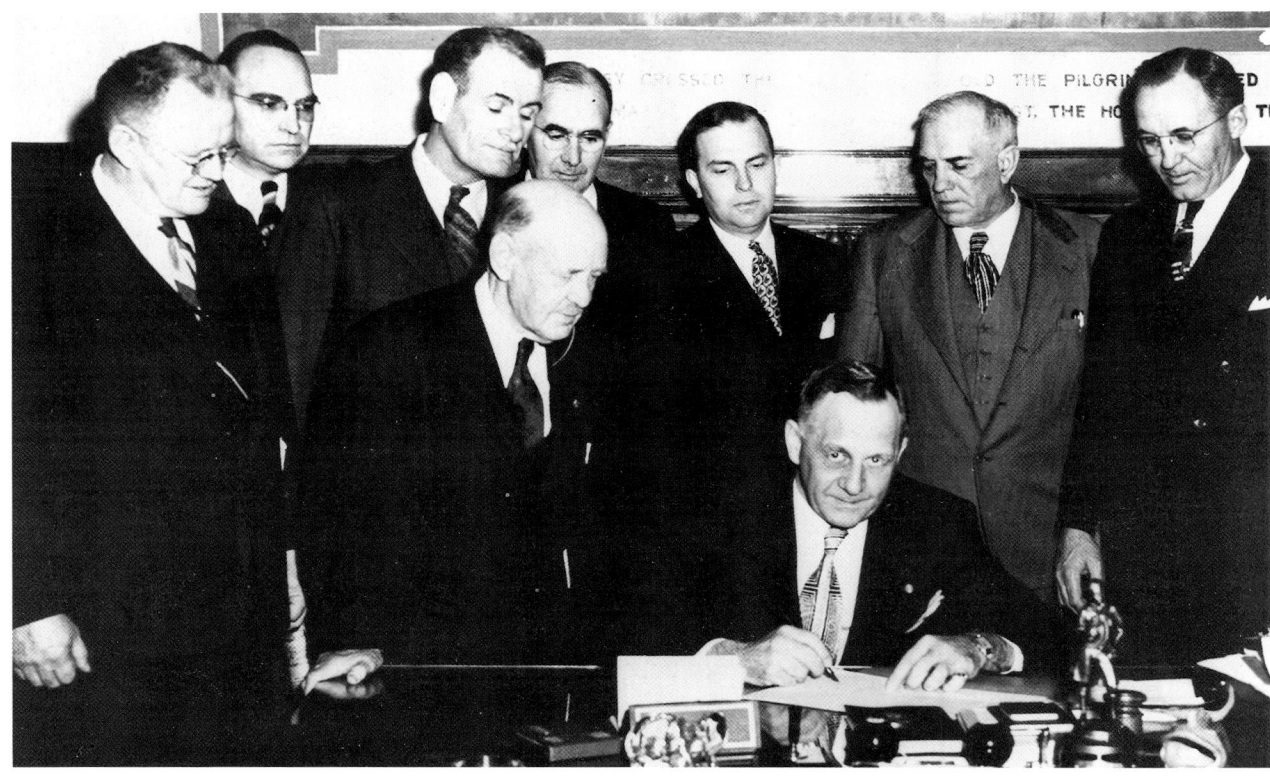

Governor Frank Carlson signing the Rural Health Program for Kansas, February 18, 1949.

On February 18, 1949, the Honorable Frank Carlson, then governor of Kansas, signed the bill "Rural Health Program for Kansas," which had been passed by both houses of the legislature. It was the purpose of that bill to provide major expansion of the University of Kansas Medical Center in order that more doctors, nurses, medical technicians and other ancillary personnel might be trained to alleviate a serious and growing shortage of such personnel in the state.

This Rural Health Program has become of major historical interest not only in Kansas but in the entire United States. The foreward-looking attitude of Kansas legislators has focused the eyes of the nation upon this state. This one bill has literally made the name Kansas synonymous with medical progress throughout the United States. The health plan it outlines has served as a stimulus for many other states to plan toward the solution of their rural health problems. That the program has been successful is an acknowledged fact.

—W. Clarke Wescoe, M.D., dean, "The University of Kansas School of Medicine, A Progress Report," *The Journal of the Kansas Medical Society*, February 1953.

Well, after two or three years I found myself absolutely fascinated with what I was doing. Because, I suddenly discovered that this was just not pushing papers around, this is the whole business of people. Dealing with people, identifying them, motivating them, having some dreams, some ideas, moving in that direction. That's when the whole Rural Health Program developed. I conceived that because I saw that that was a problem out in the state. I then figured out a way to tie the building program into the rural health program. More doctors and programs and getting them out and getting the legislature to support that, because the legislature had some money. The state had some money that had built up during the war that they couldn't spend and I got first in line and I discovered I was a pretty good politician.—Interview with Franklin D. Murphy, January 19, 1990.

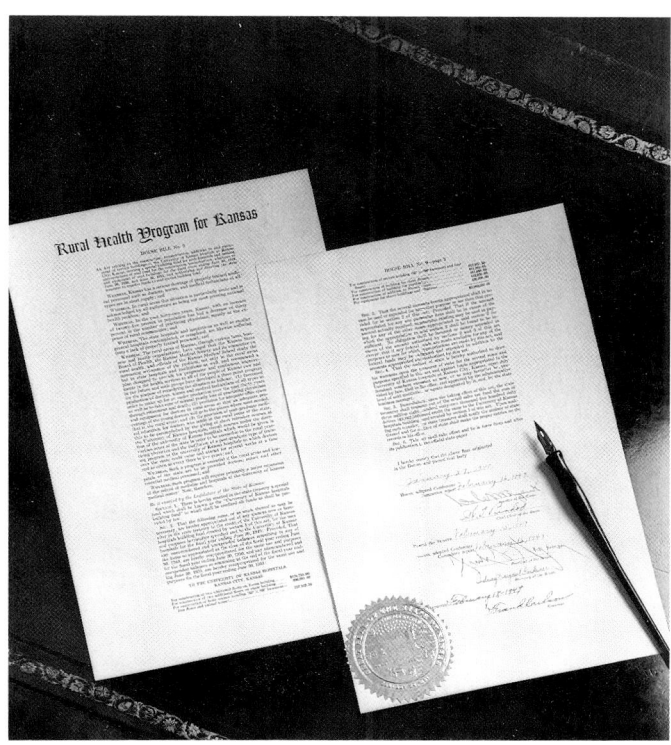

The document that launched the Kansas Rural Health Program, with the pen that Governor Carlson used in the signing.

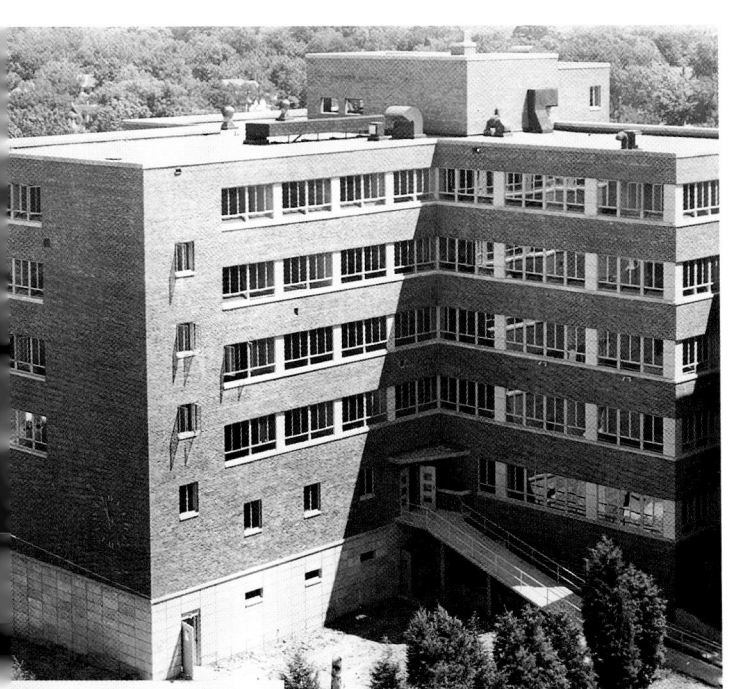

Wahl Hall, completed in 1953.

When Harry Roswell Wahl became Acting Dean of the University of Kansas School of Medicine in 1924, the fortunes of the Medical School were at its lowest ebb and the task of Dean most formidable. Undaunted, he took over and has steered the course of the Medical School with skill, prudence, and sanity. Now, on his resignation after twenty-five years of devoted service, he has the satisfaction of seeing the school past the rocks and rapids, and in calm waters.

Suetonius, the Roman historian, remarked that Augustus Caesar found Rome a city built of brick and left it one built of marble. Wahl took over an institution on a new site with one building and left it with ten. He taught by work and example that the physician should not only be skilled in his profession but should have an understanding heart. He trained generations of medical students in pathology, the basis of clinical medicine and surgery, and educated a veritable family of pathologists. These students and disciples will remain an even more lasting monument to Harry Roswell Wahl, than the imposing buildings erected during his administration.
—*Jayhawker MD*, 1949.

July 14, 1951, one day after the catastrophic flood inundated Kansas City, K.U.M.C. mobilized its resources to administer typhoid toxoid to thousands of disaster stricken people.

Day after day, until August 1, they lined up for protection against the disease which claimed so many lives in the 1903 flood.

Junior and senior medical students worked in two-hour shifts of 5 each; student nurses worked overtime, as did clerks and typists; staff men and hospital employees gave time for supervision and organization of the immunization drive.

Interns and residents were spotted at strategic points in the flood area for the purpose of giving first-aid treatment and minor therapy to the thousands of homeless victims.

When the final count was made, a total of 41,709 typhoid shots had been given to some 16,000 people; not a single case of typhoid fever was reported in greater Kansas City.
—*Jayhawker MD*, 1952.

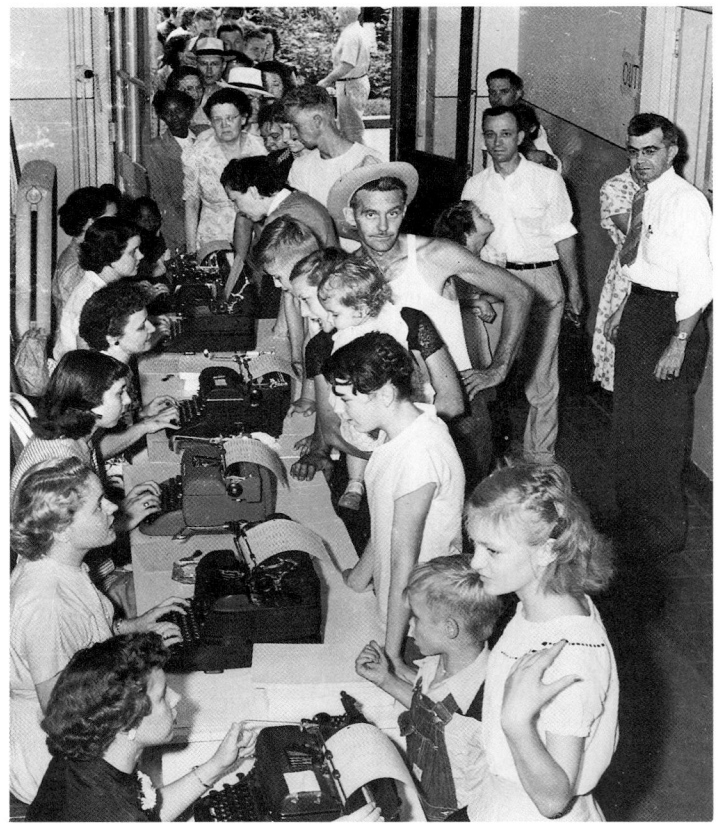

People line up for typhoid inoculations at the Medical Center following the 1951 flood.

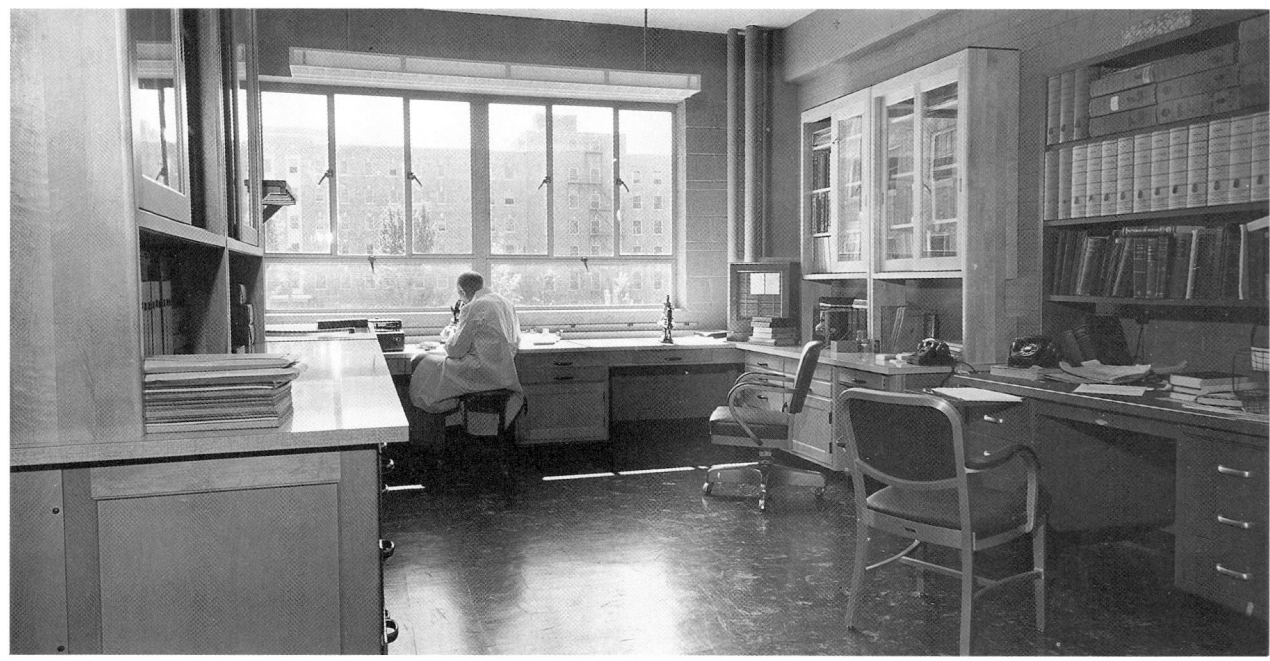

Dr. Wahl at work following his retirement as dean.

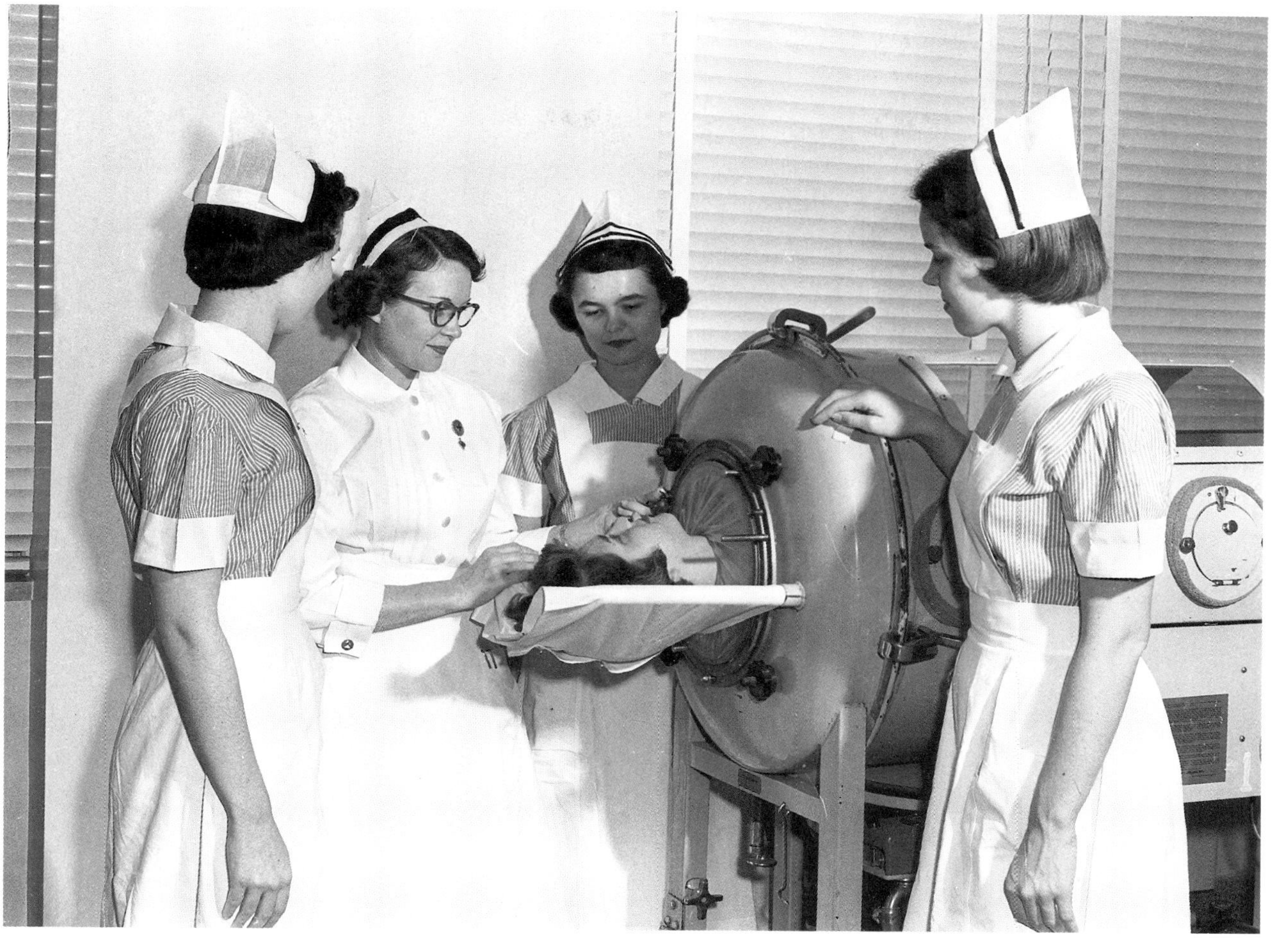

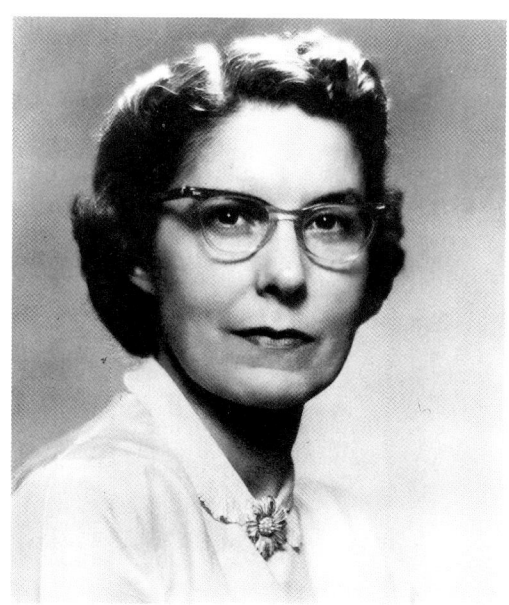

A common experience: student nurses and their instructor watch over a polio victim, ca. 1955.

E. Jean Hill, R.N., M.S., director of nursing, 1949–1963.

It is the considered opinion of many of us that our nursing program will not really flower until it is established as a separate entity from the School of Medicine. It needs leadership and it needs leadership badly. Its enrollments exceed those of several of our University schools. Those of us primarily involved in the problems of medical education can advise but hardly adequately administer nursing education as well. Nursing under the present circumstances is almost a "step-child." If we are to pursue our course and continue to train and educate for this profession, then we should do it well.
—University of Kansas Medical Center Biennial Report, 1954–1956.

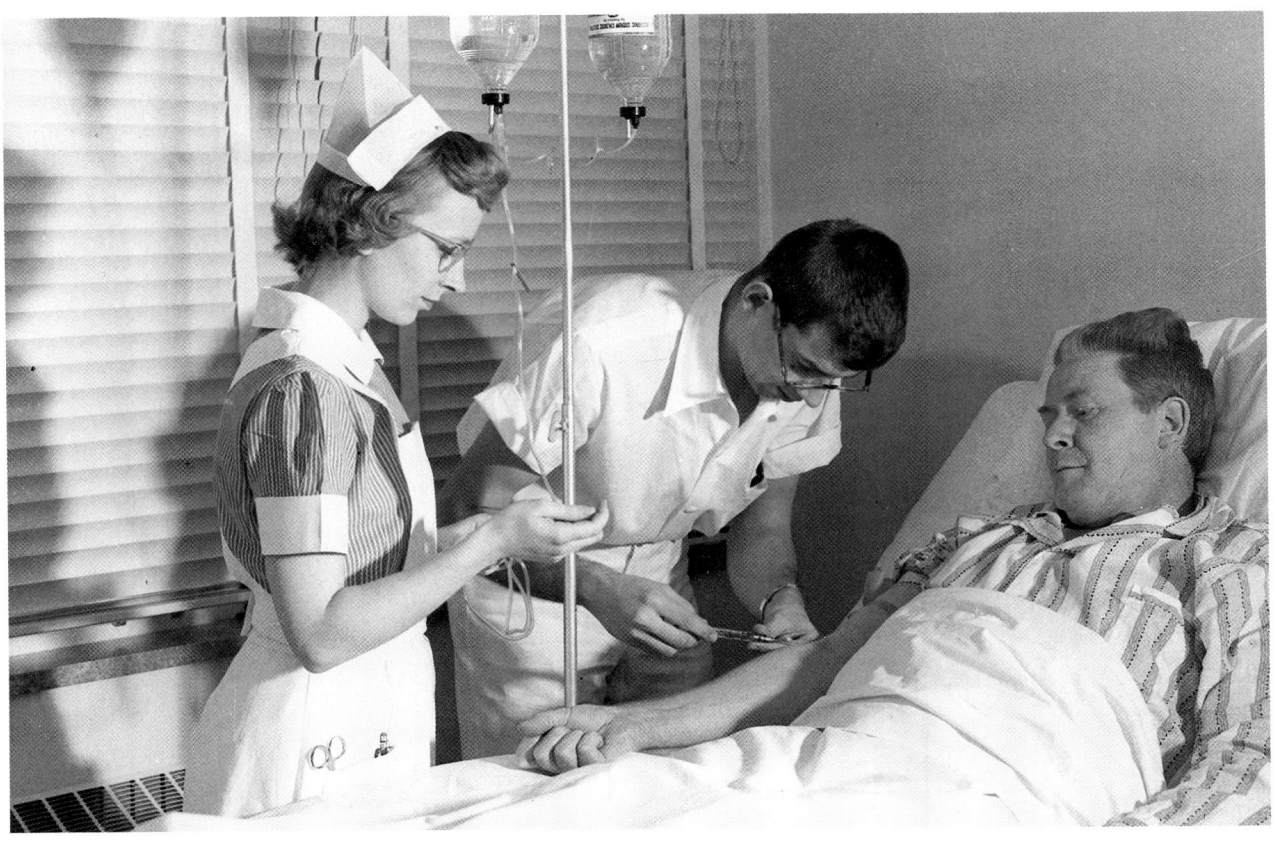

A patient receiving an injection, late 1950s.

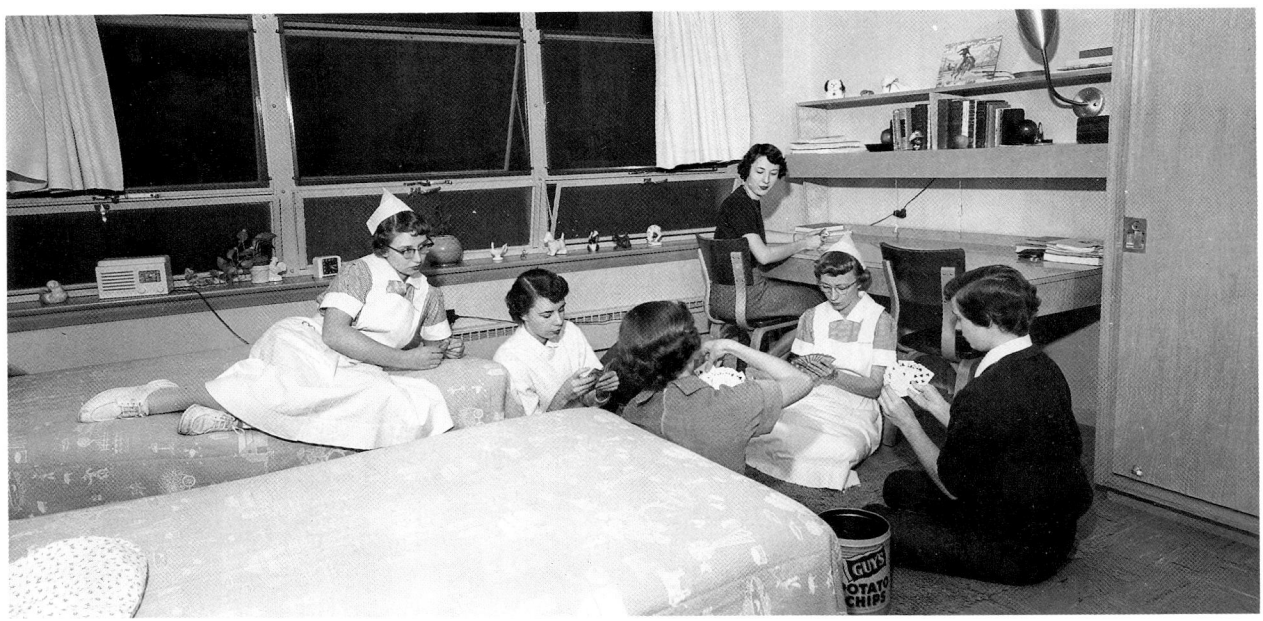

Off-duty student nurses enjoying an evening's entertainment in their quarters in the Nurses' Residence, ca. 1954.

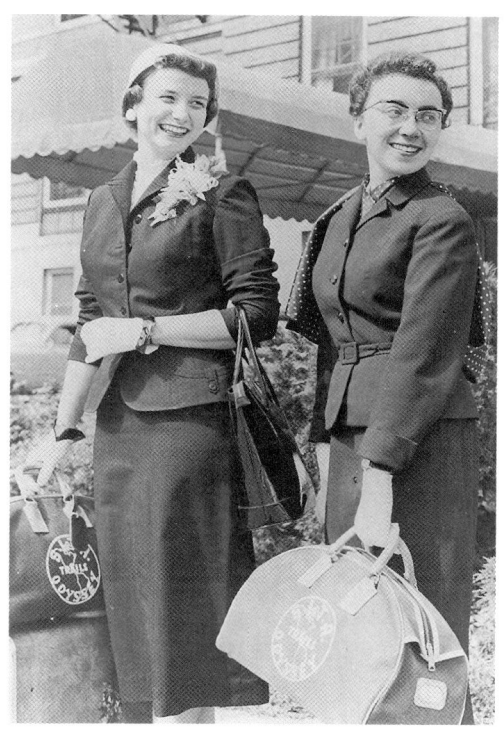

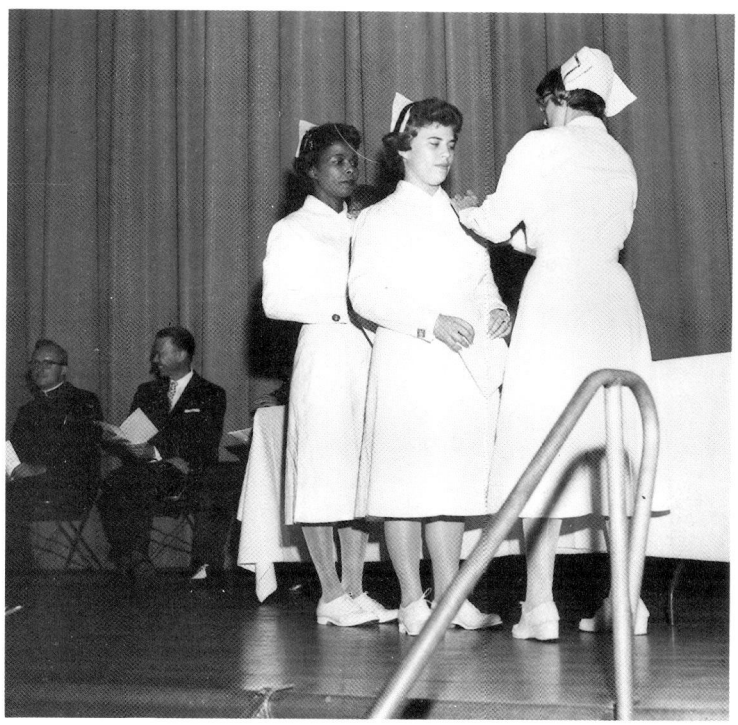

Irma Lou Kolterman and Wanda Stalcup leaving the Medical Center for an international meeting of student nurses in Rome, Italy, April 1957.

The August 6, 1959, pinning ceremony.

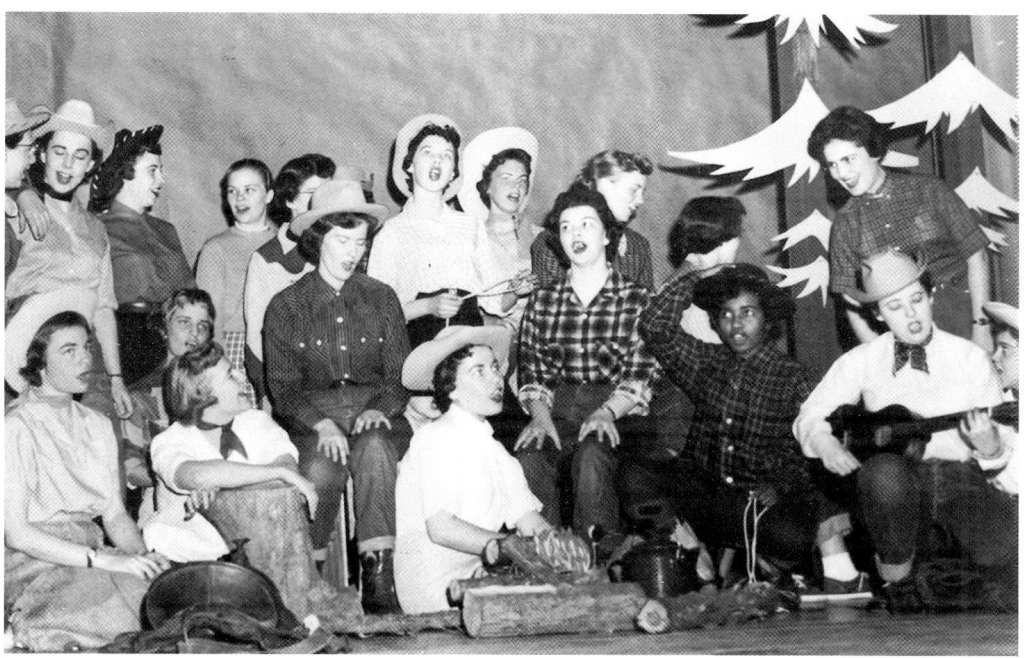

Caduceus Capers, an annual event of the Department of Nursing, was planned and performed by nursing students during the 1950s and 1960s.

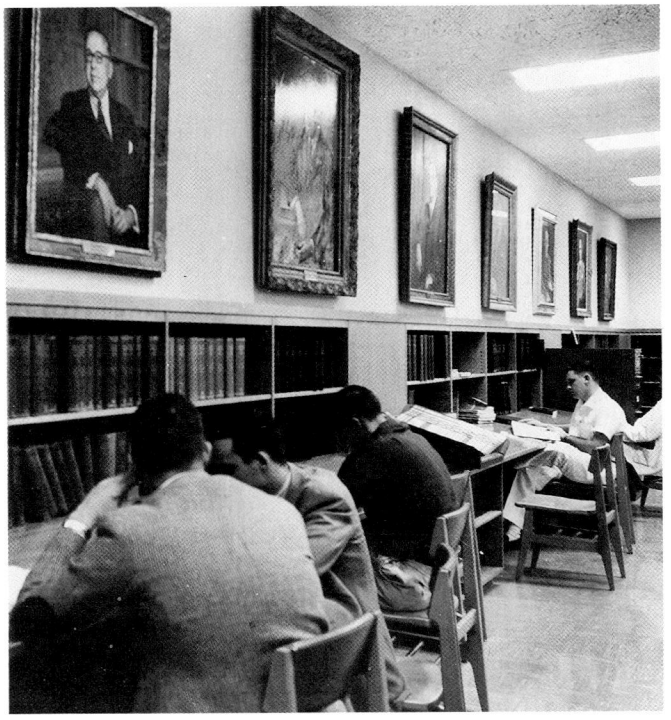

Students studying in the new library, late 1950s.

Today the University of Kansas School of Medicine stands as a first-class institution of medical learning. Under its influence come yearly many young men and women in all branches of medical activity, and from it each year are disgorged the finished products—the doctors, the nurses, and the many types of medical technical personnel—to care for the health needs of the people of Kansas and this great Mid-Western area. It is providing postgraduate medical training yearly for hundreds of doctors. Members of its faculty are participating increasingly in many fields of medical research. Truly the University of Kansas School of Medicine is a going and effective institution.
—Franklin D. Murphy, M.D., in *Jayhawker MD*, 1949.

The University of Kansas School of Medicine again had the largest enrollment by physicians in refresher, circuit and continuation postgraduate courses of any school in the United States and Canada during the school year 1954–55. The department of postgraduate medical education had 2,034 doctors enrolled for courses, 894 of this number from out-of-state. Enrollees came from 34 states, the territory of Hawaii, Canada and Thailand. In addition to the doctors, 978 nurses, technicians and lay people attended courses. The department has maintained this position of leadership in total enrollment for the past four years.
—*Topics*, March 1956.

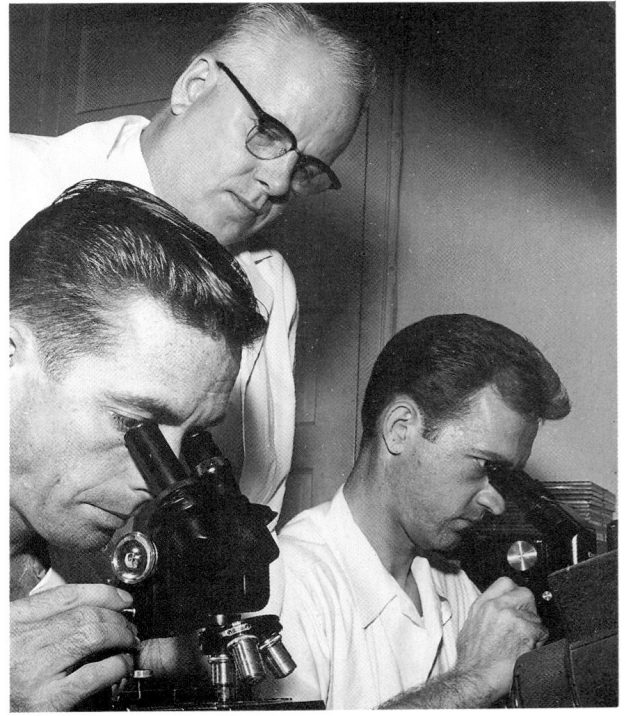

Postgraduate studies: Dr. Sloan Wilson, professor of medicine, works with Dr. Robert P. Hudson, resident, and Dr. David Shivel, ca. 1958.

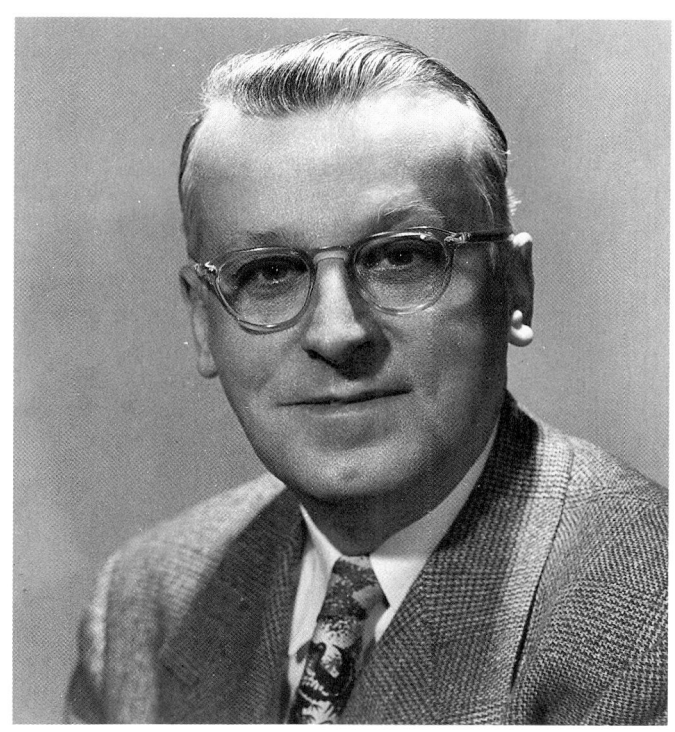

Edward H. Hashinger, M.D., acting dean of the Medical School from 1951 to 1952.

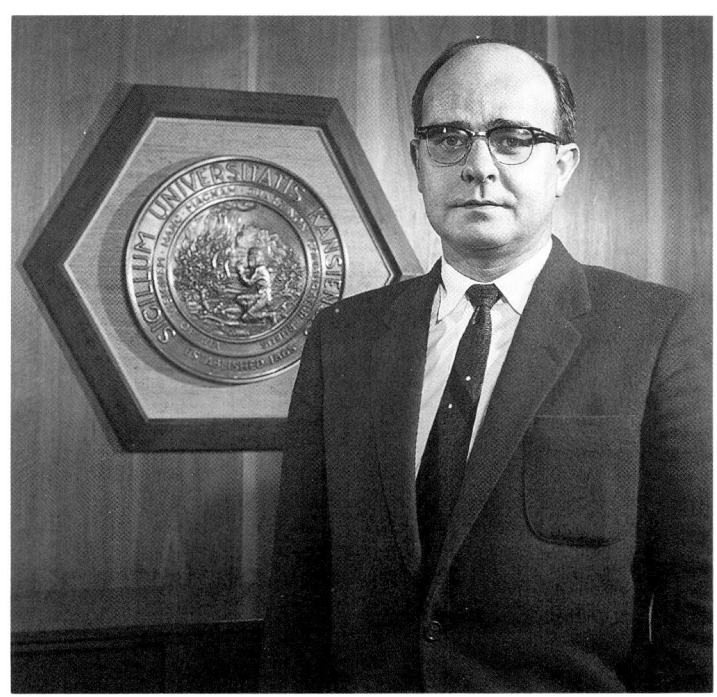

W. Clarke Wescoe, M.D., dean and director of the Medical Center, 1952–1960.

It is my firm purpose to strengthen and solidify the programs that were put into effect by my predecessors. We have gained, in a short time, a nationwide reputation for being the medical school to watch for bigger things; we must produce, for the country and our state are looking to us. Our greatest interest is, and must be, the training of more good physicians, nurses and other medical personnel to fill the needs of Kansas.
—W. Clarke Wescoe, M.D., dean, in Kansas University School of Medicine and Medical Center *Bulletin,* August 1952.

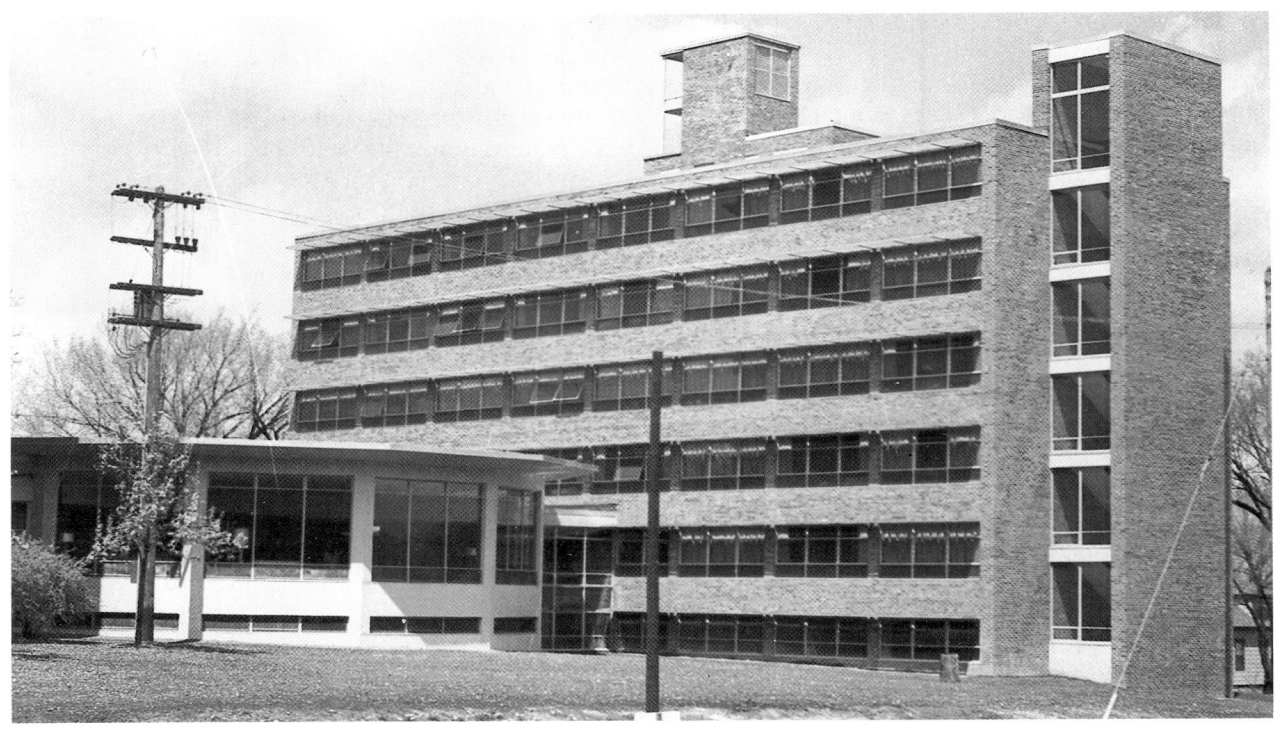

Nurses' Residence after its completion in 1953.

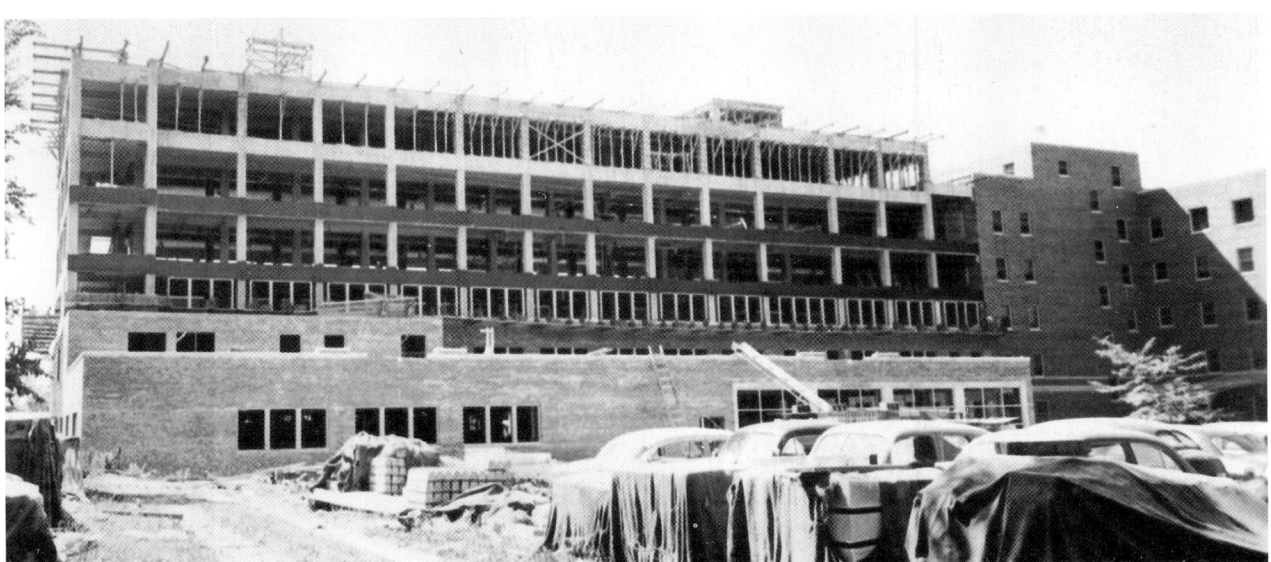

Construction of F Building, 1953.

Since the close of World War II, the people of Kansas, through their legislative representatives, have appropriated more than 5 1/2 million dollars for the expansion of the University of Kansas Medical Center. These appropriations represent substantially more money than has been put into the Medical Center since its establishment. Already these dollars are being translated into new and well-equipped teaching units, all designed for the purpose of making more and better doctors, nurses, and technicians for the state. The responsibility of arousing the interest required to support these legislative appropriations belongs to many diverse individuals and groups in our state, including representatives of agriculture, industry, government, and the medical profession itself. This program of expansion and development has in truth been a project by the people and for the people and has begun to reflect just credit on the enlightened citizens of Kansas.—*Jayhawker MD*, 1951.

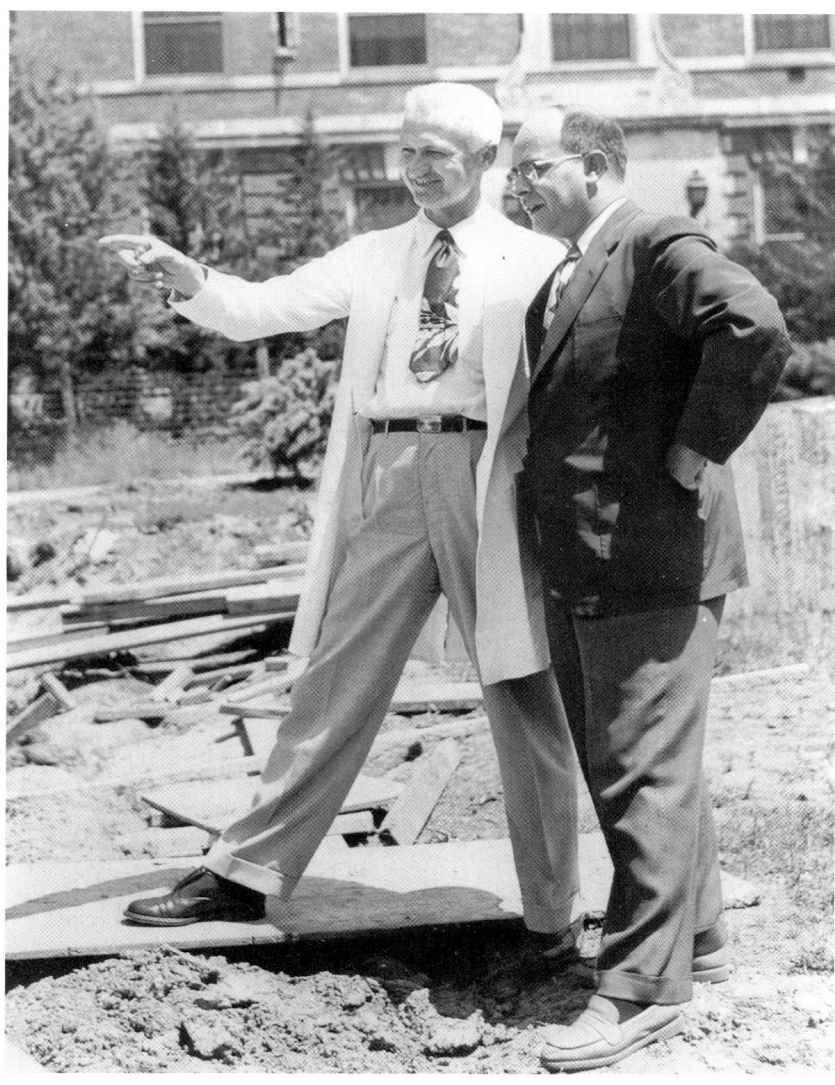

Assistant Dean Vernon Wilson, M.D., and Dean Wescoe, at the site of the new Library Building, 1956.

In succeeding Dr. Murphy at the medical school Dr. Wescoe has carried forward the boom in new buildings, enlarged staff, research projects and improved teaching methods. Two solid revisions have been emphasized particularly—the expansion of post-graduate teaching and the integration of the physiology of the body system with the teaching of anatomy to undergraduates.

Under Wescoe the K.U. school has emerged among the top layer of American medical schools in its instruction of doctors out in practice, keeping them informed on how to apply new advances to their treatments. The number of these courses and physicians who flock to them, at the K.U. center, has set new records among medical schools.—*Kansas City Star*, July 1, 1956.

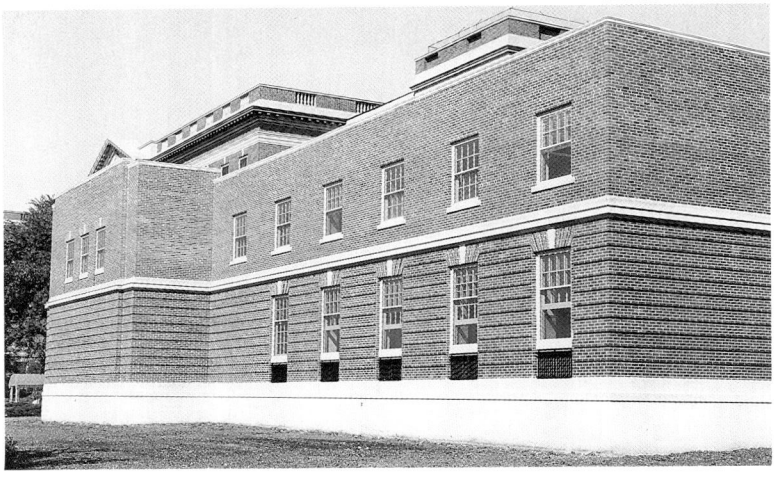

The completed Library Building, 1957.

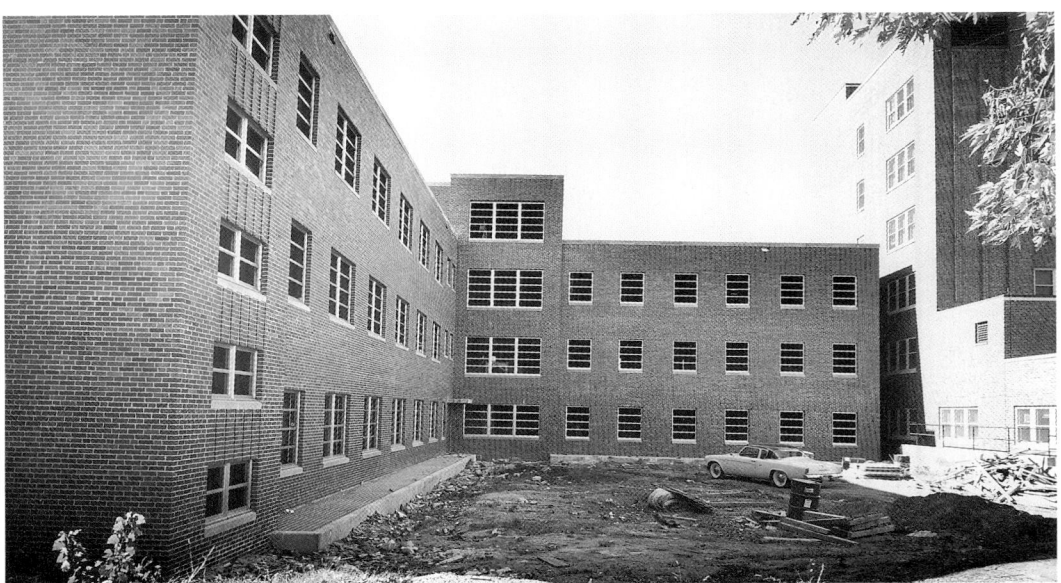

The Psychiatry Building opened in 1957.

You have been privileged to be students in the University of Kansas School of Medicine during the period of its greatest and most vigorous growth. You have been the heart of this school in the days when it grew from being one of many to the point where it has become the focus of national and international attention. You have lived in an atmosphere where construction has practically been the watchword; during your residence you have seen our school double its physical dimensions. Your school has never been stronger. We are entering a period, of necessity, where physical growth will come more slowly and where the gains of the last few years will become more firmly consolidated. Academically, of course, spiritually and research-wise, growth will continue apace.—*Jayhawker MD*, 1953.

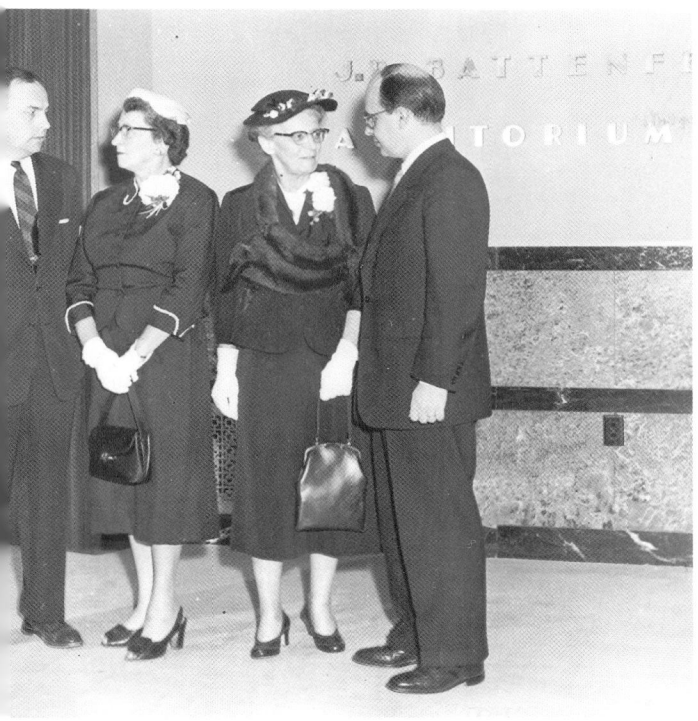

Dr. Franklin D. Murphy and Dr. W. Clarke Wescoe, dean, with Mrs. E. H. Hashinger and Mrs. C. B. Francisco at the dedication of the Student Center and Battenfeld Auditorium, April 4, 1954.

The long-needed Student Center at the University of Kansas Medical Center became complete reality on Sunday, April 4, in the dedication of the completed building, the magnificent Battenfeld Memorial Auditorium and the C. B. Francisco Memorial Lounge.

The Battenfeld Memorial Auditorium is the only one at the KU Medical Center that can seat the entire student body and faculty simultaneously. Beautifully equipped with 924 theater seats, full theater lighting, staging, and projection booth, it can accommodate any type of program. The stage backdrop . . . is a reproduction of the Temple of Aesculapius on the Island of Cos off Asia Minor, where the practice of scientific medicine began with Hippocrates.
—Kansas University School of Medicine and Medical Center *Bulletin,* June 1954.

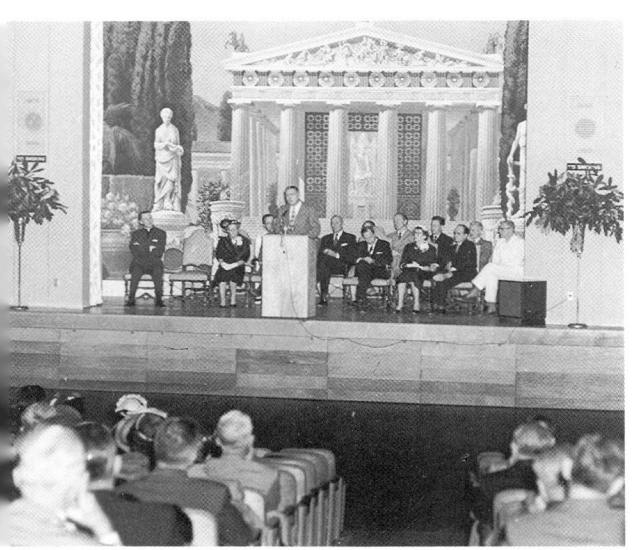

Galen Tice, M.D., professor of radiology, speaking at the dedication of the Student Center.

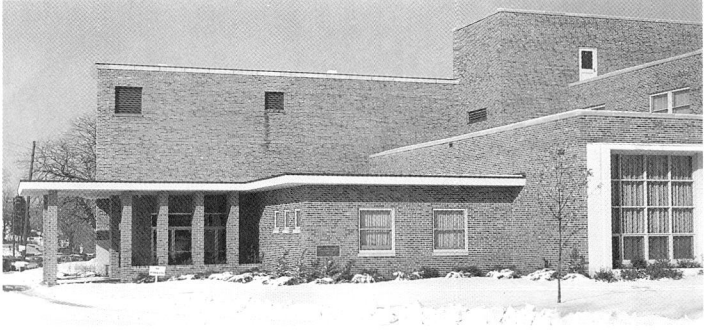

The Student Center was occupied in 1954 and expanded in 1963.

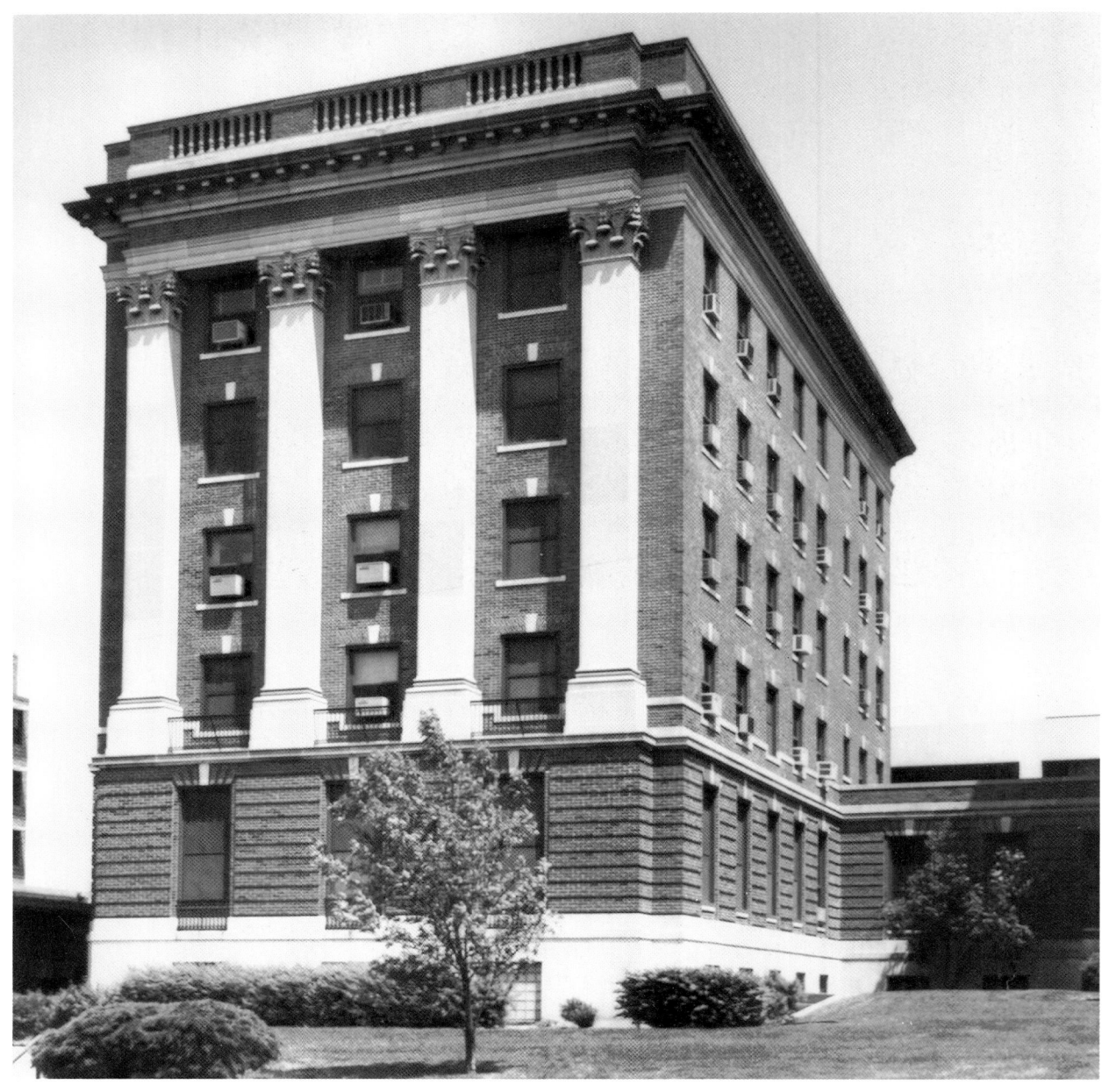

Hinch Hall during the 1950s.

Living in Hinch Hall and using our meal tickets in the cafeteria gave us few occasions or reasons to leave the confines of the medical center. Concerts and other programs were held in Battenfeld Auditorium in the student center, which also contained the bookstore and could be reached through a convenient tunnel. We ventured out as little as possible, especially during the winter months. While walking through the tunnel on a January evening, it came as quite a shock to realize that we had not been outdoors for weeks. It seemed that we were becoming a bit mole-like in our behavior.—Grace E. Holmes, M.D., "The Year Hinch Hall Went Coed," unpublished manuscript, January 1989.

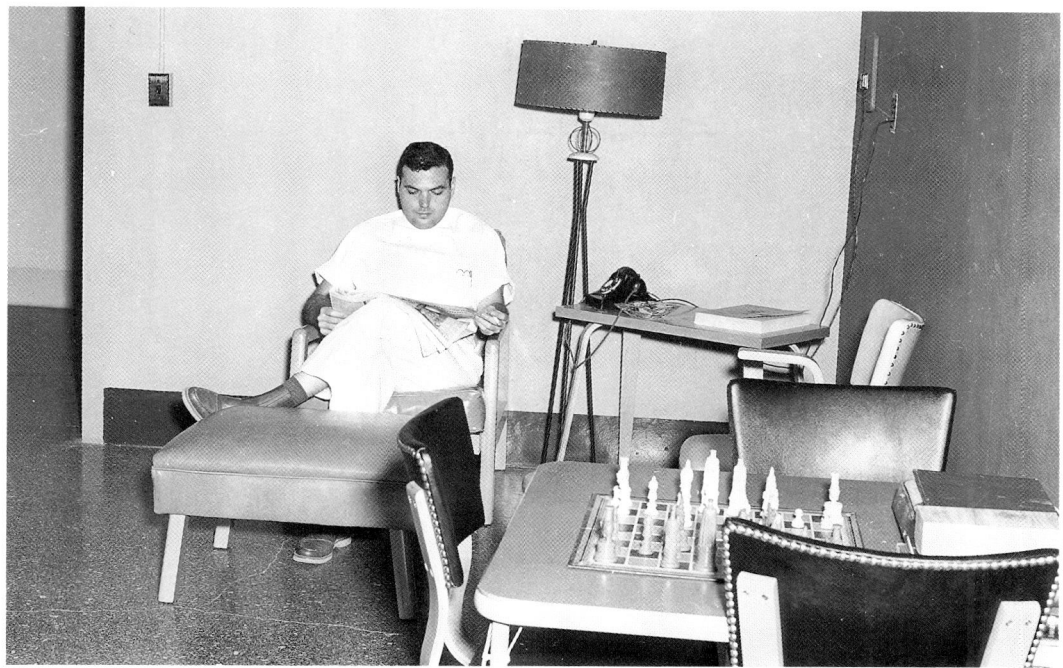

Interns' quarters, August 1954.

The internship moved along slowly though we often wondered whether it would ever end. As others can attest, the internship year seems like several years crammed into one. We were learning much about medicine and were impressed with the friendliness of Kansans and specifically with the interest and kindness generally shown to house staff by the senior staff. We were fortunate to work with Gunnar Proud on ENT and his entourage of residents including Ferd Kirchner and Yogi Williams, Bill Valk in Urology and John Foret, one of his many residents, Galen Tice and Don Germann in Radiology. . . .

Though times and personnel change, hospital facilities enlarge, modernize and become updated, and medical science, skills and therapies revolutionize, patients don't really change nor does the physician-patient relationship. Caring about patients was stressed and impressed on us during that internship in "the early days." Even in these modern times the same ingredients are still basic to house staff training at KUMC. Maybe that's why it doesn't seem so long ago.
—Grace E. Holmes, M.D., "A KUMC Internship," unpublished manuscript, January 1989.

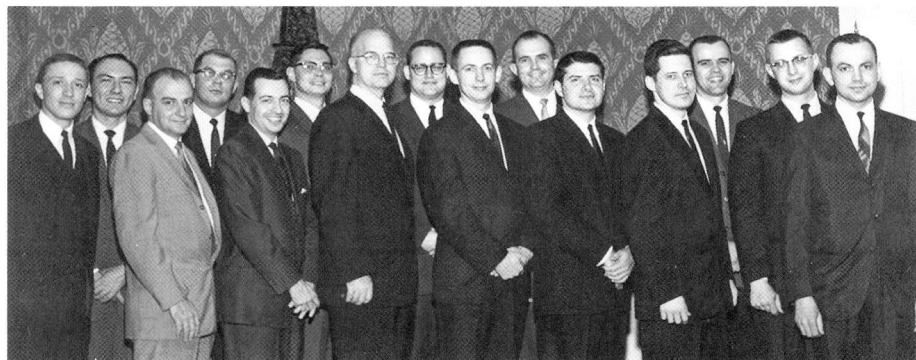

Surgery residents group with Frank Allbritten, Jr., M.D., chairman of surgery.

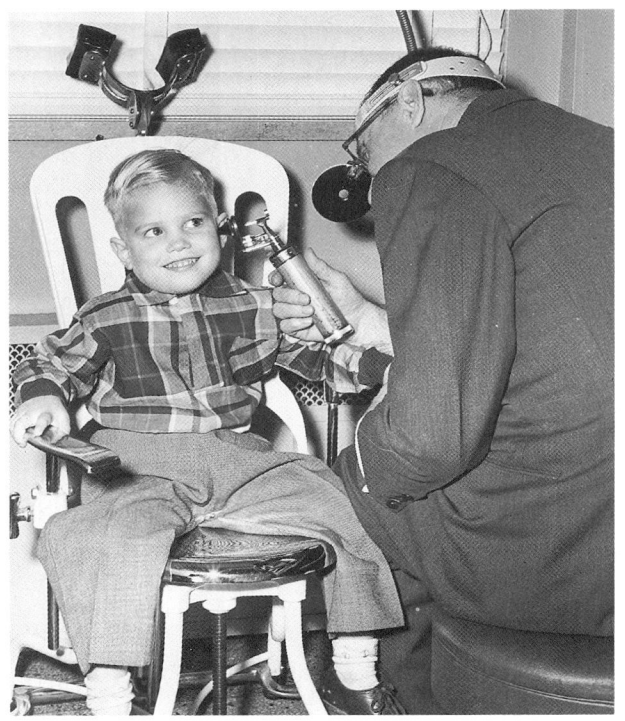

In the spring of 1949 the Department of Hearing and Speech of the University of Kansas Medical Center was established by a special grant of the Kansas Legislature. The grant made four specific requirements—that a pre-school be established at the Medical Center, that the Department of Audiology be continued, that a Parent Training Session should be started, and that provisions should be made for a teacher training program. This grant was made to coordinate the programs of several groups working independently in the State of Kansas and the Greater Kansas City Area.—June Miller, M.A., "Hearing and Speech Program at the University of Kansas Medical Center," *American Annals of the Deaf,* May 1951.

Hearing and Speech Department, 1950s.

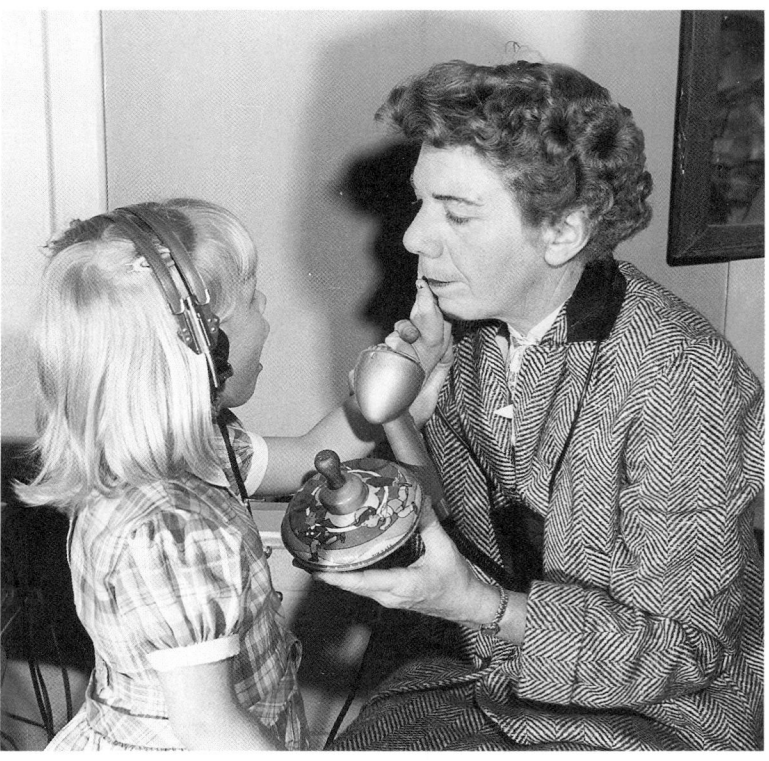

Young patient being examined in the Hearing and Speech Department by Dr. June Miller, ca. 1955.

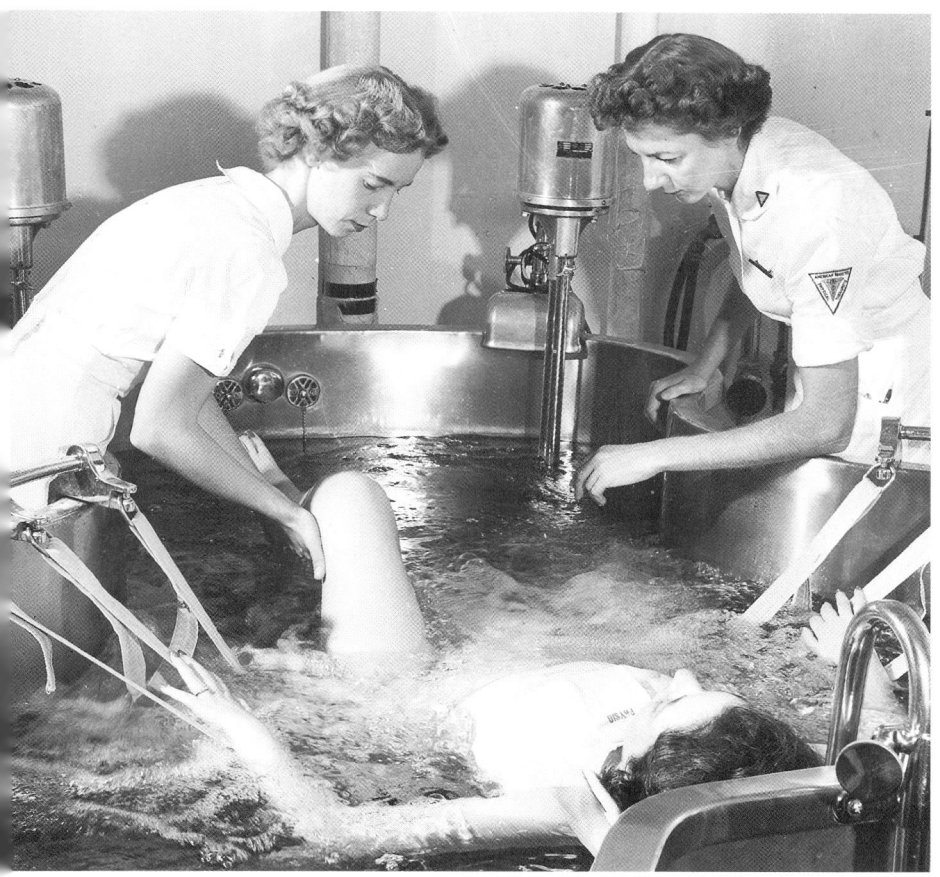

Physical Therapy's hydrotherapy tank.

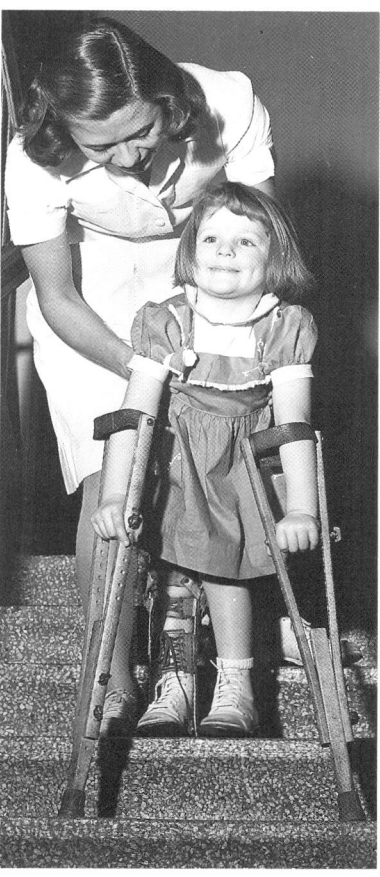

Physical therapist helping a patient
negotiate the stairs, ca. 1955.

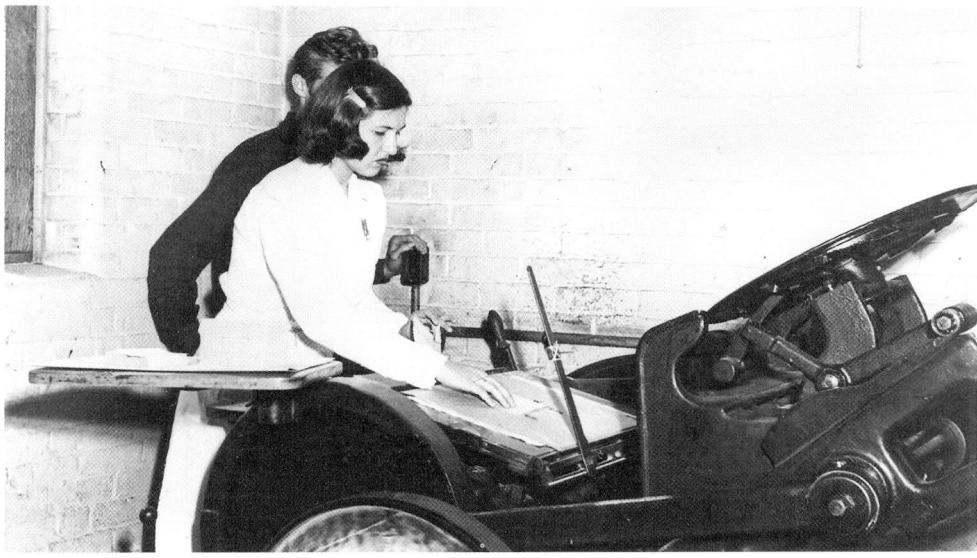

Occupational Therapy, 1951.

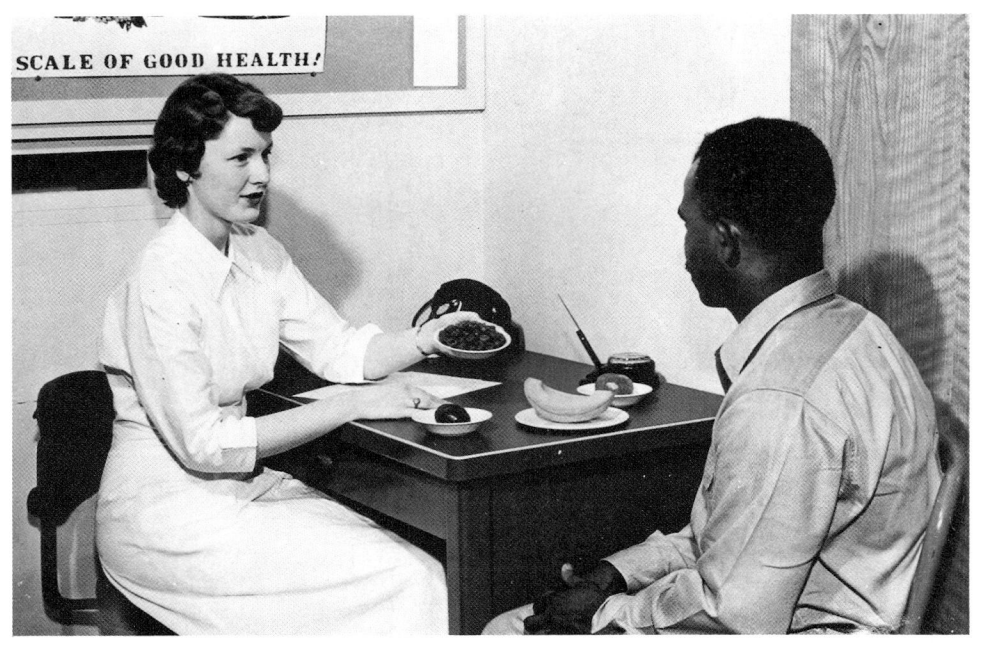

Nutritional counseling, 1950s.

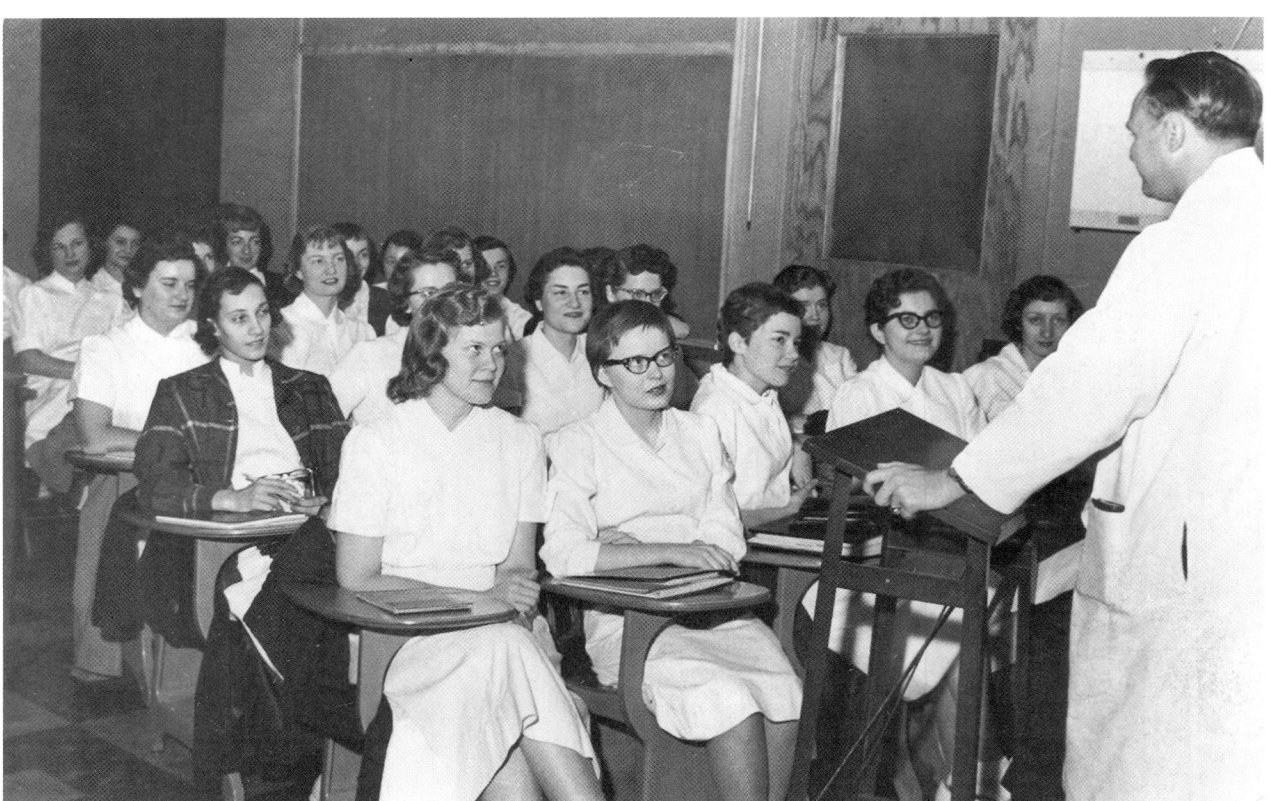

A laboratory technician class, 1950s.

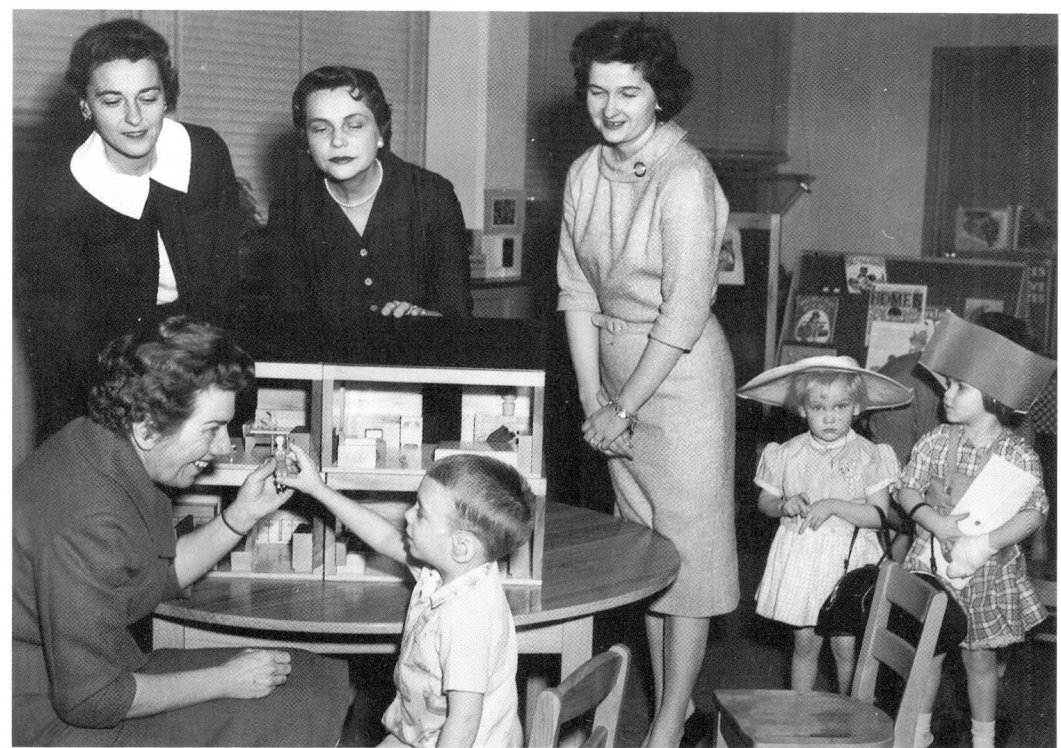

The Children's Rehabilitation Unit, ca. 1960.

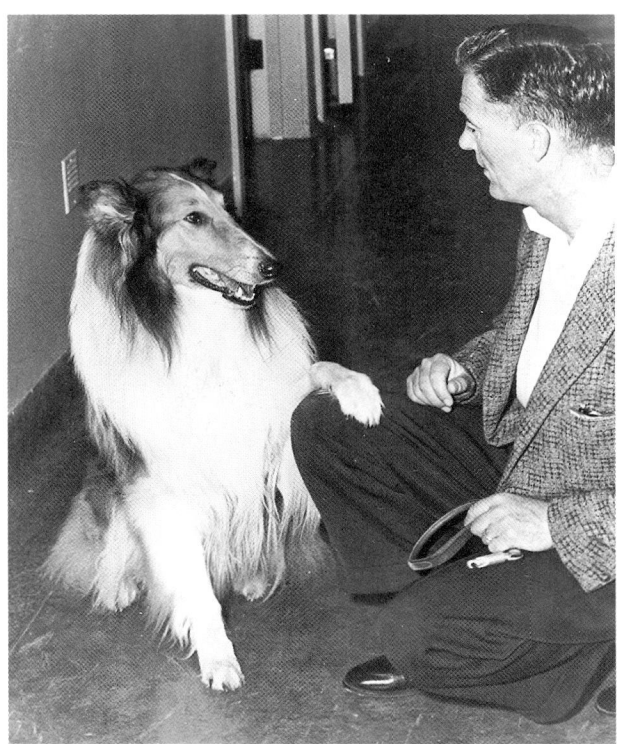

Lassie and trainer Jack Weatherwax visit pediatrics,
May 17, 1957.

Lassie, famous TV personality, came to Kansas City to appear in a show in the Municipal Stadium. Thanks to our Gray Ladies a special appearance was made at KUMC May 17 in the pediatrics area. The kids got a big treat out of seeing the famous collie go through his (Lassie is a male) paces under the watchful eye of his trainer and half-owner Jack Weatherwax of Hollywood. There are now two Lassies—the original, now 17 and retired, Lassie, Jr. and his son Laddie, who made the trip to become used to public appearances and to learn his future trade! It was a big day for our young patients.
—*Topics*, June 1957.

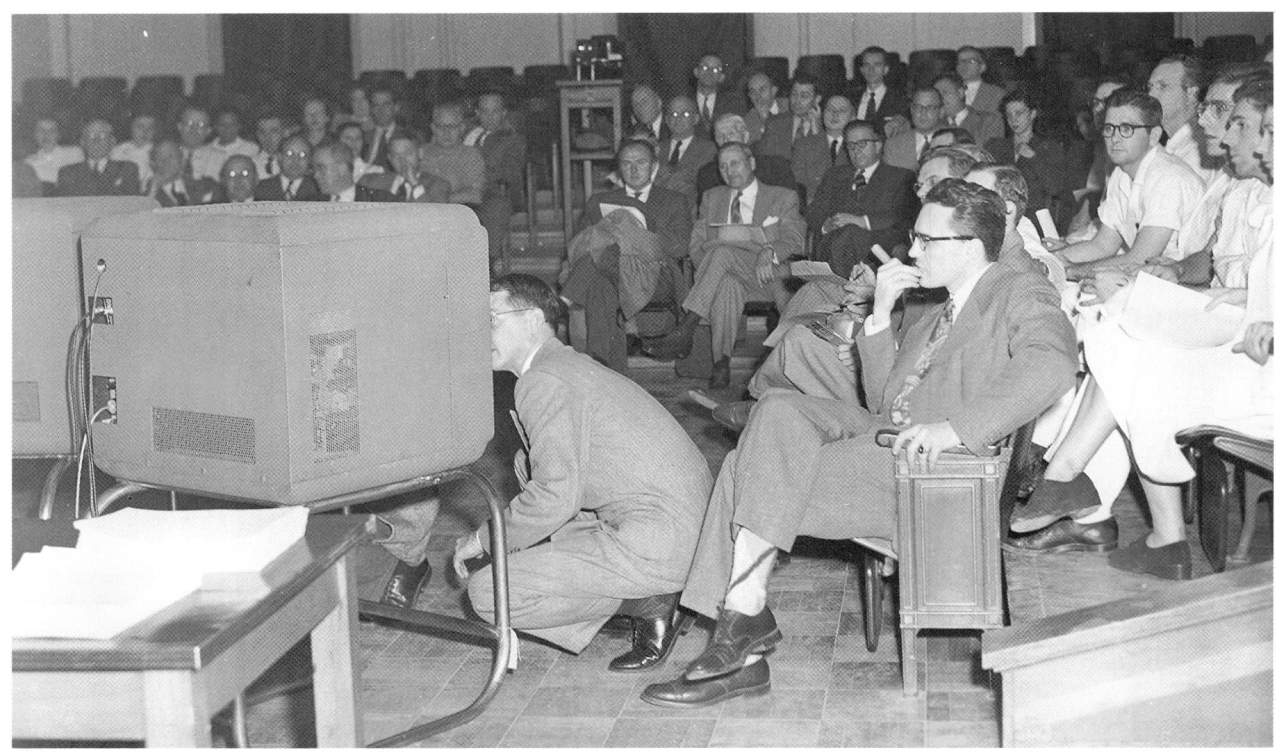

Early use of television in the classroom, 1950s.

Magnified pictures of the operating site, combined with eye and ear observations of techniques around the operating table have revived the amphitheater as a teaching device. This can be called a "super immediacy" in medical education. The real patient, plus the real setting, plus television, makes it possible for a gallery audience to see what before only one or two might see. —*Topics*, January 1955.

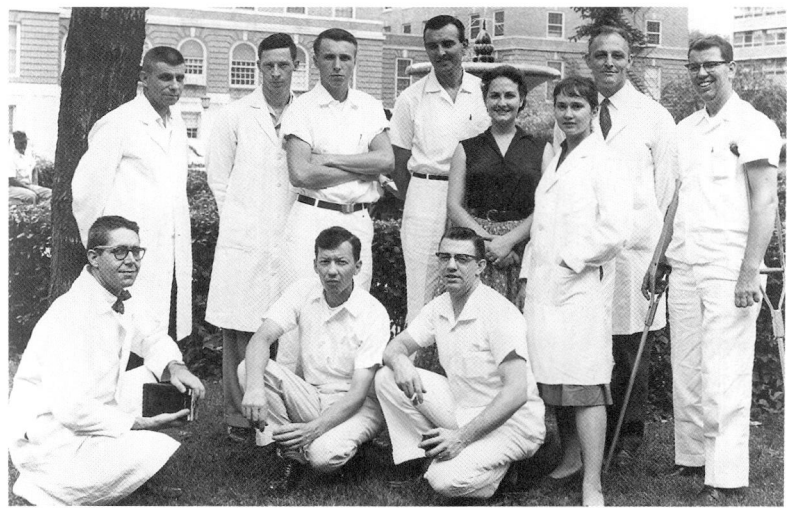

Members of the Medical Communications Department, ca. 1961. Burton Johnson is at the far right.

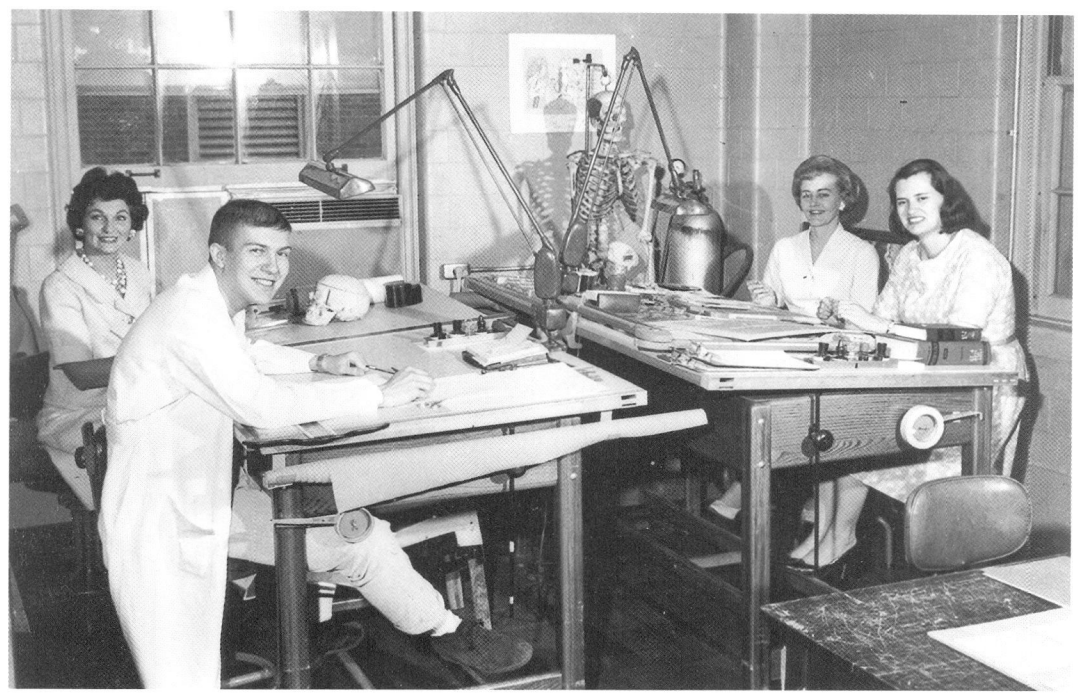

Medical illustrators Beverly Sherril, John Jensen, Virginia Hartley, and Joanne Clifford, ca. 1960.

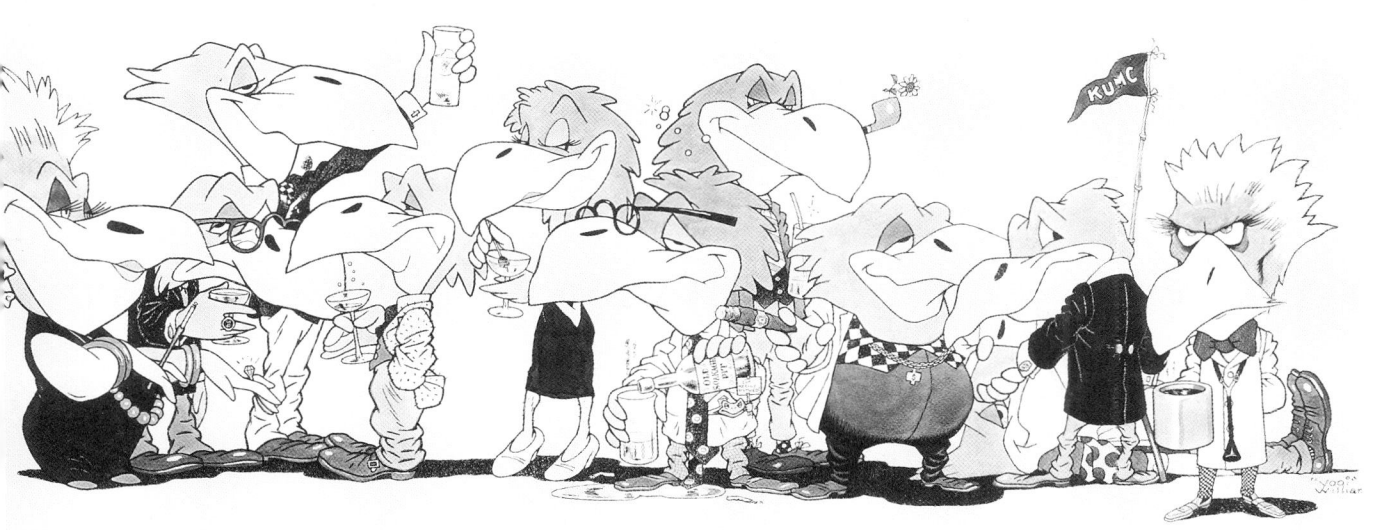

Medical Center faculty as portrayed by Gene "Yogi" Williams, M.D., for the class of 1954 reunion.

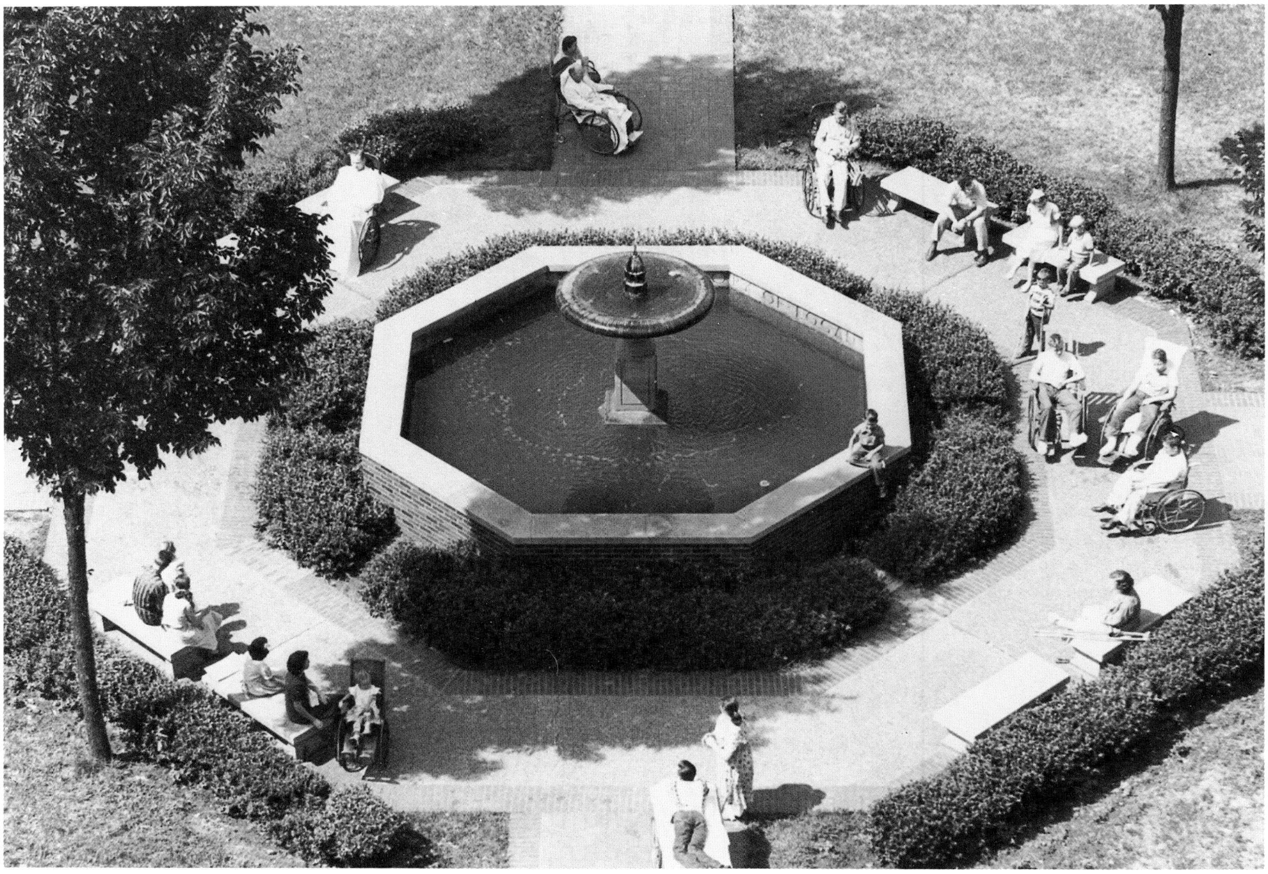

A summer scene at the Clendening Fountain in the 1950s.

Although the fountain's primary purpose is a memorial to Dr. Clendening, it serves many people at KUMC in various ways. It's a pass through area between buildings. On spring and summer days it is a refreshing oasis in the middle of the hospital area. In the wintertime when the trees, shrubbery and fountain are covered with snow, it makes a beautiful setting for a large Christmas tree. In all seasons it provides a "view of the outside" to hospitalized patients who can watch from the corridor windows.—*Topics,* June 1956.

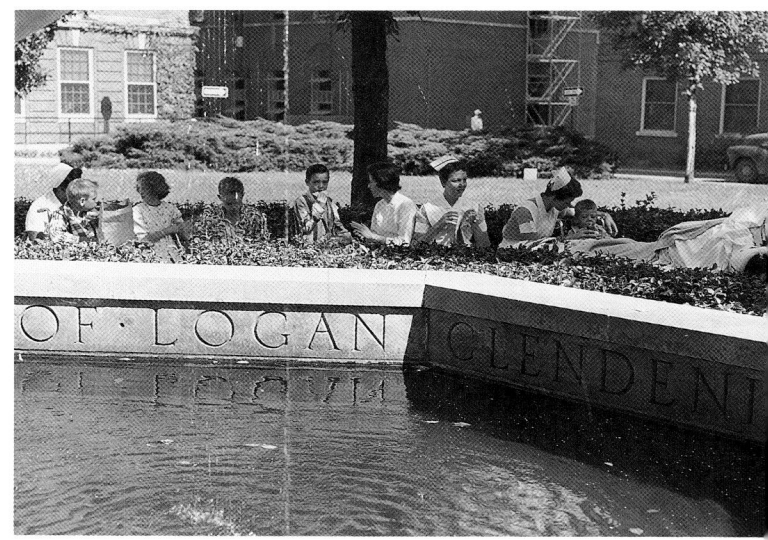

Children enjoying the sun, ca. 1955.

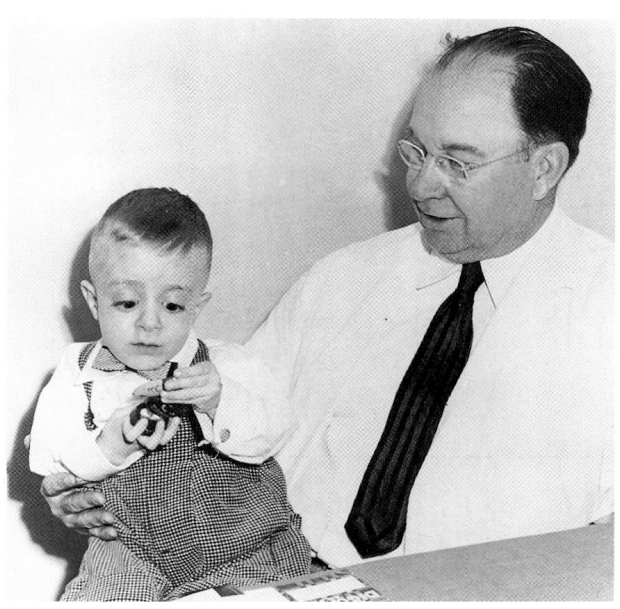

James B. Weaver, M.D., chairman of the Department of Orthopaedics with a patient, ca. 1960.

Medical care is close to the heart of every man, woman and child of this country, and if the people cannot get the leadership to resolve their medical problems from us they must turn elsewhere. If we are to furnish the leadership we must be realistic and we must not develop a mass paranoia which reflects itself in an automatic objection to every idea of change in the way we train physicians and in the problems of medical prepayment protection.

The medical school deans and faculty must come out of their ivory towers and find out what the practicing physicians as well as the people of the country need. The practicing physician on the other hand, through the medium of organized medicine, must deeply and seriously concern himself with the problem of provision of adequate facilities to train more doctors, to train them better and to guarantee post-graduate experience for all men in the practice of medicine.—Franklin D. Murphy, M.D., dean, to Ralph H. Pino, M.D., August 13, 1948.

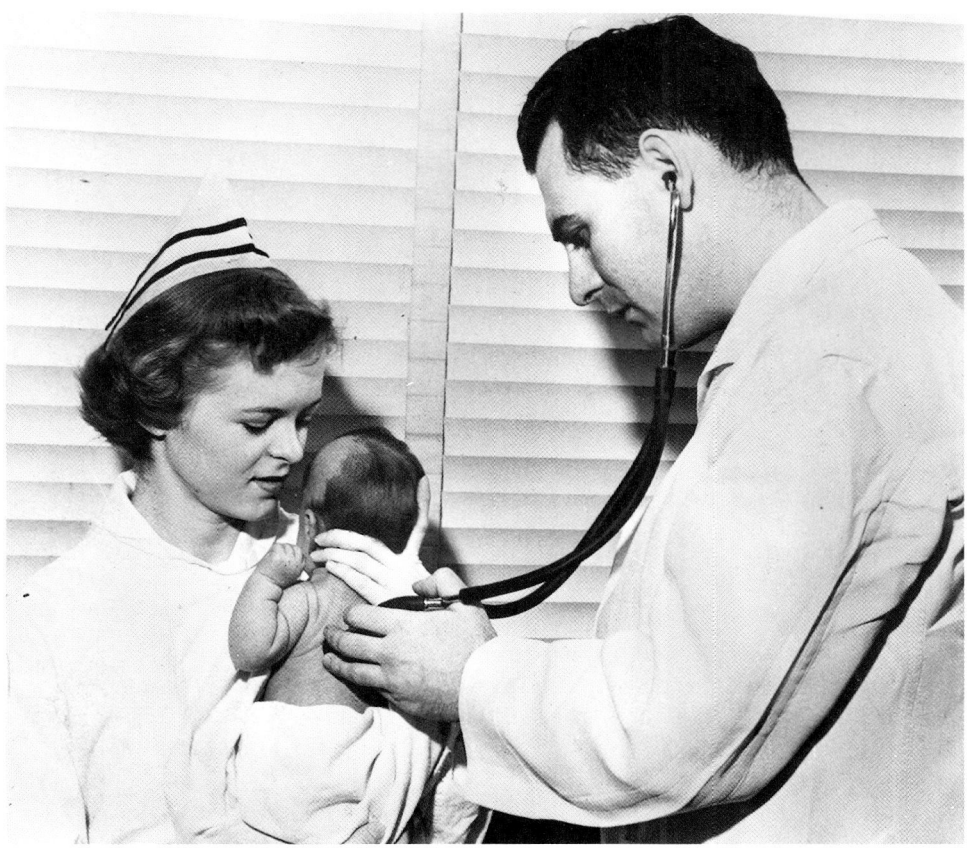

A doctor and nurse examining a baby, ca. 1960.

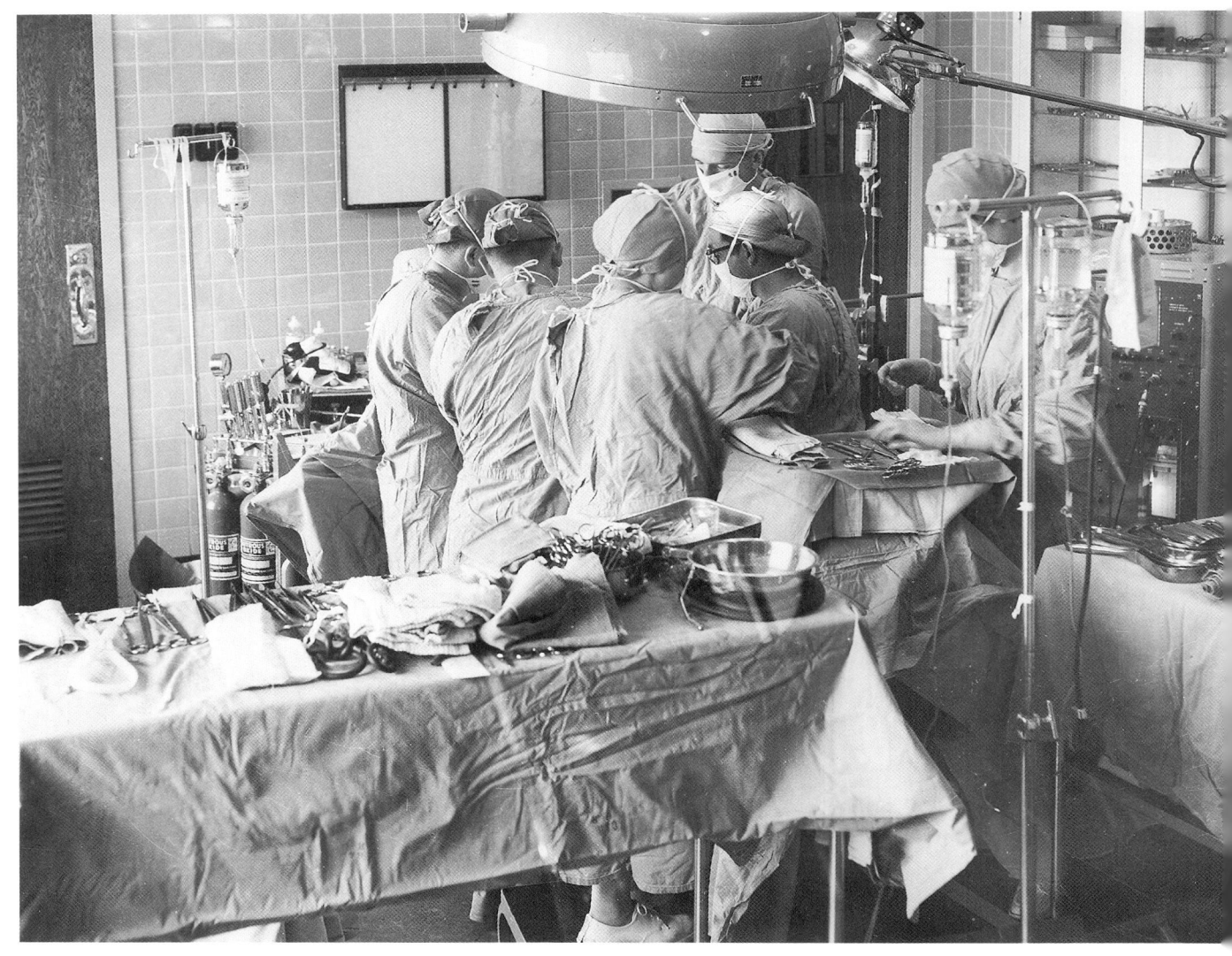

Surgery in July 1956.

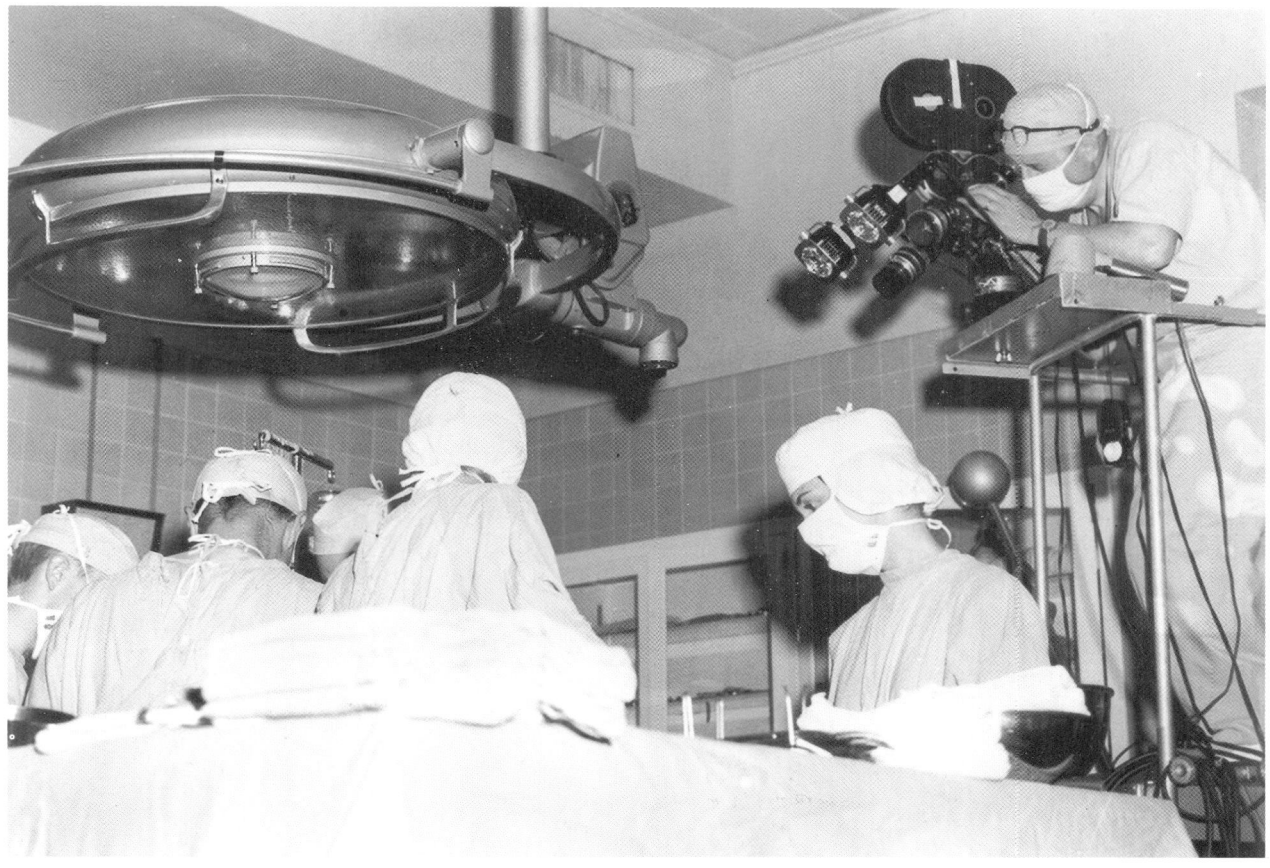

Medical photography in the operating room, late 1950s.

We need many more good doctors, but not one more poorly trained doctor. Producing more top doctors is a challenge to our profession, but more so to the American people, who should and must provide the money needed to do it.

The growth of specialties in medicine will increase, not decrease, because the science of medicine is so complex. At the same time the role of the general practitioner grows in importance. The family doctor is the guide in the treatment choices, and when he is both competent and honest he calls in specialists as they are needed. The good doctor, general practitioner or specialist, is one who knows when he must call in experts in various fields, the better to serve his patient.
—*Kansas City Star*, July 1, 1956.

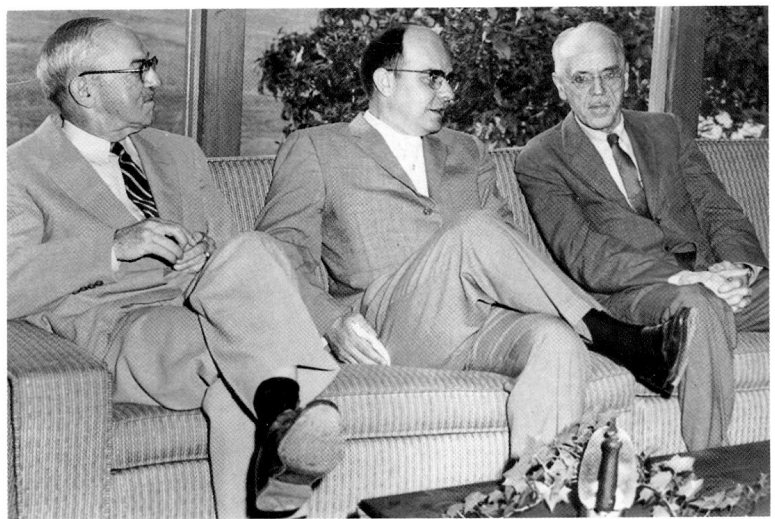

Disease often shapes men's lives. From the day of his birth to the day of his death, man is engaged in a constant struggle against disease, trying to prevent disease or, when it appears, trying to overcome it. Since the beginning of history, nations, which are aggregates of men, have carried on this same struggle. Disease has caused the migration of people, has conquered armies, depopulated nations, changed the course of history.—Ralph H. Major, M.D., *Jayhawker MD*, 1962.

Drs. Ralph H. Major, W. Clarke Wescoe, and Paul Dudley White (President Eisenhower's cardiologist), ca. 1960.

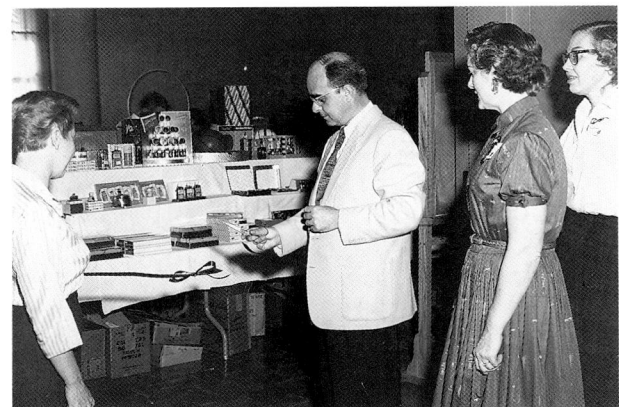

Dr. Wescoe at ribbon-cutting ceremony for the Medical Center Auxiliary gift shop, October 30, 1957.

Dedicated in ceremonies December 4, 1955, was the Lacy Haynes Cardiovascular Research Laboratory.

Two of the laboratory's rooms are devoted to human diagnostic and research studies in blue babies and congenital heart disease; a cardiac catheterization room and a procedure room where laboratory tests will be carried out. The third room is a conference room for training medical students and resident physicians in the use of the stethoscope in examining the heart; electronic stethoscopes built into each seat will permit as many as twenty students to hear the same heart sounds simultaneously.
—*Kansas University School of Medicine and Medical Center Bulletin*, February 1956.

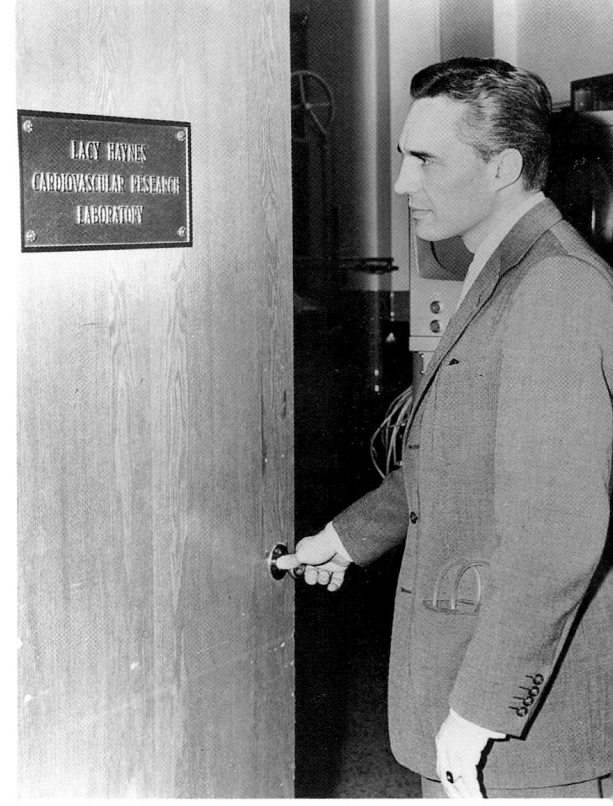

E. Grey Dimond, M.D., chairman of the Department of Medicine, at the dedication of the Lacy Haynes Cardiovascular Research Laboratory, December 4, 1956.

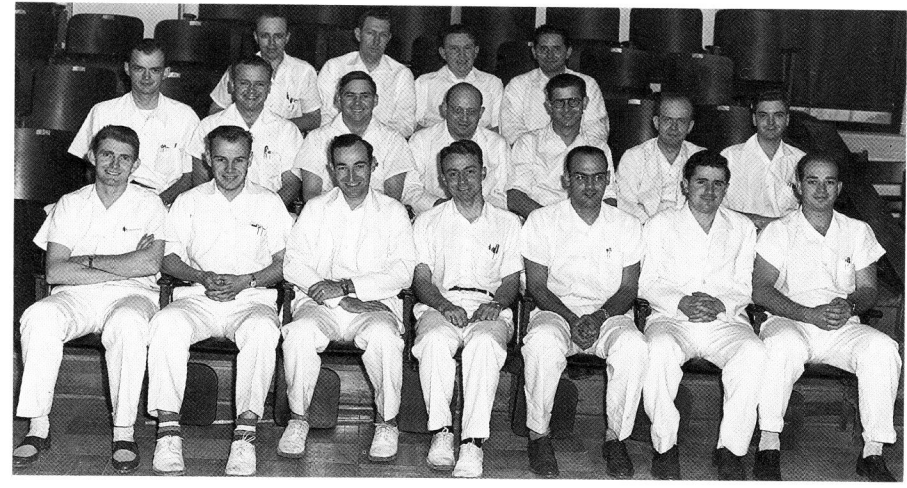

Cardiovascular Department personnel, 1951.

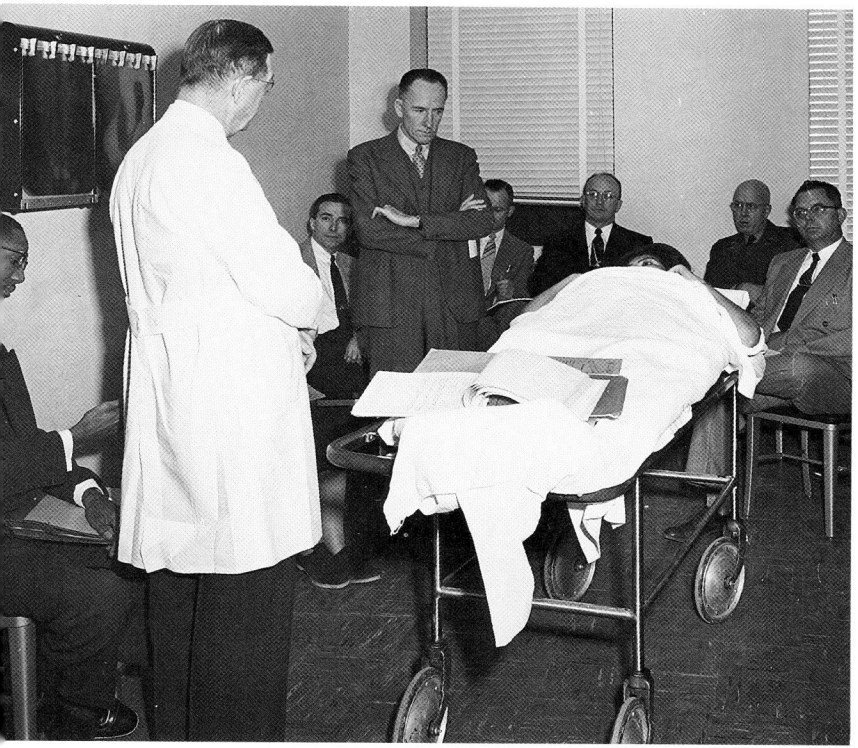

Thomas G. Orr, M.D., professor of surgery, conducts a postgraduate demonstration, 1950s.

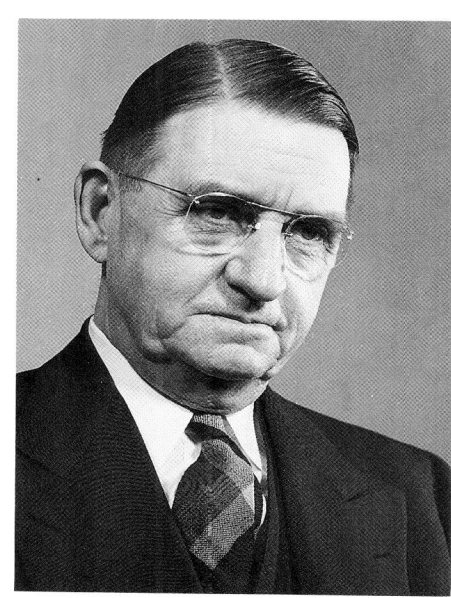

Dr. Orr, late 1950s.

I never, never called the older ones—Tom Orr, Ralph Major, Harry Wahl—never would I call them by their first names. It was always Dr. Major, Dr. Wahl, Dr. Orr, Dr. Curran, Dr. Dennie, etc. Never would I do anything but. The same was true in Lawrence. When I went to Lawrence, there were professors that had been my professors when I was a student. . . . Now, the younger ones were always of course . . . first names.—Interview with Franklin D. Murphy, M.D., January 19, 1990.

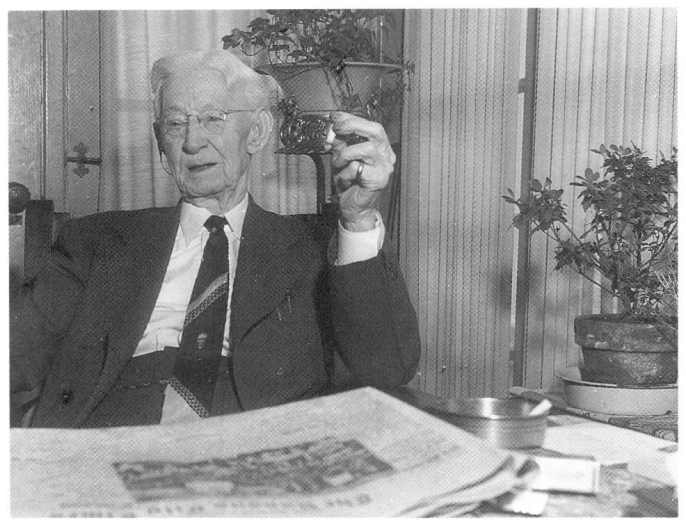

The profession of medicine has achieved its very high position today mainly because of its scientific discoveries—so much so that one may be caught with the idea that science is all there is to the practice of medicine. If so, then our scientific knowledge may outrun our philosophy and our excessive anxiety over the health of the body may replace preoccupation with the welfare of the soul. We must be remindful that the practice of medicine has to deal with human personality, human hopes and fears, and human failings as well as concern for the human body.—Edward H. Hashinger, M.D., "The Practice of Medicine," unpublished manuscript, October 2, 1957.

George M. Gray, M.D., professor emeritus of surgery and one of the founders of the medical school, 1957. Dr. Gray died in 1958 at the age of 102.

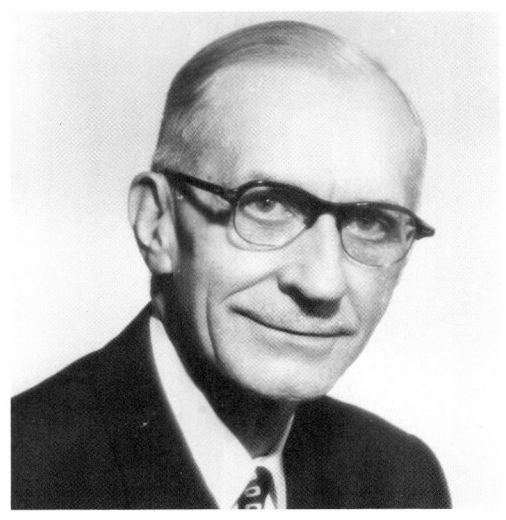

Frank R. Teachenor, M.D., a leader in the development of neurosurgery in the Kansas City area, ca. 1953.

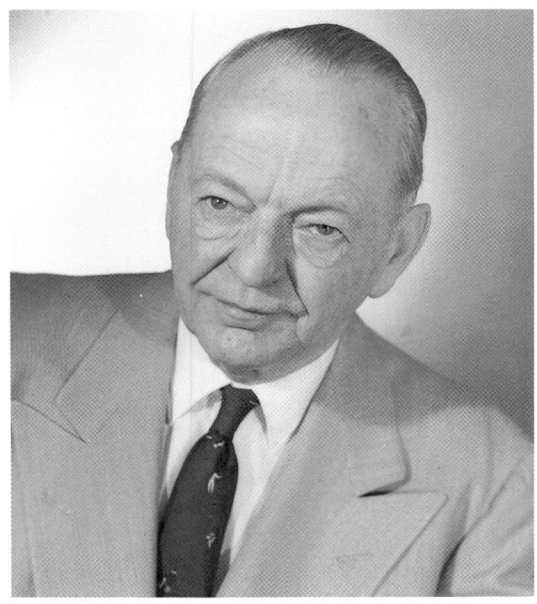

Leroy A. Calkins, M.D., professor and chairman of Obstetrics and Gynecology, 1929–1959.

The influence of the K.U. center should be placed on integrative efforts so that all well-trained doctors in the area can put their efforts to best combined advantage.

Hospitals can work together, private or public, for the raising of standards. Where one special facility can better do the work of scattered ones there should be one. In Kansas City an example of such a need is one center for child patients, instead of wards for children in scattered hospitals. . . .

The K.U. center as the area's teaching hub is interested in getting this integration, surely if slowly, in the belief it will give more patients better service at the least cost.—*Kansas City Star,* July 1, 1956.

When I came here, research space was minimal. . . . We worked in the basement, next to a furnace room, and there was no air conditioning. . . . So we stripped down most of the time and did our research in our underwear.

When we operated there was no air conditioning either, so I often put an ice collar around my neck.—Gunnar O. Proud, M.D., *Wyandotte County Star*, July 6, 1983.

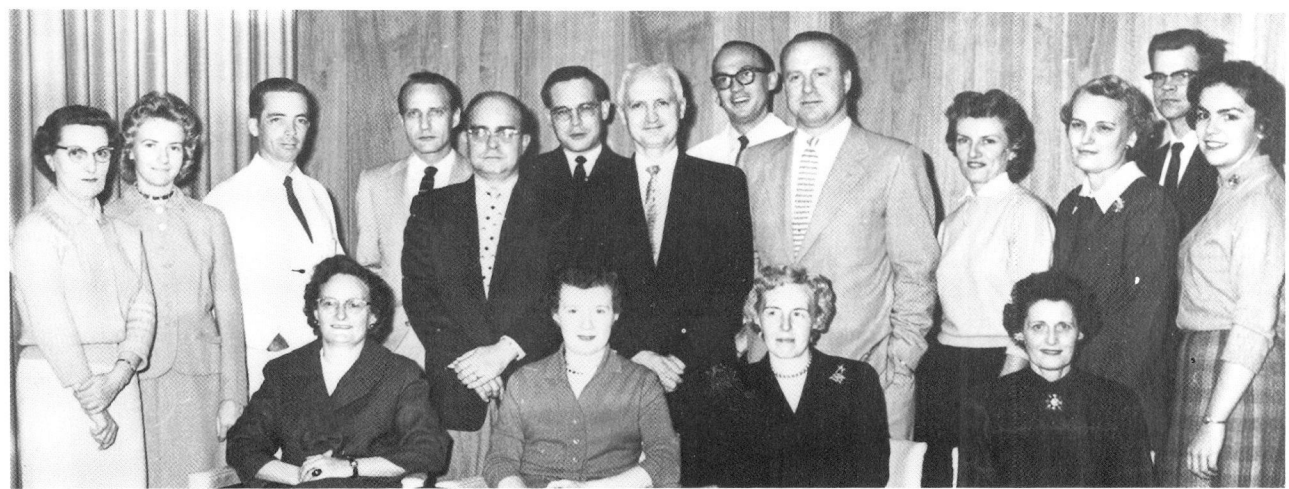

University of Kansas Medical Center administration, ca. 1960.

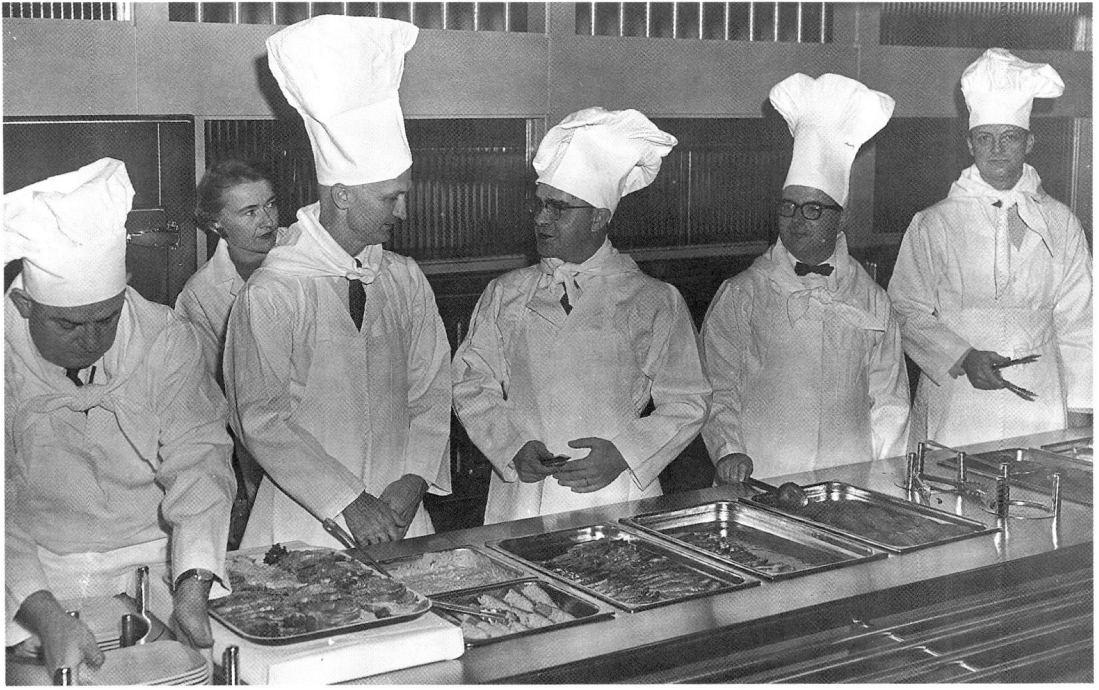

Faculty servers at the 1957 Christmas party.

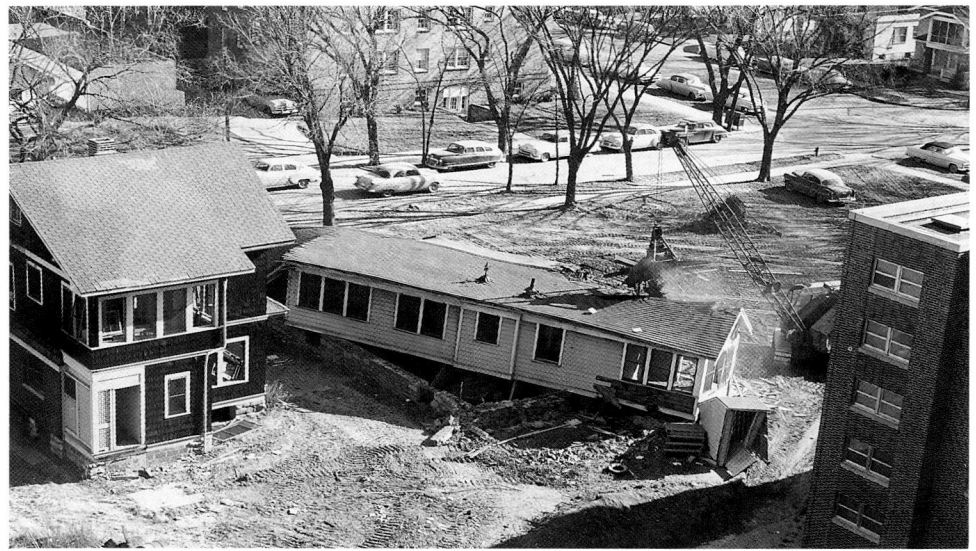

The last of the cottages: the demolition of vacant neighborhood houses for additional Medical Center construction, January 1957.

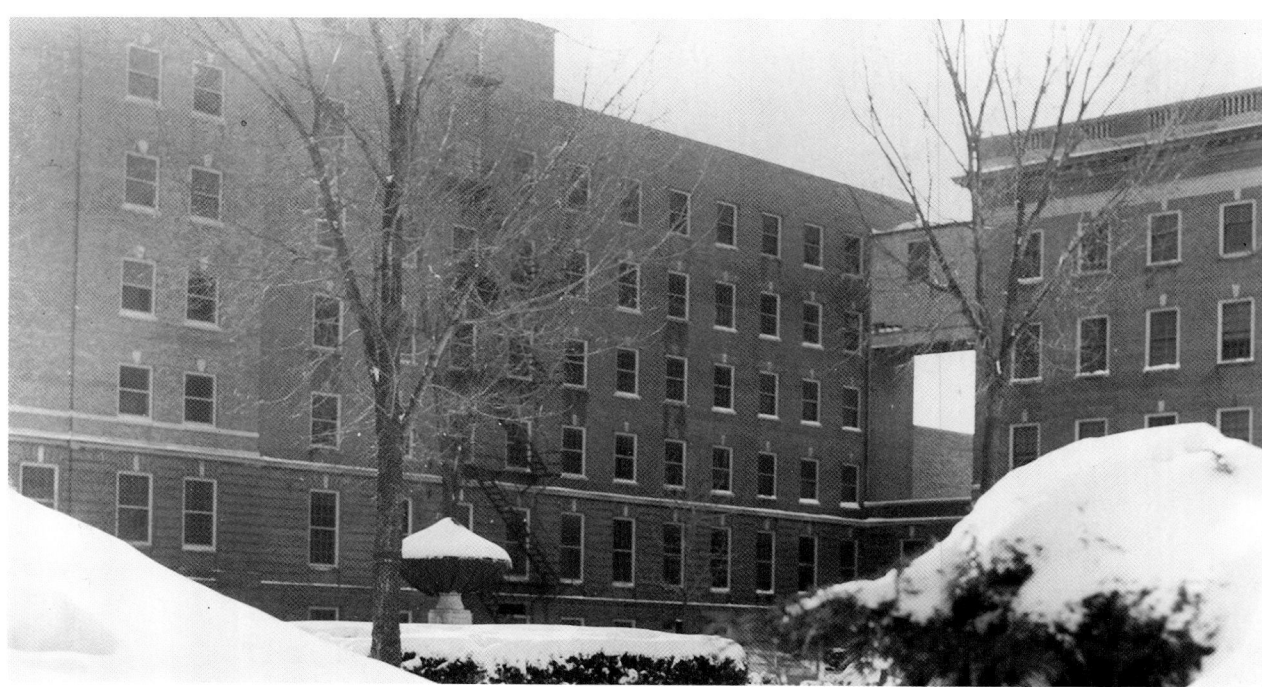

The Clendening fountain during the 1958 blizzard.

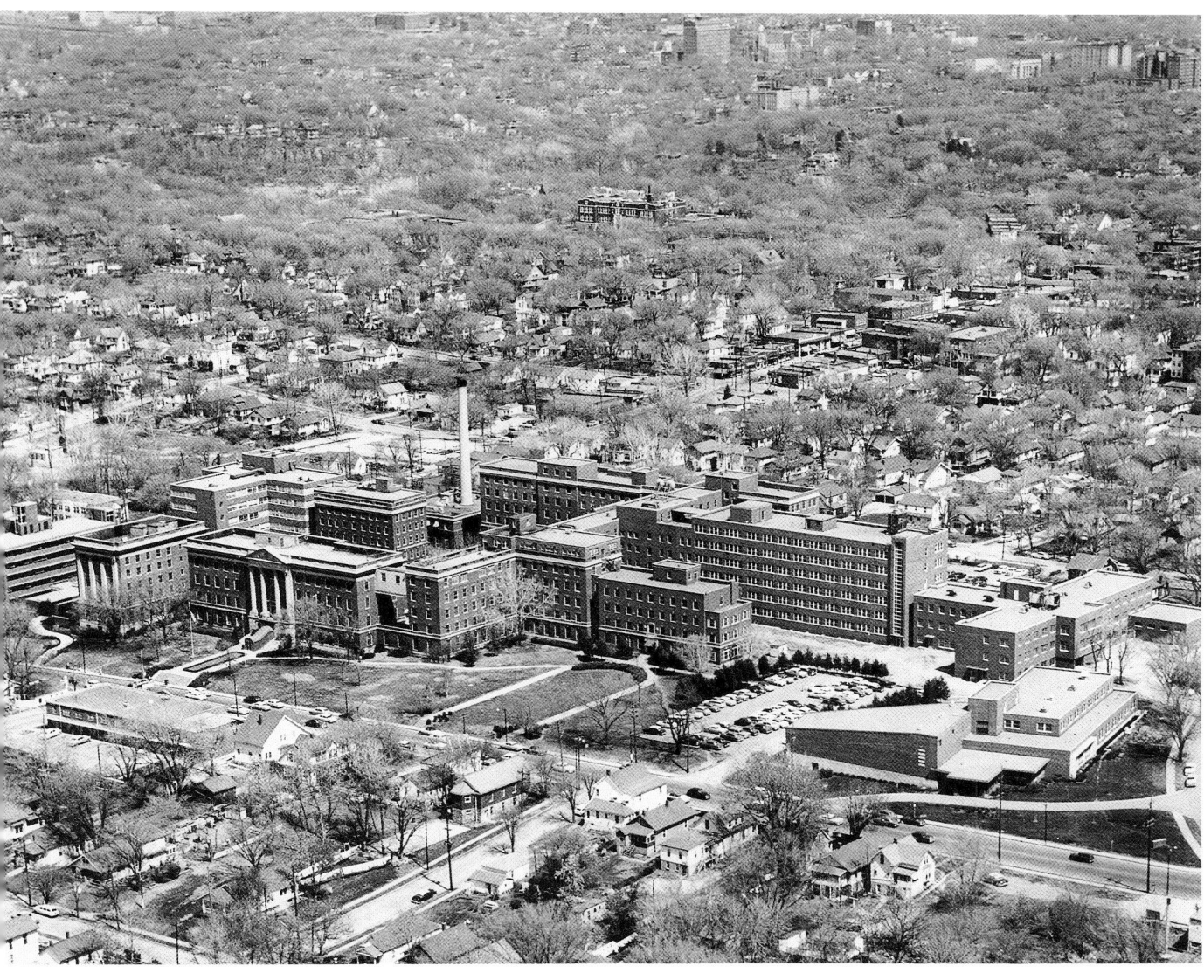

A 1955 aerial view of the University of Kansas Medical Center.

Who, Bob, remembering our pitiful beginnings in 1905—seven rooms on the second floor of an old flat building at Seventh Street and Central Avenue, Kansas City, Kansas, and the basement of the old Medico-Chi Building on Independence Avenue, Kansas City, Missouri, and observing what we now have on the Kern tract—who, I say, could have envisioned such a metamorphosis! Truly, in spite of the vicissitudes of outrageous fortune, the varied mutations of our progress have moved in mysterious ways her wonders to perform.
—Don Carlos Guffey, M.D., to Robert McE. Schauffler, M.D., February 5, 1957.

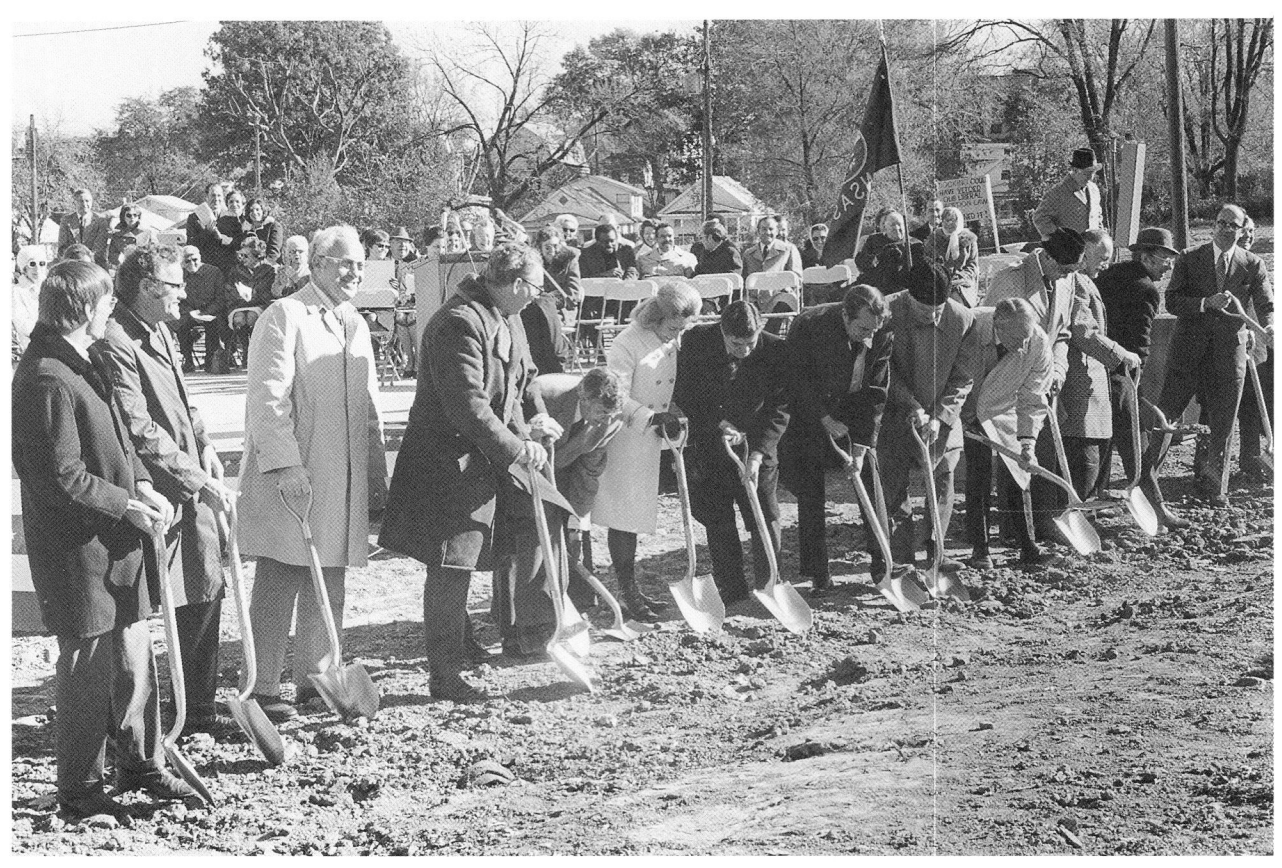

Groundbreaking ceremony for the new University of Kansas Hospital, November 10, 1973.

6

A Period of Great Change in Medicine

During the 1960s and 1970s, frequent high-level administrative changes occurred at the University of Kansas Medical Center. Temporary and appointed officials came and went almost as a matter of course. They held a variety of formal titles—provost and dean, acting vice chancellor, and vice chancellor for health affairs—until 1974, when the University of Kansas Board of Regents settled on the designation of executive vice chancellor. Counting W. Clarke Wescoe, who left in 1960, as had Franklin D. Murphy before him, to become chancellor of the University of Kansas, the medical school had nine head administrators in less than twenty years. Considered against Harry R. Wahl's twenty-four year tenure, the attrition rate appeared alarming.

Yet the administrative changes related less to the selection process than to attendant conditions. Some men held acting positions: Russell C. Mills, Ph.D., for three months in 1966; Charles E. Brackett, Jr., M.D., for eleven months in 1970-1971; and David W. Robinson, M.D., for nine months in 1975-1976. After their short terms as acting executive vice chancellor, Mills, Brackett, and Robinson assumed other responsiblities at the Medical Center. Of the appointed leaders, C. Arden Miller, M.D., served from 1960 to 1966; George A. Wolf, Jr., M.D., from 1966 to 1970; William O. Rieke, M.D., from 1971 to 1975; and Robert B. Kugel, M.D., in 1976 and 1977. David Waxman, M.D., served as deputy executive vice chancellor for a short period, then became executive vice chancellor in 1977, holding the post for the next six years.

Unlike other periods in the history of the University of Kansas Medical Center, no single individual—a Hoxie, a Wahl, or a Murphy—defined institutional development. Even so, the Medical Center continued to expand and progress. One reason for the continued change was the acceptance throughout Kansas of the Medical Center as an established institution, one that no longer depended for survival on how well a given administrator dealt with the legislature. Of course, the ability of medical leaders to make needs known and to lobby effectively still counted, but the old days of strict monetary restraints and continual justification for the existence of the school had ended. Despite the administrative turnover, the Medical Center advanced in size and prestige at a steady and impressive rate.

The leaders of the school found themselves involved with tasks that they had never expected to perform during their days of medical training. "I don't know how many Rotary Clubs and Kiwanis and Lions and all of these others that I addressed, there were scores, literally, around the state that I spoke to," Dr. Rieke recalled. "I travelled very, very widely, always in an attempt to uplift and bring new support, and I thought that it was successful. I think that when time came for the legislature to help us in terms of authorizing bonding authority for the new hospital that these things at least had some positive role in the decision, but there was a lot of energy in those things." Dr. Wolf remembered spending an unpleasant and hectic night in a motel room across Rainbow Boulevard from the Medical Center at a negotiating session with representatives of striking Medical Center service employees. Dealing with labor troubles and speaking before service clubs were new administrative responsibilities that evolved as the Medical Center continued to grow and gain status in Kansas.

Throughout the 1960s, the Medical Center fared well with the governor and legislature, and with Wescoe following Murphy to Lawrence, the state became accustomed to having the University of Kansas headed by a leader from the Medical Center. When Wescoe left the University of Kansas in 1969, his replacement, Laurence Chalmers, a professional education administrator who openly opposed American involvement in Vietnam, proved unpopular with many influential Kansas politicians. Consequently, some observers thought, the legislature punished the Lawrence campus at budget time, favoring the medical school. Furthermore, Chalmer's relaxed style of leadership had left the Medical Center operations virtually independent, and at one point, certain political leaders considered detaching the medical school entirely from the University of Kansas. Before anything further happened, Chalmers departed and the situation changed once again. The new chancellor, Archie R. Dykes, worked to restore the primacy of the Lawrence campus. This resulted in confrontations that contributed to Rieke's decision to resign. The short tenure as executive vice chancellor of Dr. Robert B. Kugel, a pediatrician who had hoped to revitalize the rural health programs, led to further complications. David Waxman, M.D., replaced Kugel in 1977. Yet, and it needs reiterating, the University of Kansas Medical Center was no longer a stepchild in the family of Kansas higher education.

In 1962, the first year medical program moved from Lawrence to the Rainbow campus; at long last the primary components of the medical school were consolidated in Kansas City. But to head off the possibility of a rival state-supported medical school in Wichita, the Medical Center opened a branch campus in that city in 1971. A year later, demolition crews razed the last of the old Goat Hill buildings, drawing to a close a controversial era in Kansas medical education. Important internal administrative changes reflected educational improvements at the Medical Center. Of special note were the establishment of separate schools of Allied Health and Nursing. Allied Health consolidated a number of departments, ranging from Dietetics and Nutrition to Physical and Respiratory Therapy. The School of Nursing, finally independent from the School of Medicine, swiftly advanced in status, building on groundwork laid by such administrative leaders as Martha Pitel, R.N., Hester Thurston, R.N., Mary Anne Eisenbise, R.N., and, arriving in 1975, Dean Doris Geitgey, R.N., Ed.D. Just as nurses and other health care professionals sought to improve their standing, so did support workers. Although the two minor labor disturbances had only lasted a few days, they served as further harbingers of change. Hospital support staff no longer took a

fatalistic view of traditionally poor wages, long hours, and unsatisfactory working conditions. Expansion, reorganization, and strikes illustrated the kind of changes that followed the modernization of Kansas medical education.

The Medical Center continued to enjoy a national reputation for producing competent, well-trained health care professionals. Under pressure from the legislature, most of the medical students were from Kansas, and a special effort was made to recruit qualified men and women from rural districts. As the number of students and the scope of clinical operations increased, so did the size of the faculty. The founding fathers gradually left the scene, but many of their replacements were graduates of the Medical Center.

The passing on of responsibilities from the teacher to the student afforded a high degree of continuity and stability; however, the institution also needed to attract "new blood" to keep pace with the rapid and dynamic changes in modern medicine. For example, the school's rural programs failed to adjust fast enough to the realities of rural medicine, increased medical specialization, and rising health care costs. While the School of Medicine did develop a strong Department of Family Practice, some observers considered this only a token step. The addition of a center for women's breast diseases and the Gene and Barbara Burnett Burn Center were important, as was the development of better emergency medical services, but these programs hardly represented dramatic new directions calculated to set national standards. The regional preceptorship workshops continued to be important. However, many talented faculty, especially those educated outside Kansas, stayed only a few years and then left to make names elsewhere. The lack of emphasis on research, reflected by inadequate laboratory space and minimal outside funding, hindered the expansion of the Medical Center in relation to other comparable institutions and made it difficult to attract nationally recognized academicians. Administrative instability delayed solutions to well-identified educational and research problems.

Meanwhile, the Rainbow campus continued to expand. The Spencer Memorial Chapel opened in 1965 and the Applegate Energy Center in 1973. Two large structures, Orr-Major and Wahl Hall East, added needed classroom and some research space. The hospital and clinics underwent several enlargements, but remained scattered and cramped. The Medical Center continued to rely on a number of affiliated hospitals for student education. A move to consolidate clinical arrangements, along with the obvious need for more space, spurred the planning of a new hospital for the Rainbow campus. Traditionally, public buildings in Kansas were examples of no-frills architectural and fiscal austerity. Even so, during Brackett's term as acting vice chancellor, a building committee chaired by Kermit Krantz, M.D., disregarded the usual formula, proposing a hospital suitably designed to fulfill long-term requirements—in other words, a structure larger than currently needed. In the mid-1970s, a friendly governor and legislature committed Kansas to building a $65 million hospital, the most ambitious public construction project ever undertaken by state authorities. Special legislation that authorized a $25 million bond issue speeded the start of construction on the several-year project. On one hand, the greatest triumph in the development of the University of Kansas Medical Center appeared within reach. On the other, fundamental changes in American

medicine seemed to indicate, even as the new hospital moved toward completion, a need for fewer hospital beds. Some feared that the hospital, once completed, might be a "white elephant," a disaster for Kansas taxpayers.

The photographs define the changes at the University of Kansas Medical Center in the 1960s and 1970s. The last images appear of Ralph Major, M.D., Thor Jager, M.D., and other Kansas medical pioneers. Several of the faculty who would help lead the Medical Center into the 1980s are shown, among them Doris Geitgey, R.N., Ed.D., in nursing administration and Robert P. Hudson, M.D., in history of medicine. A number of photographs, some taken in conjunction with the opening of new departments, such as Family Practice and the Burnett Burn Center, illustrate the fast pace and varied activities of a modern medical school. Finally, the construction photographs of the new University of Kansas Hospital dramatize the drive of the Medical Center into a promising future, moving forward despite the risks toward national stature in American medicine.

Only when medical schools enjoy the independence that comes from adequate funds at the local level can those schools assist in shaping national programs rather than be shaped by them.—C. Arden Miller, M.D., dean, *Kansas City Star*, October 9, 1962.

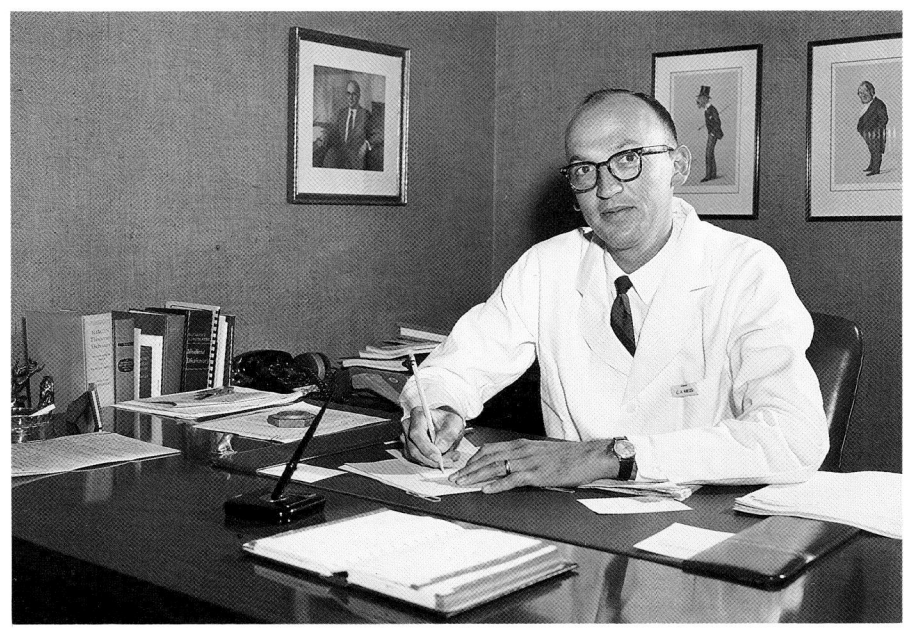

C. Arden Miller, M.D.,
provost and dean, 1960–1966.

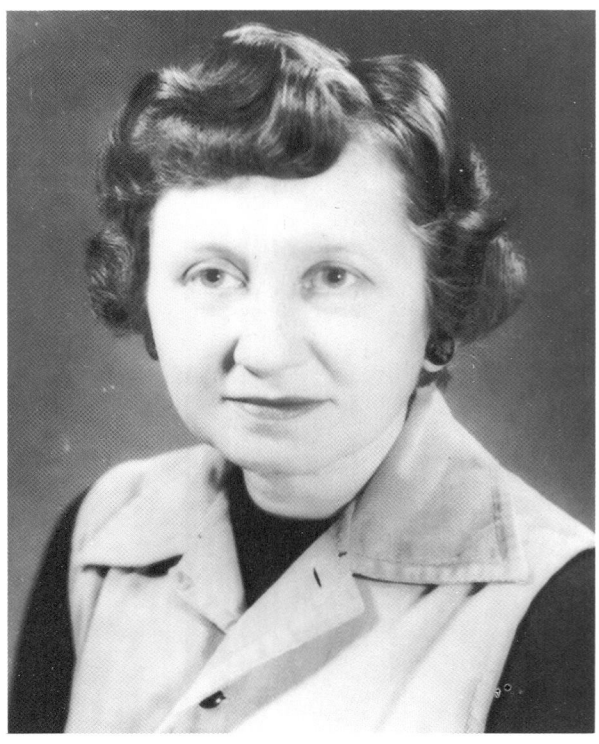

Martha Pitel, R.N., Ph.D., chairman of the School of Nursing, 1964–1969.

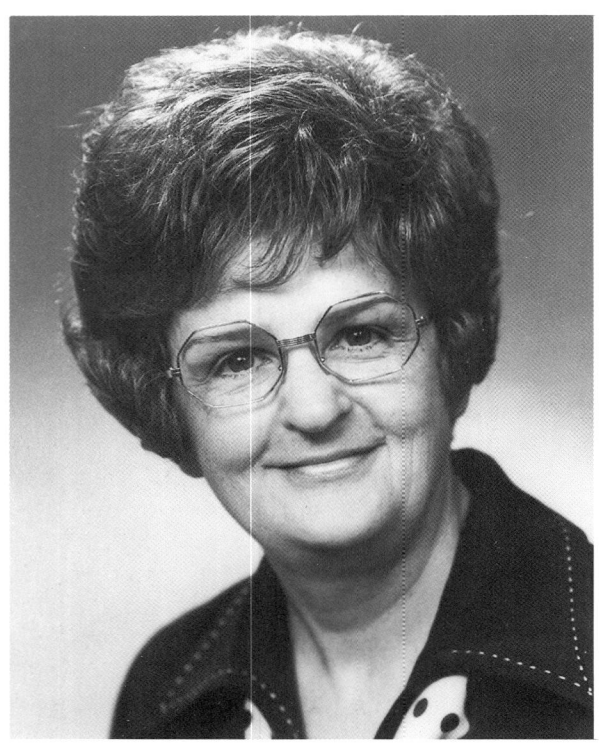

Hester Thurston, R.N., School of Nursing acting chairman, 1971–1974; acting dean, 1974–1975.

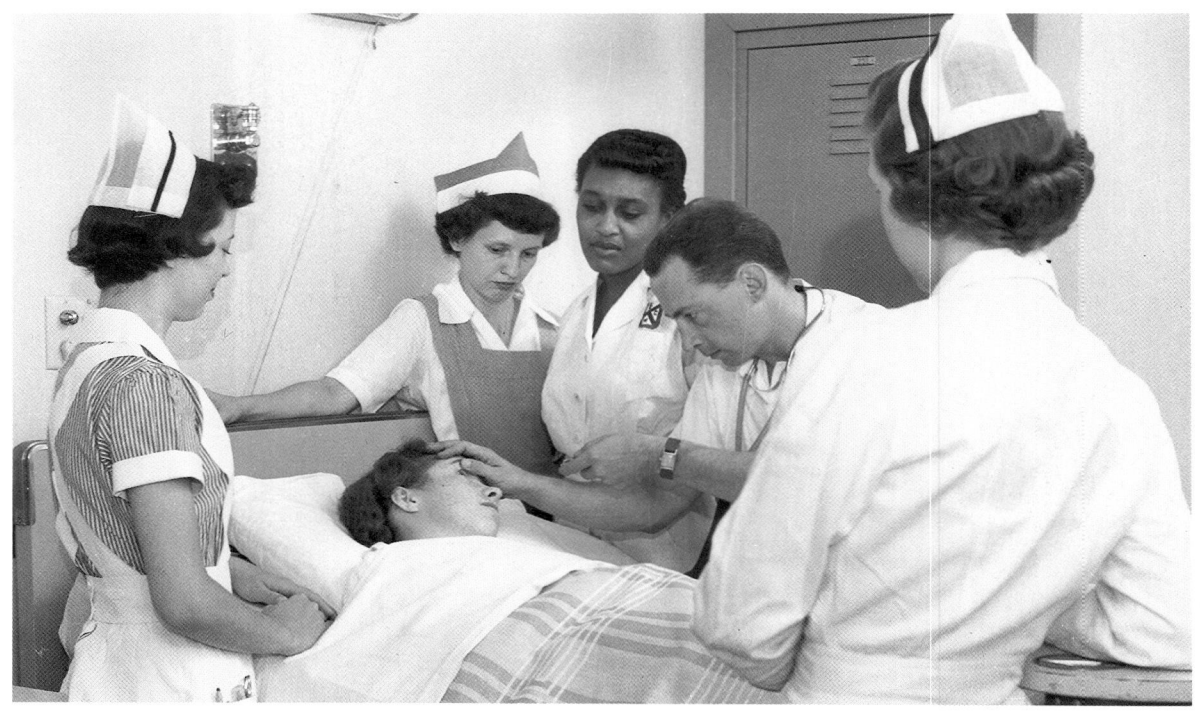

Representatives from nursing, allied health, and medicine with a patient, early 1960s.

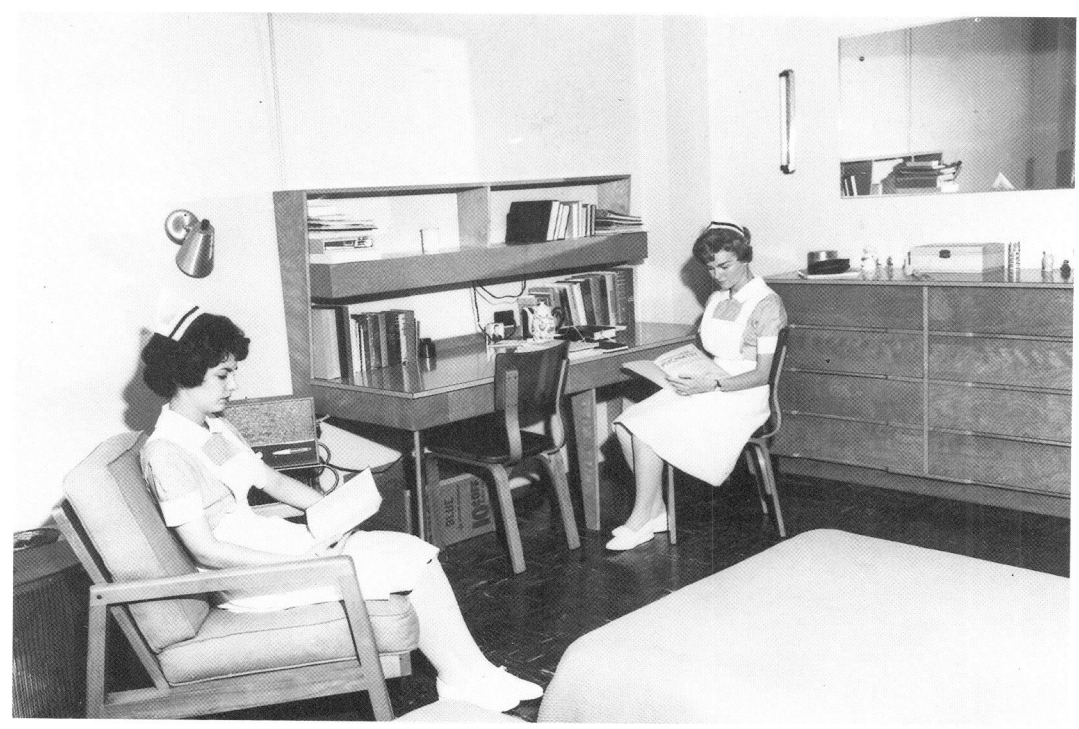

Student nurses in their quarters, early 1960s.

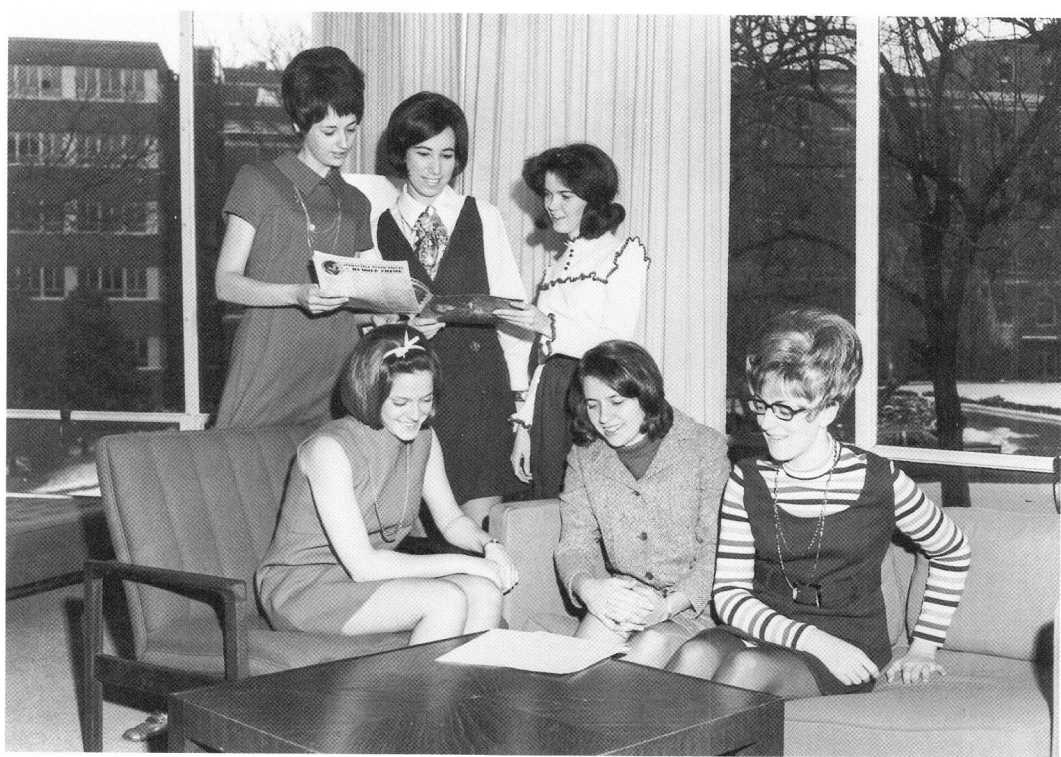

Caduceus Capers staff, March 1970.

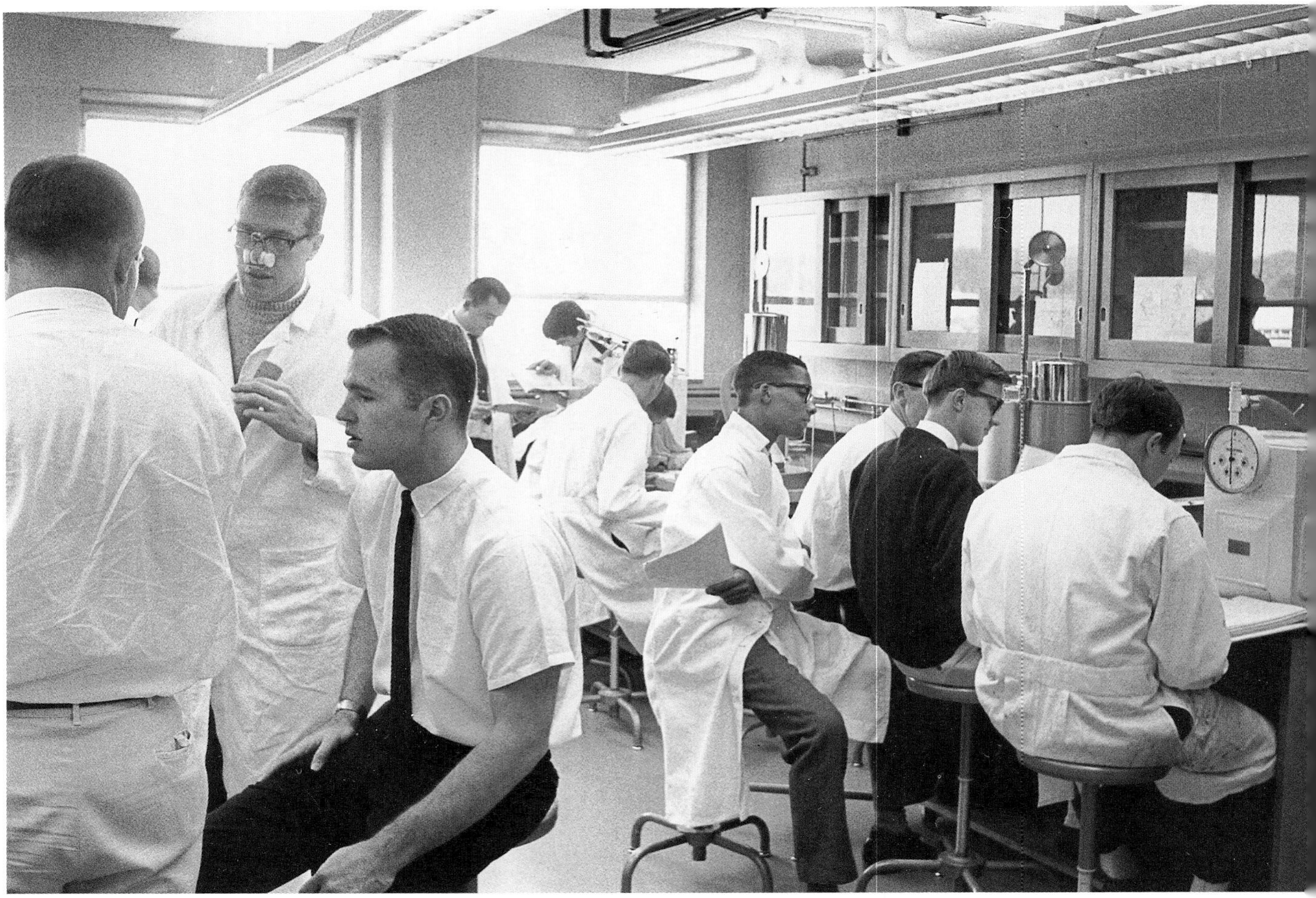

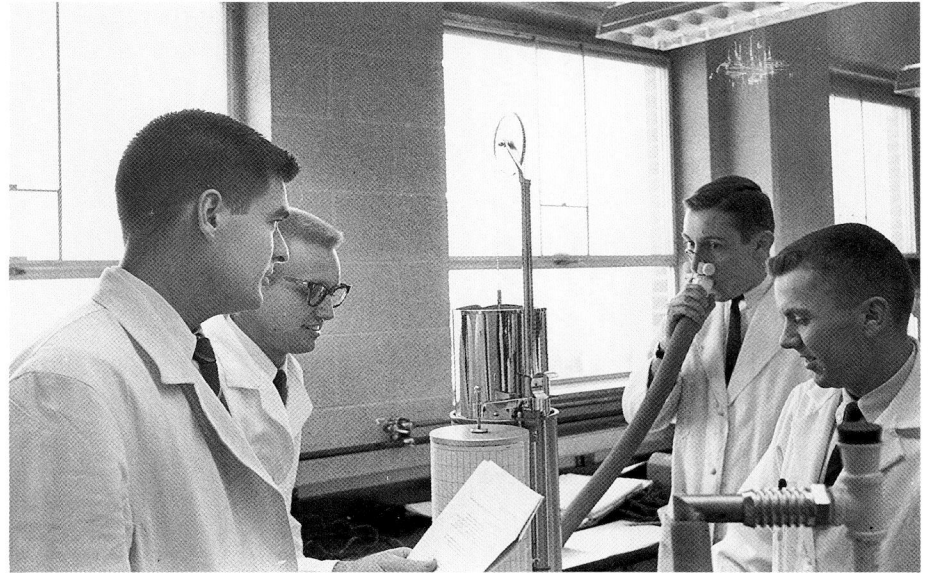

Medical student laboratory
session, 1960s.

The student's major affiliation is with the university. His major commitment is to gain from this relationship an education which will equip him to deal with the rest of society. Within the university there can be no rationale by which this dynamic, intelligent, and motivated individual can be ignored. The student should participate in the operation of the institution not only as a passive recipient of knowledge, but as an active donor of opinions, ideas, and suggestions. He should be given the responsibility of not just gaining an education, but also of helping to shape the educational process in all of its ramifications.
—William G. Bartholome, M.D., *Jayhawker MD*, 1969.

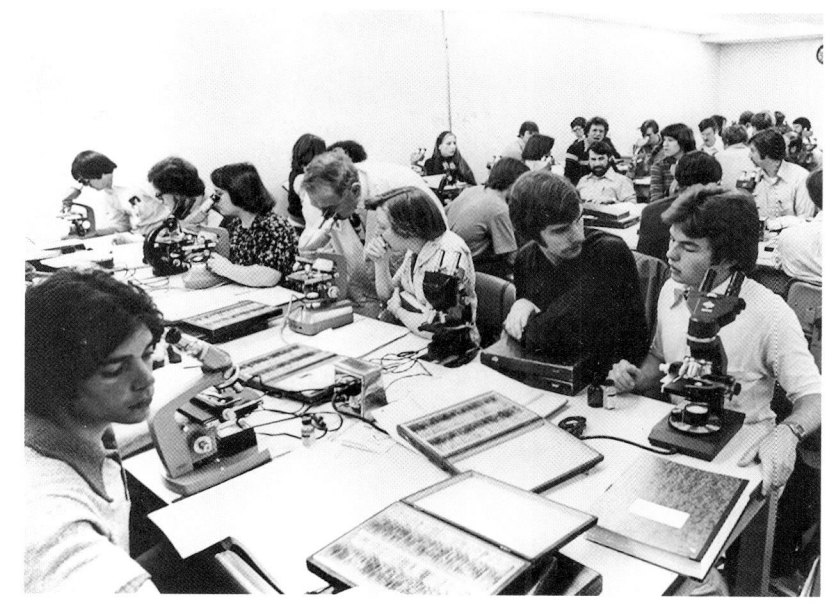

Students at work with microscopes, 1970s.

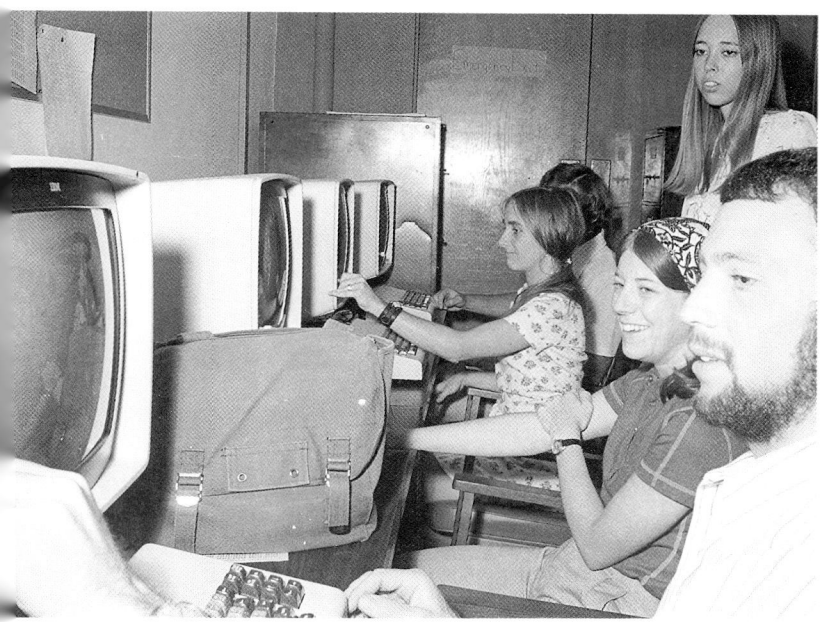

Students at computers in the Educational Resource Center, July 1975.

It appears the time has passed when a single human mind can even begin to know all that is useful in aiding patients. Already proven vital in business procedures and useful in fundamental research, computers are now moving into the areas of medical teaching, patient care and even diagnosis.

In Kansas City, the KU Medical Center and Research are the only two with computers, while a third (Baptist Memorial) has one on order.
—*The University of Kansas School of Medicine and Medical Center Bulletin*, April 1965.

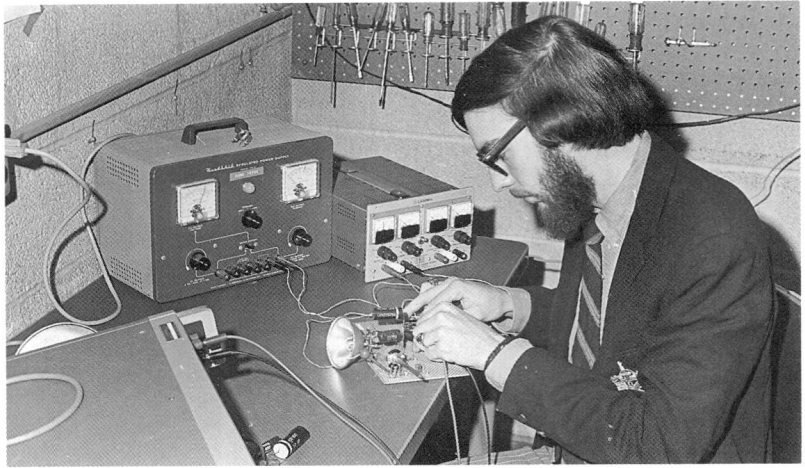

Dan Lawrence of Biomedical Engineering, January 1971.

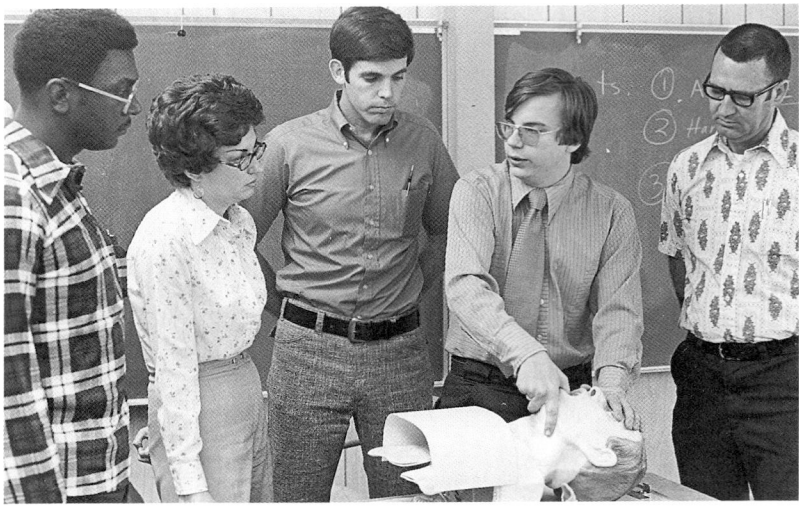

Emergency Medical Technology demonstration, April 1974.

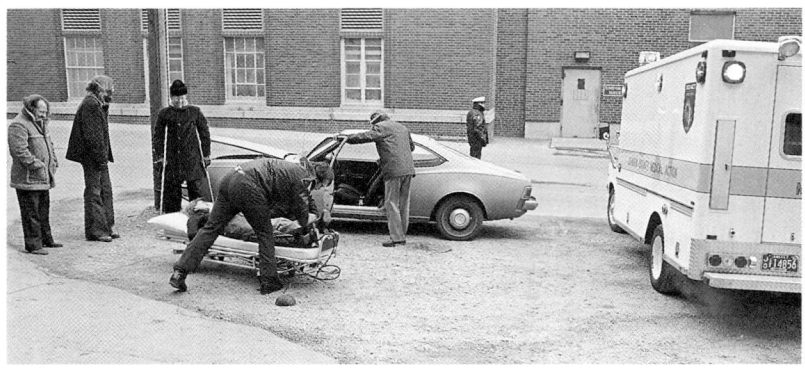

Emergency Medical Services training activities, 1977.

The highest honor a University can pay its students is the confidence that they will establish for themselves, individually or collectively, a code of behavior, a loftiness of purpose, and a seriousness of effort, that are beyond reproach and which set a higher standard of performance than officers of the University would presume to impose by fiat. This is the philosophy that has guided your University. Students are not the subject of rules and oaths. They are not even the passive recipients of teaching. They are the creative performers of a University, the pursuers of learning in a setting where knowledge is preserved and advanced. The highest honor students can pay their University is the fulfillment of their talents and ideals. The measure of this fulfillment must rest with the individual student and with his life's work.

These honors are achieved by mutual trust and by mutual dedication to learning and to service. There is a nobler symbolism in the absence of oaths and obedience than could ever be achieved by their presence. We trust that a noble symbolism is manifest when no professors are willfully killed or injured at the hands of students.
—*Jayhawker MD*, 1963.

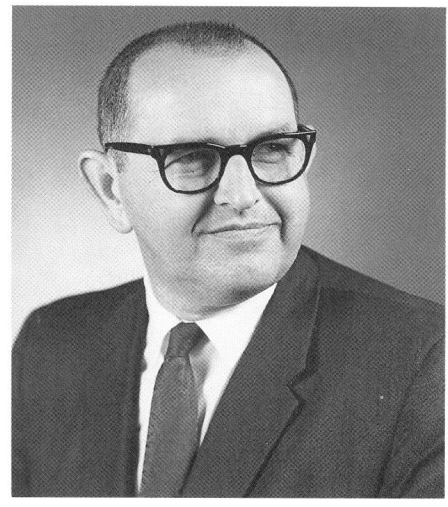

Russell C. Mills, Ph.D., acting provost and dean, 1966.

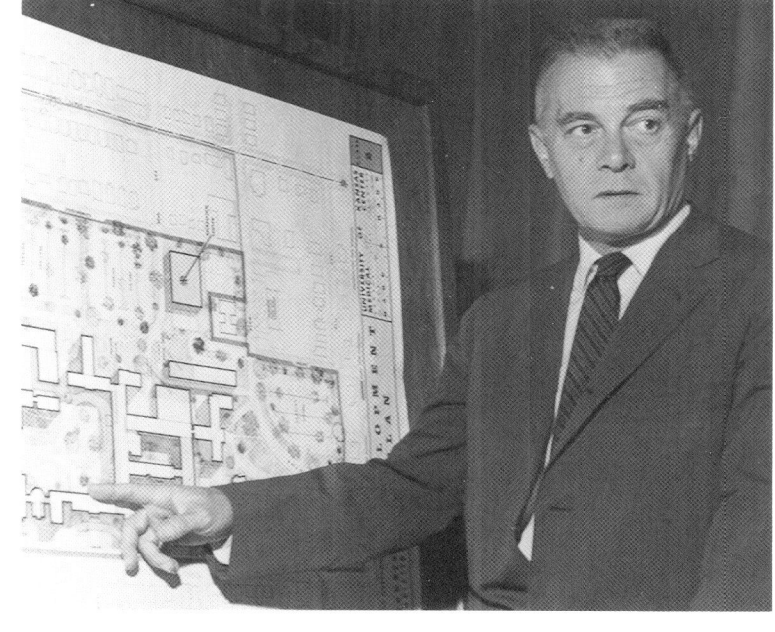

George A. Wolf, M.D., provost and dean, 1966–1970.

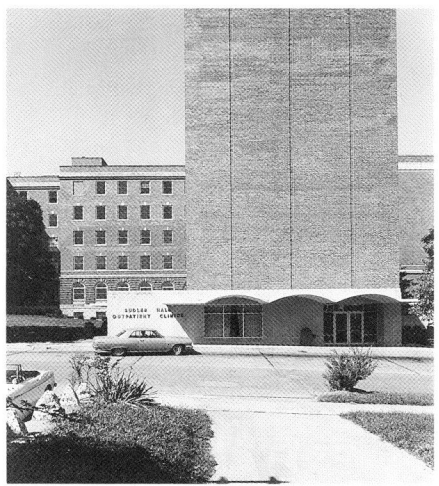

Sudler Hall outpatient clinic, 1968.

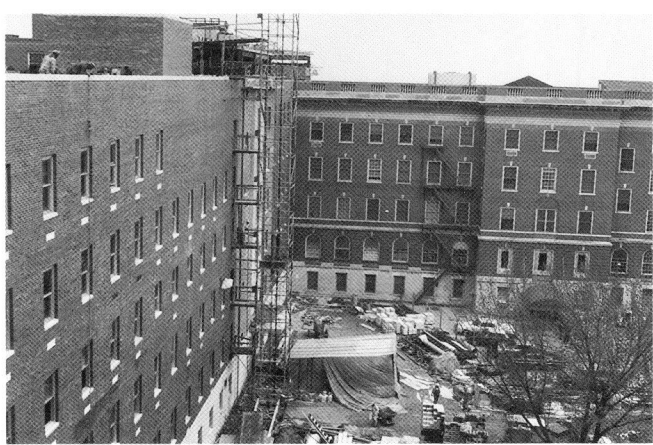

Construction activities in 1966.

We are in a period of great change in medicine generated out of concerns for social and environmental problems. There will be new emphasis on health maintenance in addition to the present emphasis on medical care. Solutions to crucial problems in patterns and systems of health care delivery as well as their financing will require determined and imaginative efforts. . . . Additionally, challenging research opportunities exist for modifying both the physical and behavioral aspects of life and for investigation of the unsolved major diseases which afflict mankind.

The complexities of the many problems relating to health care are great and are being attacked at many levels of government and communities. It is essential that you assume, in a greater way than ever before, community responsibilities in policy making. These responsibilities and needs will open additional challenging opportunities.
—*Jayhawker MD*, 1971.

147

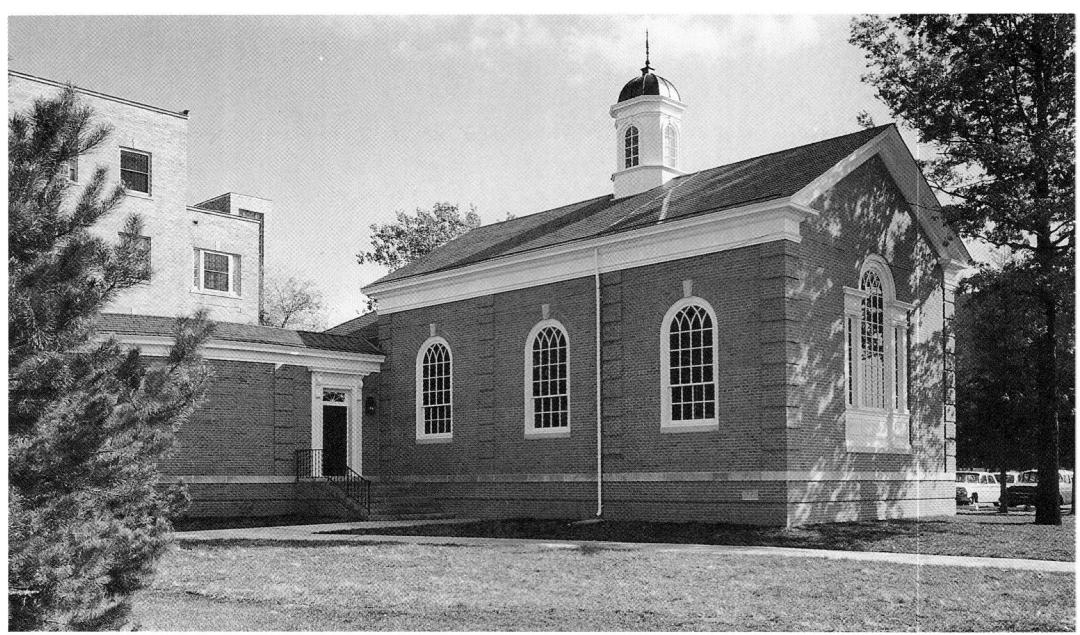

Kenneth A. Spencer Memorial Chapel, 1965.

A quiet place for respite and meditation for those who must cope publicly with fears and anxiety. A place for happiness—weddings and thanksgiving. These are needs at the University of Kansas Medical Center that could not be met by funds available for state buildings.

But the Medical Center has been given an opportunity to meet the real need of more than 10,000 patients hospitalized annually, as well as needs of the many students and staff.

This has been made possible by a gift from Mrs. Kenneth A. Spencer, honoring a more personal side of the greatness that was her late husband's. It will be dedicated in consideration of Kenneth A. Spencer's devotion to faith, and in appreciation of his personification of that which is good in humanity. It will be maintained as a non-sectarian facility.—*KU Endowment Digest*, June 1965.

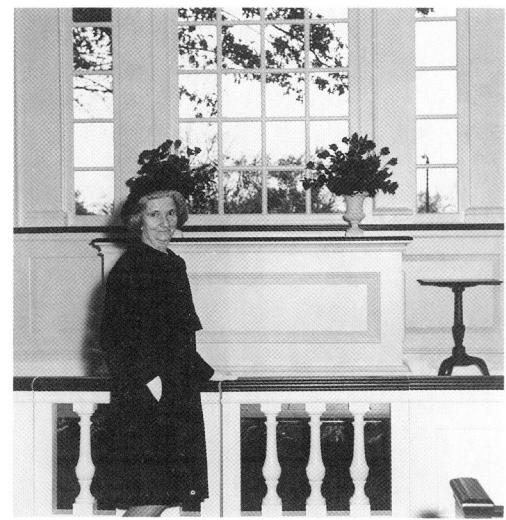

Mrs. Kenneth A. Spencer at the dedication of the chapel built in memory of her husband, October 24, 1965.

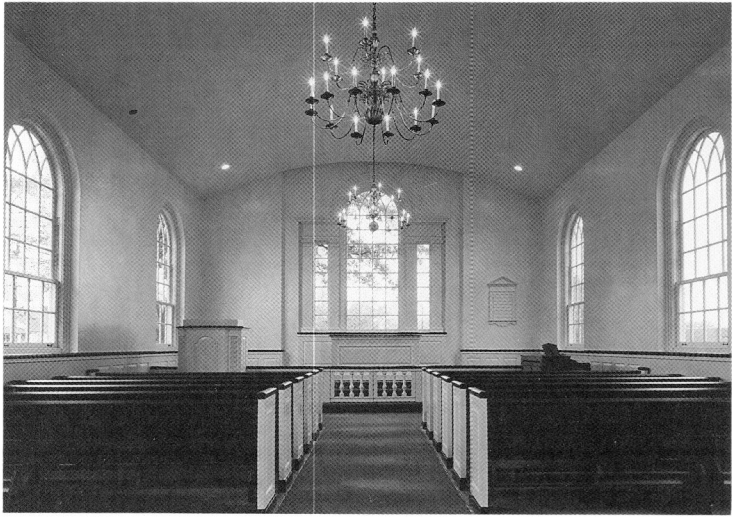

The chapel interior, 1965.

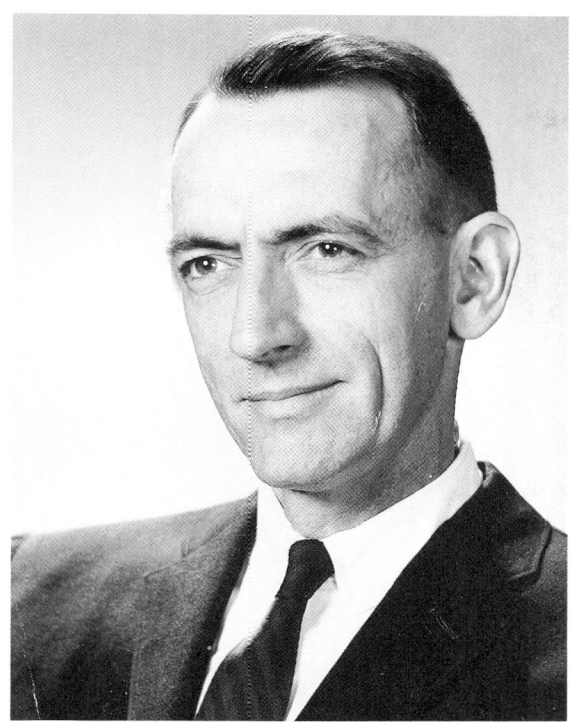

Charles E. Brackett, Jr., M.D., professor of surgery; acting executive vice chancellor, 1970–1971.

The master plan is, of necessity, general in many aspects, particularly during the stage anticipated to begin in 1974. But we can be specific in this regard— we need more land during the coming decade and we undoubtedly will need more in the future. Our present campus is now crowded with buildings and we are faced with an ever-increasing lack of parking space. The flexibility additional land provides will permit us to plan an orderly expansion of educational, research and health care facilities.

The University of Kansas Medical Center is now a community populated with four to five thousand daily; every indication points to the fact that this community will double its size during the next 20 years.
—*The University of Kansas School of Medicine and Medical Center Bulletin,* June 1964.

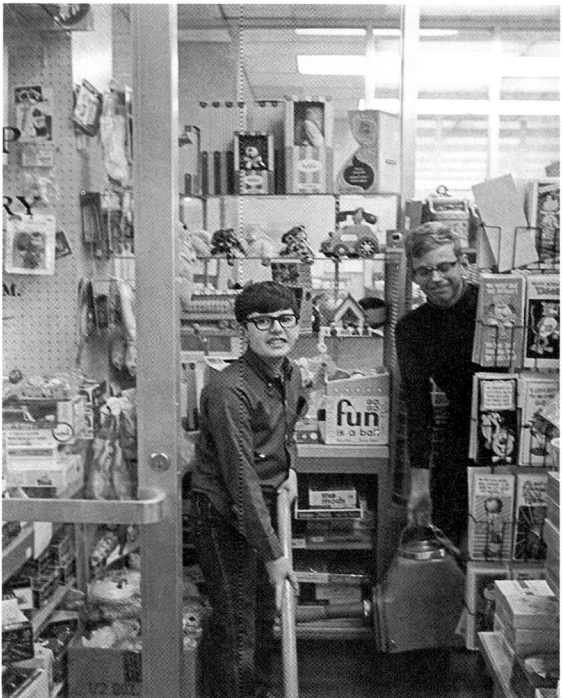

A community member helping in the gift shop during the 1969 strike.

The walkout of 400 members of the Public Service Employees Union Local 1132 AFL CIO affected everyone at KUMC in one way or another. During the shutdown of facilities, almost all personnel performed duties quite uncharacteristic of their normal jobs. Nurses mopped floors, dieticians manned the serving lines, secretaries did housekeeping duties. In addition, several community members volunteered to help out. Fortunately, all were back to work four days after the pickets went out, and KUMC began restoring operations by the week's end.—*Topics,* April 1969.

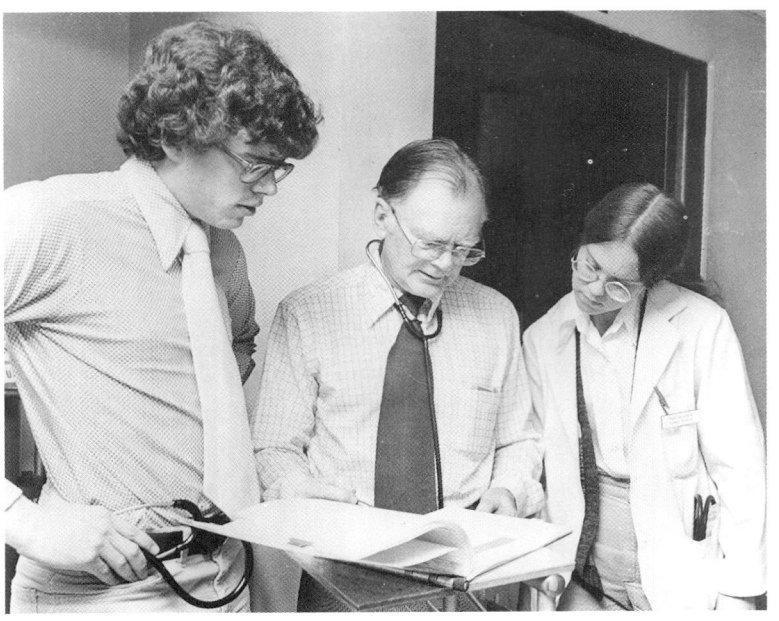

Students Jonathon Wright and Peggy McLaughlin make rounds with Dr. Francis Huston at Jefferson County Memorial Hospital in Winchester, Kansas, as part of the Medical Center's Rural Health Weekend, 1977.

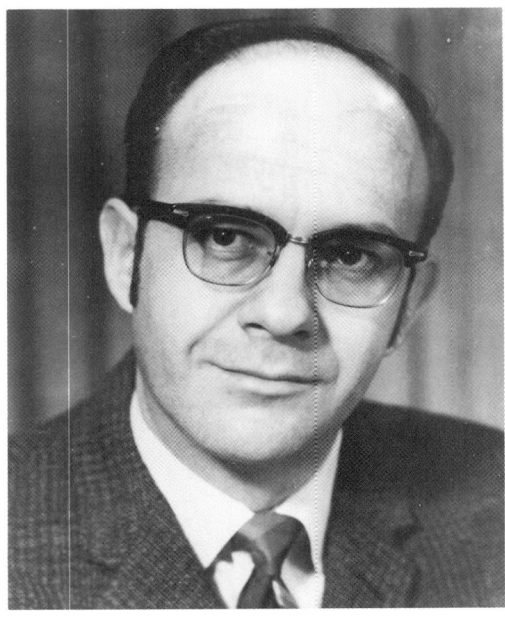

William O. Rieke, M.D., vice chancellor for health affairs, 1971–1975; executive vice chancellor, 1974–1975.

A continuing problem is the number of Kansas-educated physicians leaving the state after training.

According to the best estimates of the KU medical school, about 60 percent of its graduates opt for practice outside the borders of the Sunflower State.

The problem is complex, and both the KU medical school and the Legislature are trying to deal with it. Legislation that would in effect compel state-educated doctors to serve in Kansas for a specified period has been debated. So far, it has failed passage. New measures, perhaps less extreme, will probably be introduced this session.—*Chanute Tribune*, January 14, 1978.

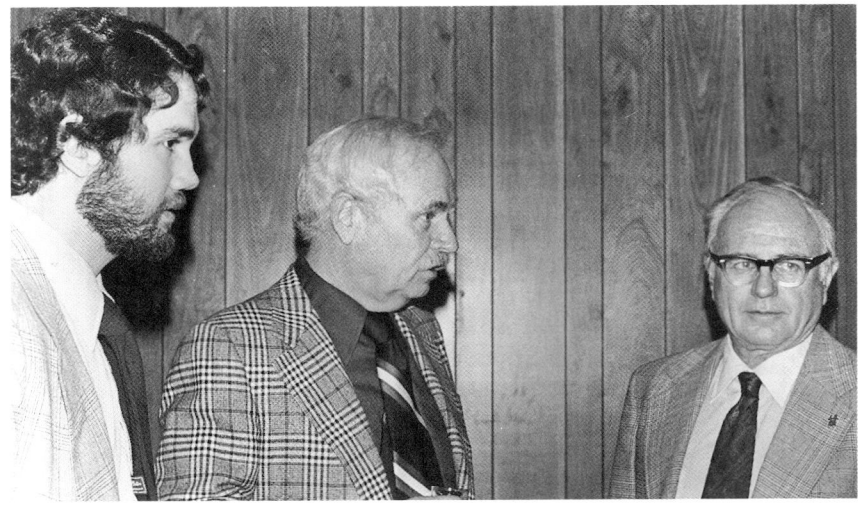

Regional Preceptorship Workshop including Larry Magee, M.D., Royal Barker, M.D., and Philip Hostetter, M.D., April 1977.

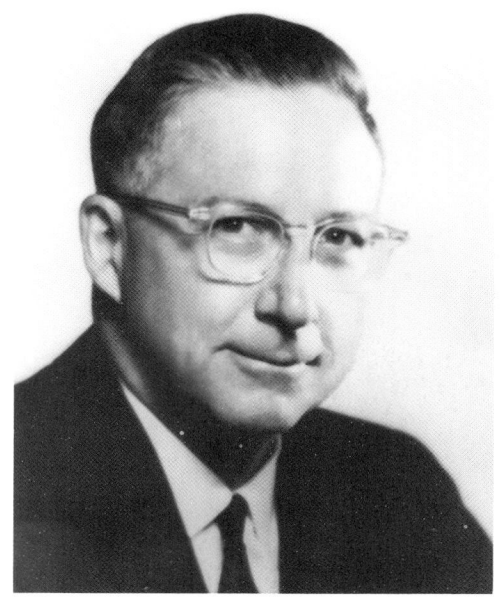

David W. Robinson, M.D., was appointed
director of the Burnett Burn Center in 1973
and served as acting executive vice chancellor
from 1975 to 1976.

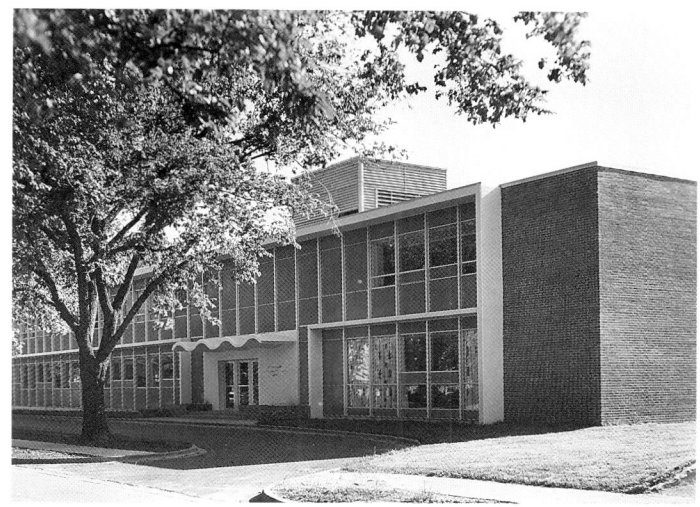

The Children's Rehabilitation Unit, ca. 1960.

Our mission is to try to meet the health care
needs of our state. It is expressed differently by
different people who have differing perceptions
about what should be emphasized most:
education, service or research. But we are
mutually agreed that our mission really is to try
to do all we can to meet the health care needs of
our state. Primarily, I believe, we are trying to
reach that goal with educational programs.

While it's not an impossible mission, it does
pose certain problems for us, and particularly
now when the emphasis both from the state
and from the federal level is on training more
family physicians and more general internists,
more general pediatricians, and more general
obstetricians—those who provide a broad
spectrum of health care—we sometimes find it
difficult to know how we can do that and still
preserve our capability to give first class tertiary
health care.—William O. Rieke, M.D., *From
Where I Sit,* University of Kansas Medical
Center brochure, 1973.

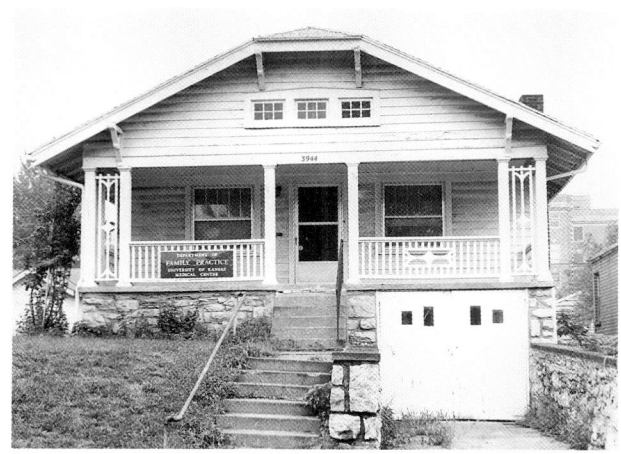

The Department of Family Practice's first office, 1970.

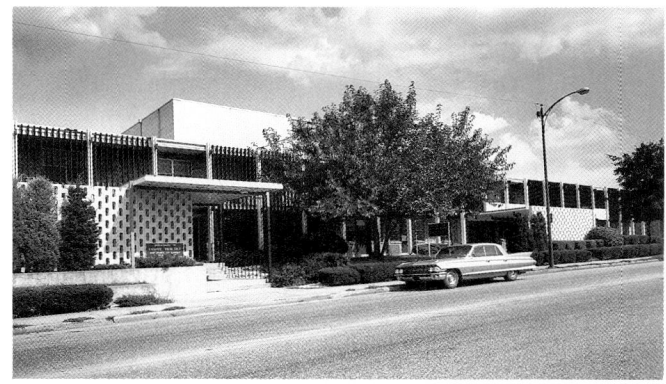

Family Practice's new quarters, 1973.

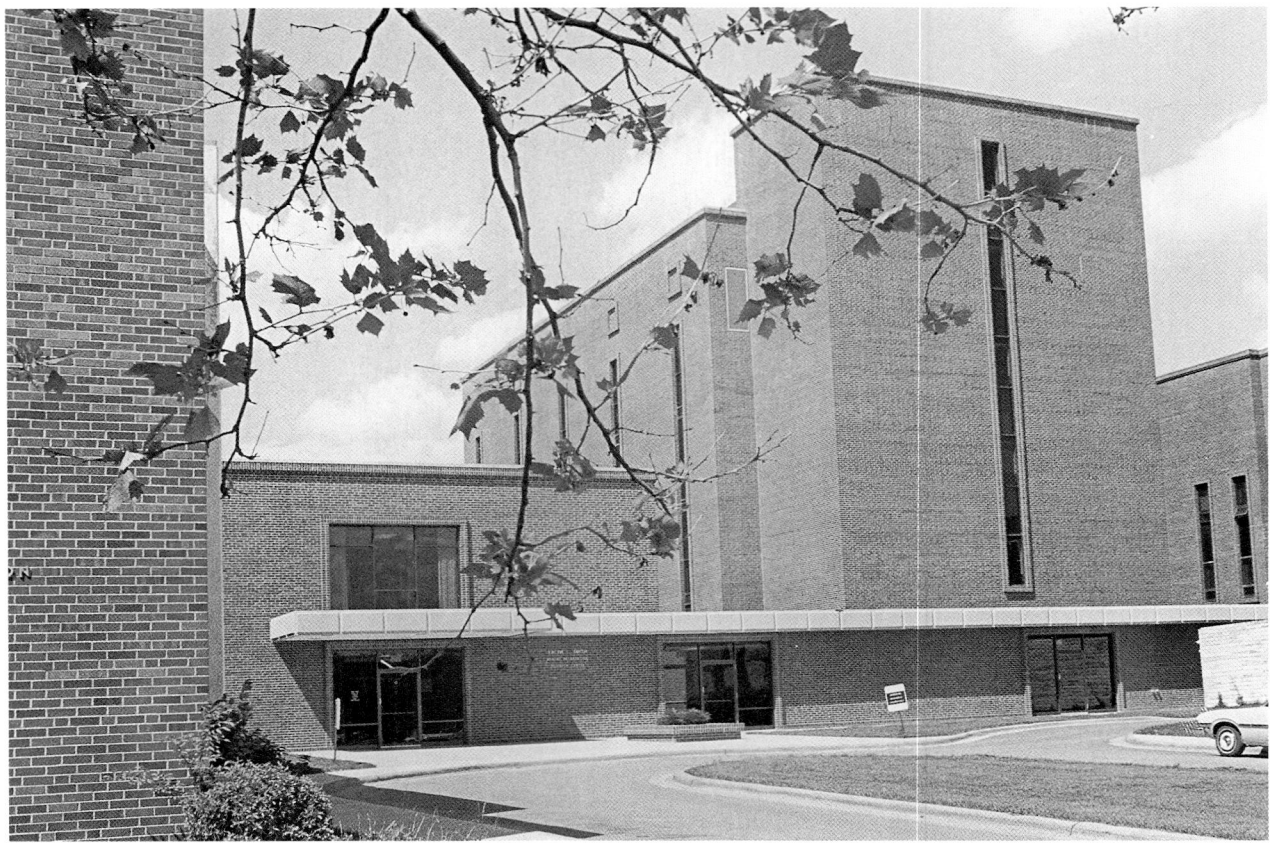

The R. L. Smith Building, 1973.

As you know, there has been an intense program, architectural and fiscal planning, in our Center since March of 1972 when the Legislature authorized a major expansion for KUMC by granting the Regents authority to issue up to $64 million in revenue bonds. These planning efforts which have been intensely supported by so many of you as well as by outside consultants of a variety of types have been exceptionally productive and successful. We have increased the size of our medical class, begun the development of a new clinical branch of the medical school in Wichita, made plans to reorganize our program in nursing education and started programs of affiliated medical education in other communities in Kansas.

I believe it is most important that everyone recognize with genuine appreciation that a recommended appropriation of this amount is *without precedence* in the history of Kansas and that this places a special obligation on each of us to do our utmost to meet the health care needs of our state in every way possible.— Memo, William O. Rieke, M.D., to All Personnel, January 10, 1973.

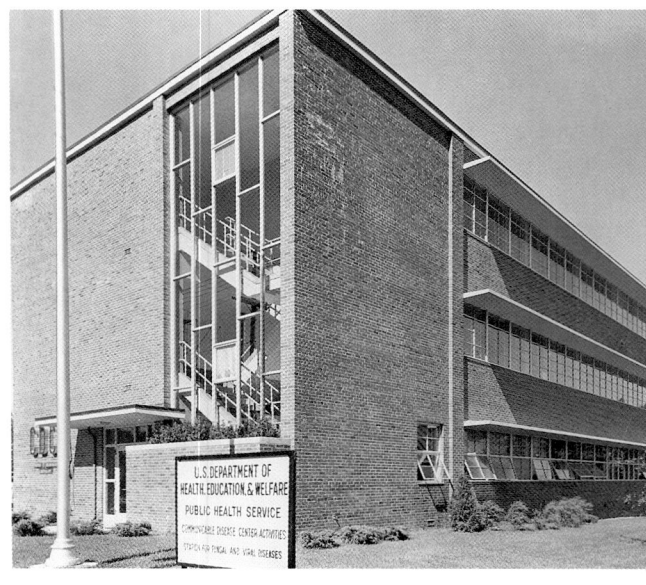

Breidenthal Laboratory, site of the Public Health Service's Communicable Disease Center in the 1970s.

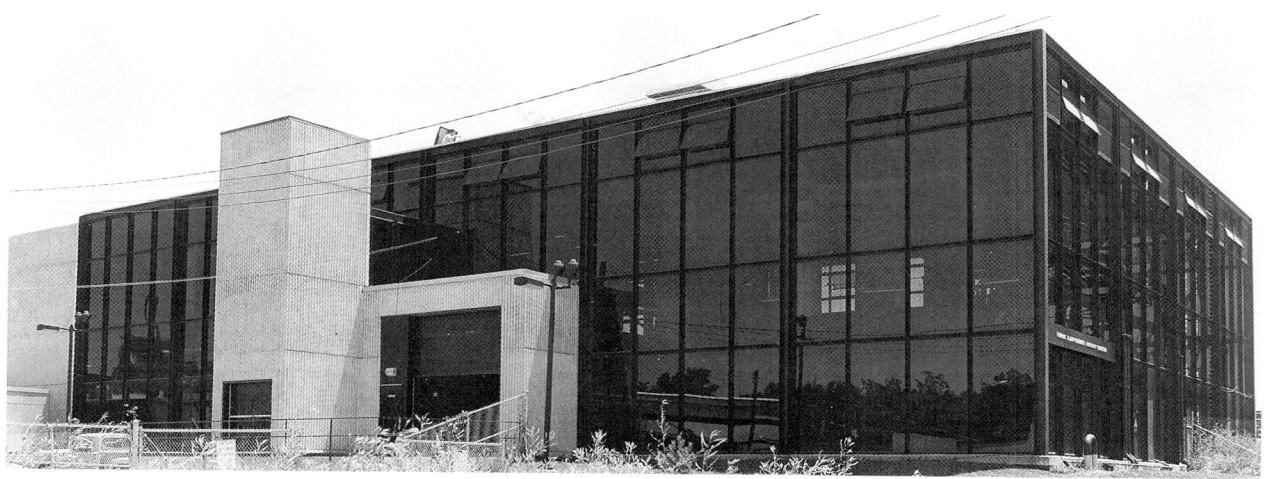

The Applegate Energy Center, completed in 1973.

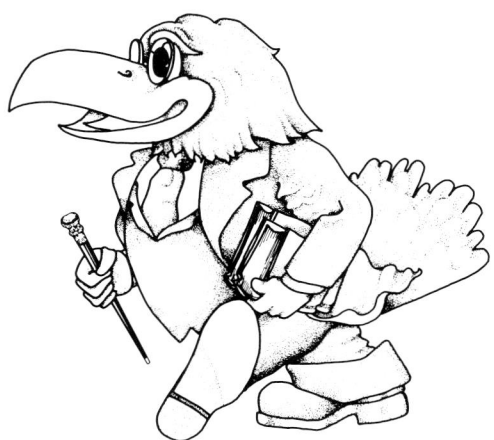

Jay Doc by Larry Howell, ca. 1974.

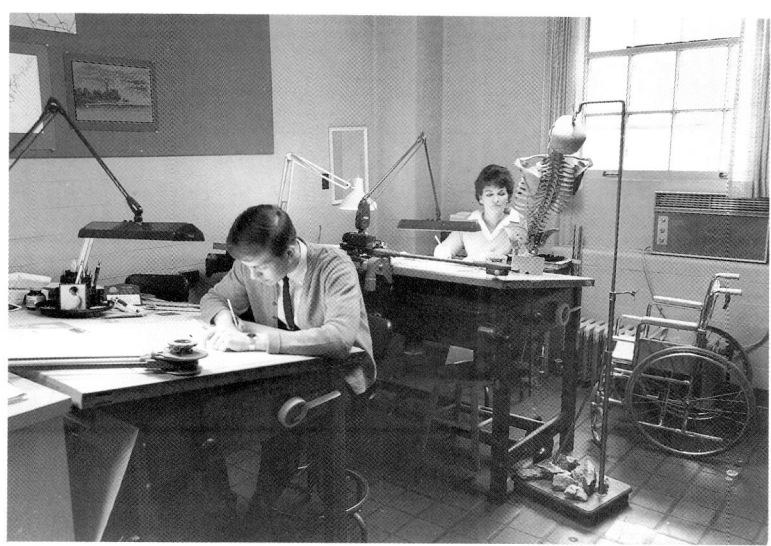

Medical illustrators, December 1964.

The faculty believes that the Department of Nursing Education can and should provide for improvement in the health care of citizens through the preparation of professional nursing practitioners, through participation in activities in the community, in educational and professional organizations and through research in the process of nursing.

The faculty believes that the professional nurse is one who is capable of giving comprehensive nursing care and is able to work effectively with other members of the health team in analyzing problem situations and implementing effective programs of action. She must be self-directing, capable of logical, critical thinking, sensitive to expressions of human need and capable of establishing meaningful relationships with people. The faculty supports the concept that the professional nurse must be responsible for giving direct patient care of a quality that promotes an optimum progression of the patient toward health or personal welfare.—Self-Evaluation Report, Department of Nursing Education, University of Kansas School of Medicine, November 15, 1962.

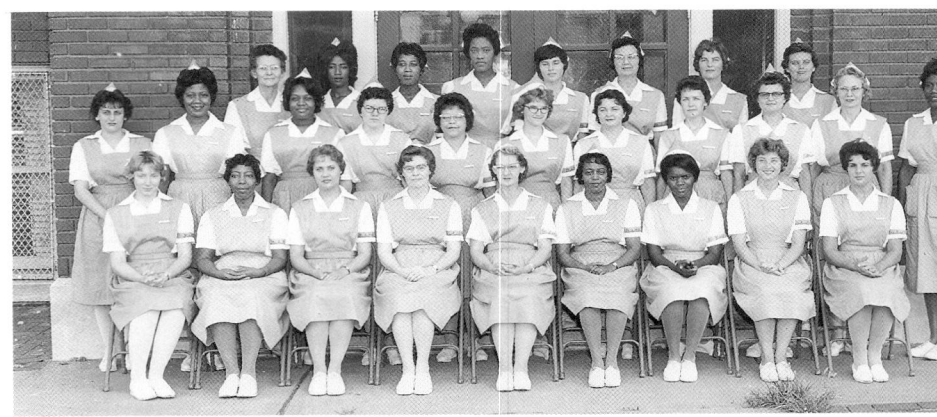

The Florence Nightingale School of Practical Nursing, 1963.

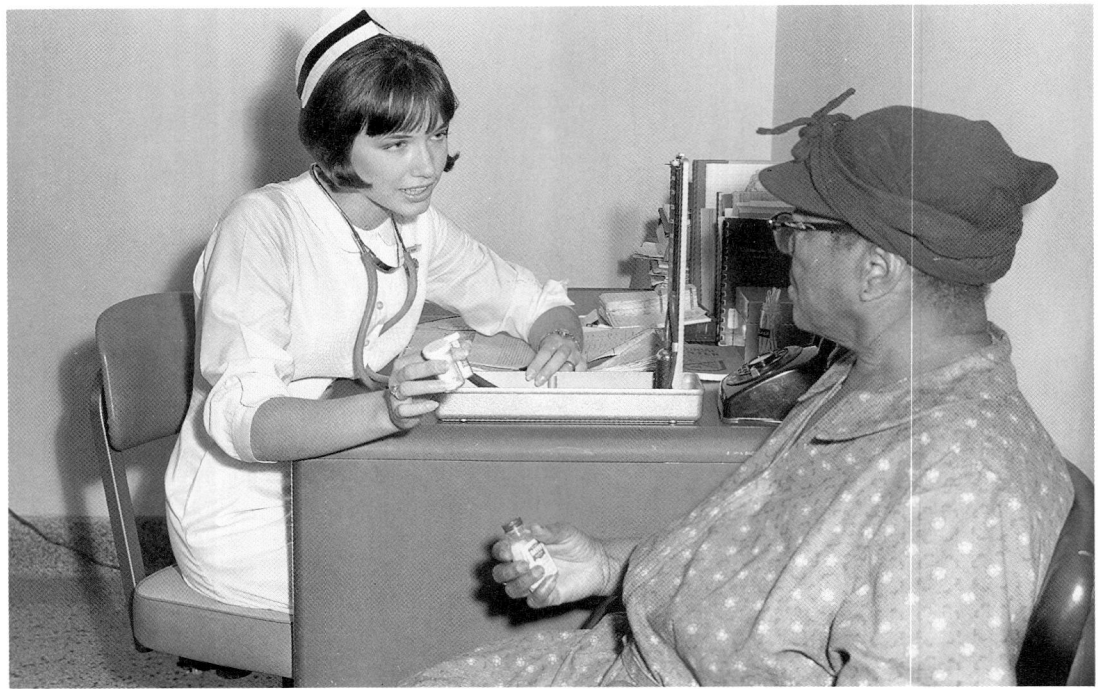

A nurse advising a patient on medication, October 1966.

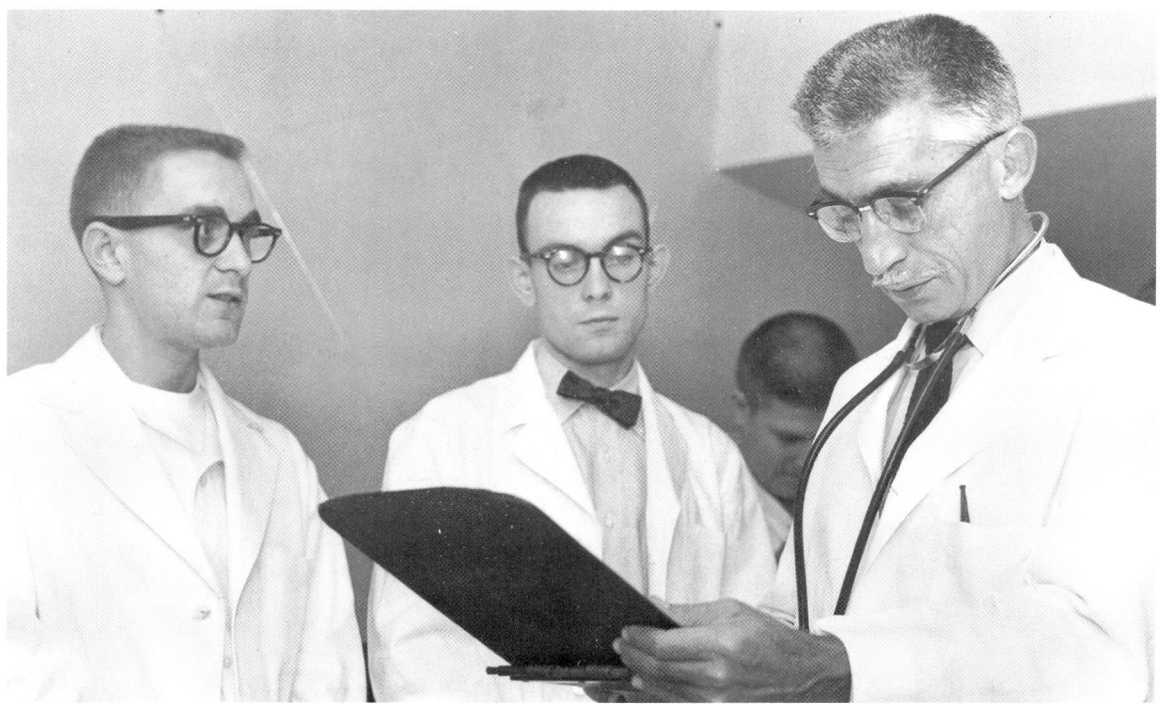

Mahlon Delp, M.D., with students, late 1970s.

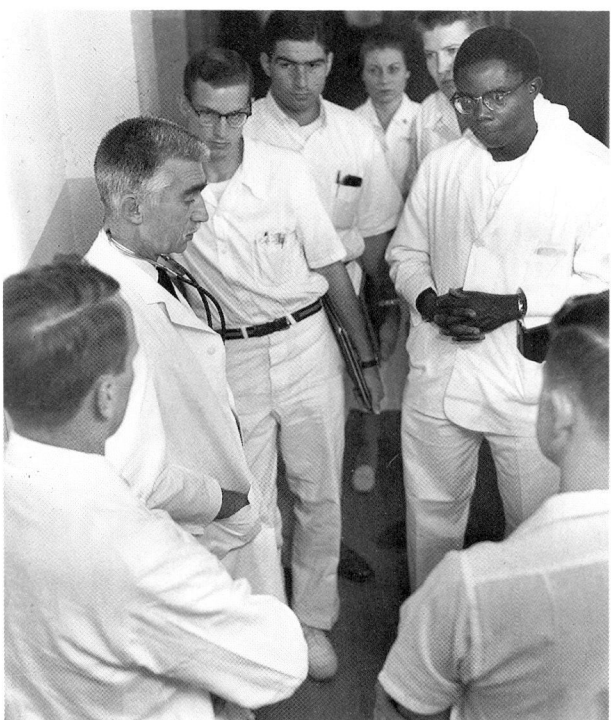

Dr. Delp conversing with graduate students, late 1970s.

The teacher's impact on his students is difficult to assess and impossible to quantitate. It is significant that Doctor Delp's students appreciate him more with the passage of time. This suggests he succeeds in teaching not facts alone, but attitudes and philosophy—the nebulous, but very real art if you will.
—Robert P. Hudson, M.D., *Jayhawker MD,* 1969.

When we arrived here we were awestruck and humbled by the vast red brick monolith that surrounded us. We struggled under the load of fifteen hundred page textbooks and we wondered if it would ever end. We faced anatomy, biochem and path and we conquered them all; finding in the process they were just words strung together. We learned that medicine is people—from the teaching to the learning; from the hoping to the caring. We found PEOPLE were why we were here.—*Jayhawker MD,* 1973.

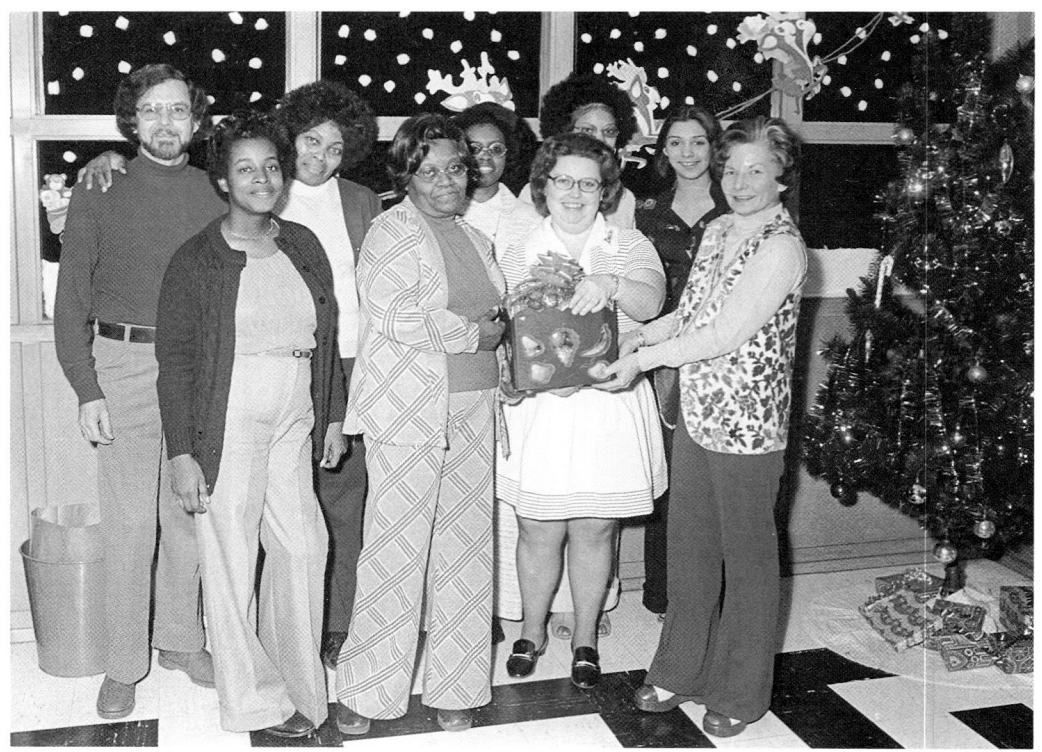

The library staff, Christmas 1974.

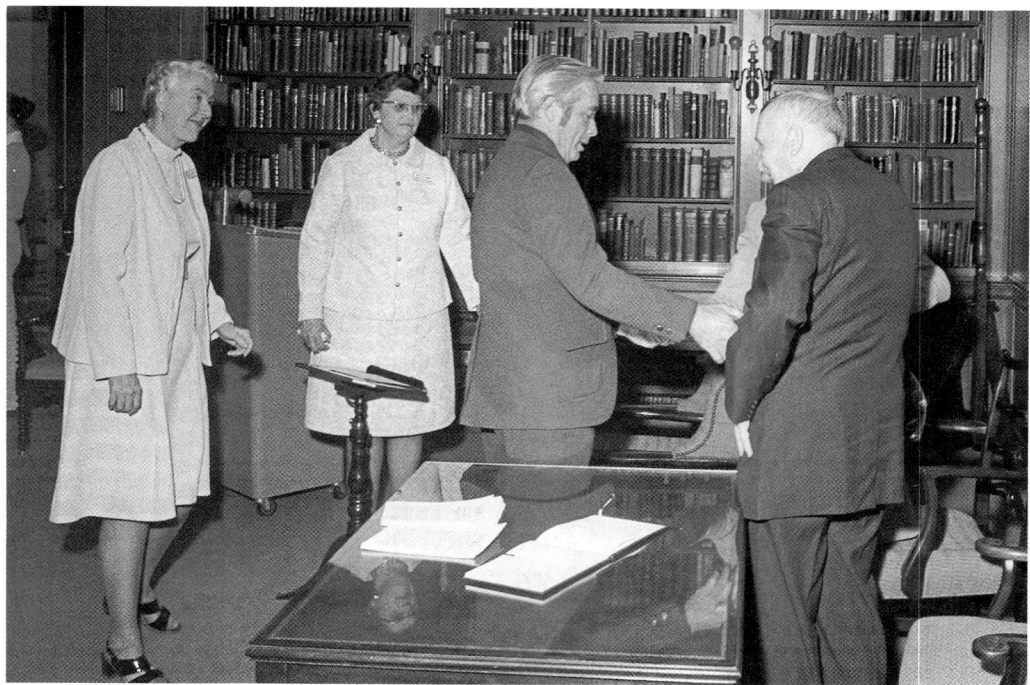

Robert P. Hudson, M.D., with Thor Jager, M.D., during the dedication of the Jager Room in the History and Philosophy of Medicine Department, 1974. Bea Jackson and Lena Downing look on.

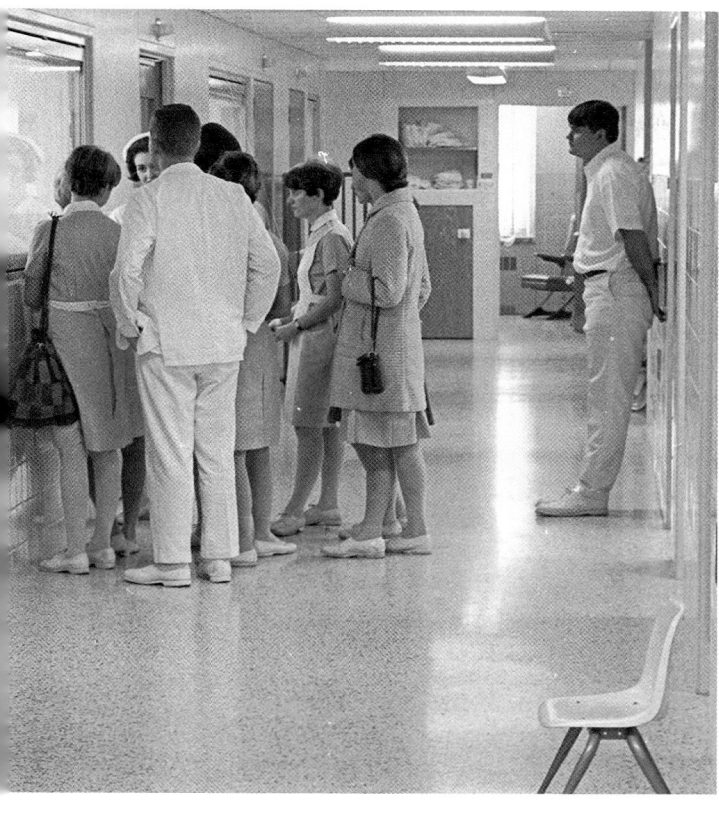

Opening of the new pediatric addition to L Building, 1968.

Too often people tend to pay attention only to day-to-day events and overlook long range progress and activities of an institution such as the University of Kansas Medical Center. True, KUMC in recent months has had its share of difficulties from a strike by housekeeping employees to a construction halt to a disagreement in the heart surgery department. But through it all, the administration at KUMC has been more than cooperative with the media to keep the public informed on the status of various situations.

At the same time KUMC has continued to take care of sick people and educate new doctors, nurses and others in allied health fields.

All these and other factors have contributed to improving KUMC which is so important not only to Kansas City, Kan., because of its location here, but also to the entire state which is so desperately in need of qualified health care personnel.
—*Kansas City Kansan*, May 29, 1974.

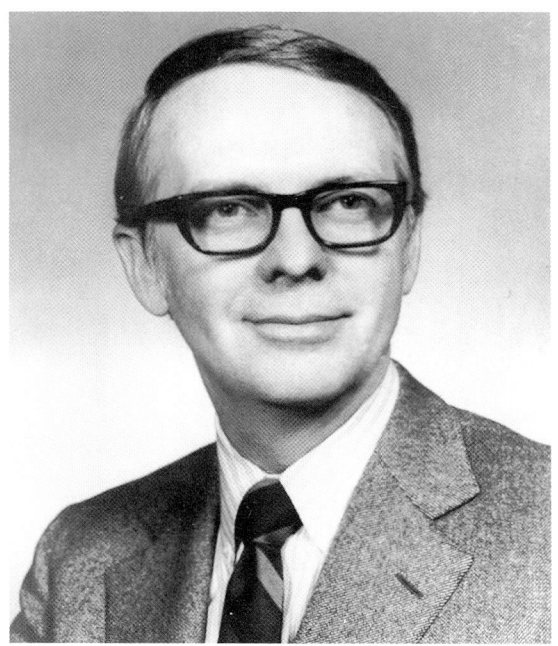

Robert B. Kugel, M.D., executive vice chancellor, 1976–1977.

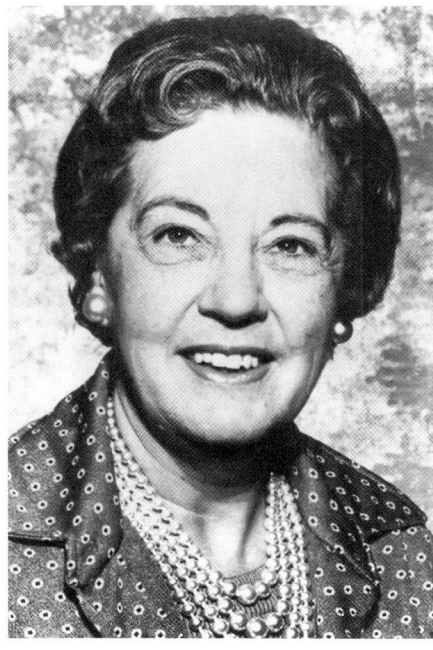

Doris A. Geitgey, R.N., Ed.D., dean of the School of Nursing, 1975–1988.

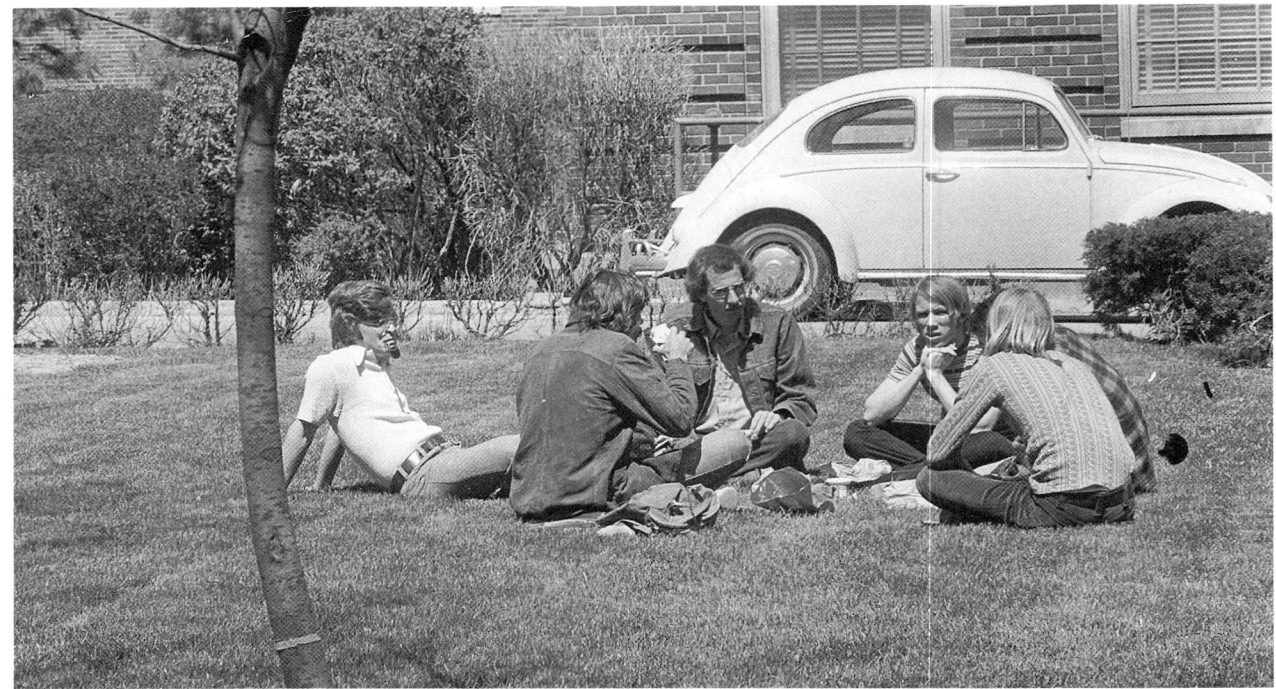

Students relaxing in the sun, ca. 1972.

During our clinical years, we as medical students are provided with the opportunity to "live in the Ward." Yet these first clinical steps are uncertain. Intimidated by our own ignorance and inexperience, we seek help in translating a mass of medical knowledge into daily practice. And it is from the housestaff that we seek this help. It is from them that we learn by example, and it is their privilege to teach us "the art of medicine."
—*Jayhawker MD*, 1976.

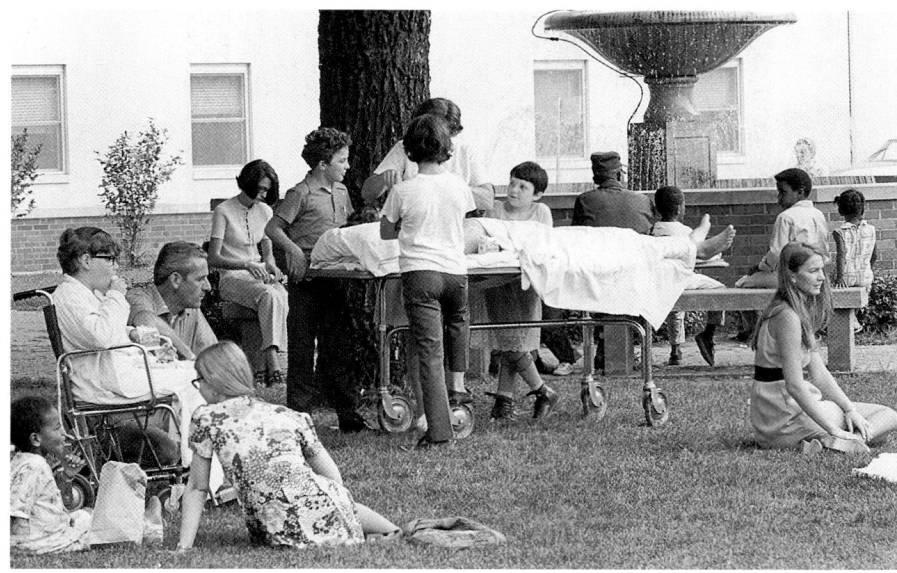

Pediatric patients at the Clendening fountain, summer 1971.

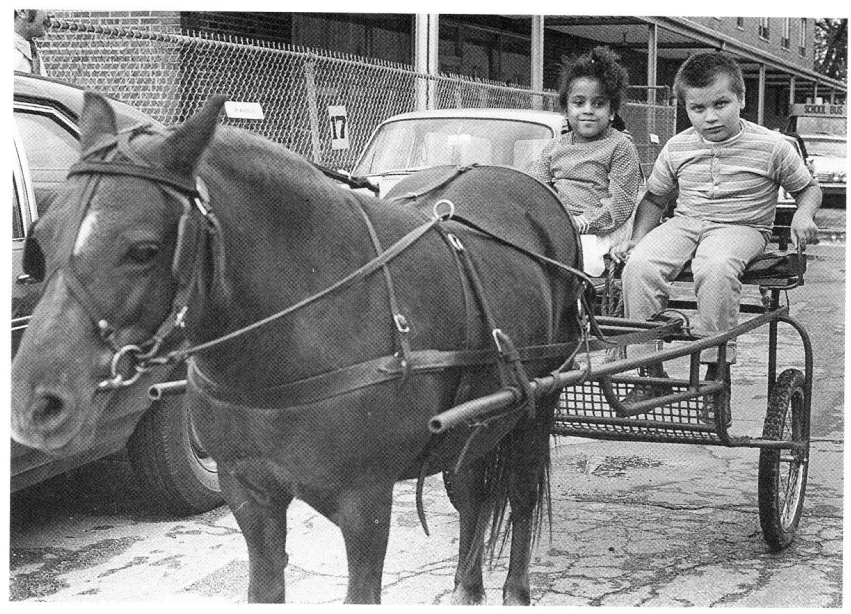

Children's rehabilitation students enjoying a pony and cart ride, June 2, 1971.

Ponies and carts entertained Children's Rehabilitation Unit students June 2. Roy Grandon, storekeeper in purchasing, brought his ponies from his home in Louisburg to give the children an afternoon outing.
—*Topics*, July 1971.

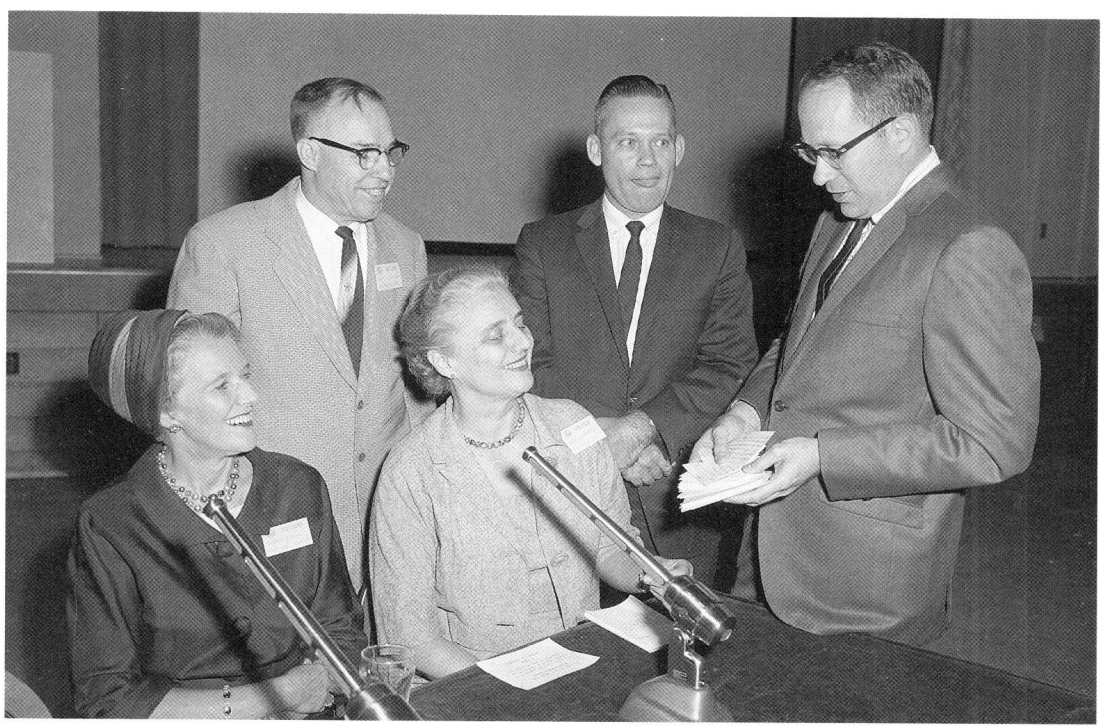

Participants in the 1964 School Health Symposium. Seated, left to right: Evelyn Duvall, M.D., and Mary Calderone, M.D. Standing, left to right: Lester A. Kirkendall, M.D., Charles Watkins, Charles E. Lewis, M.D.

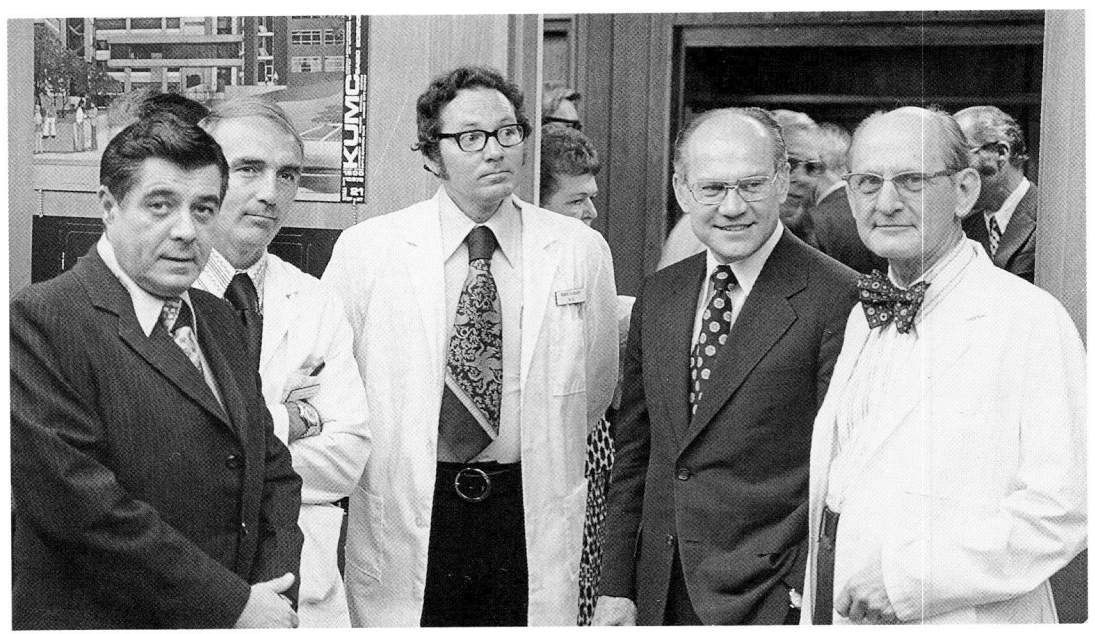

Governor Robert Docking, Loren J. Humphrey, M.D., and Robert Boudet, M.D., Chancellor Archie R. Dykes, and Vice Chancellor for Faculty and Academic Affairs E. B. Brown, Jr., Ph.D., at the opening of the Center for Breast Diseases, September 1973.

The lives of twelve women have been saved or prolonged because of early detection of breast cancer following an examination at the Detection Center for Breast Diseases at the University of Kansas Medical Center, according to Dr. Robert Boudet, assistant director for the center.

The KU Center was opened in September as one of six centers funded by a combined $8 million grant from the American Cancer Society and the National Health Institute.—*Kansas City Kansan*, April 25, 1974.

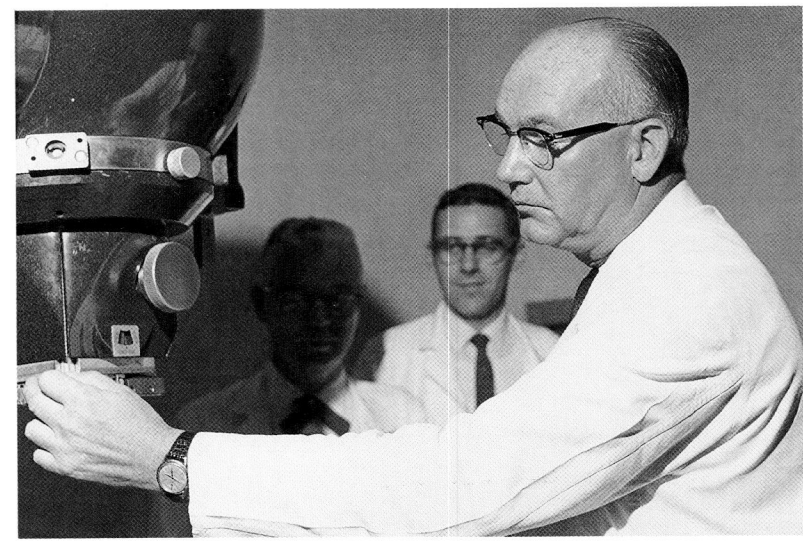

George A. Cowan, M.D., chief, Section of Therapeutic Radiology, 1968.

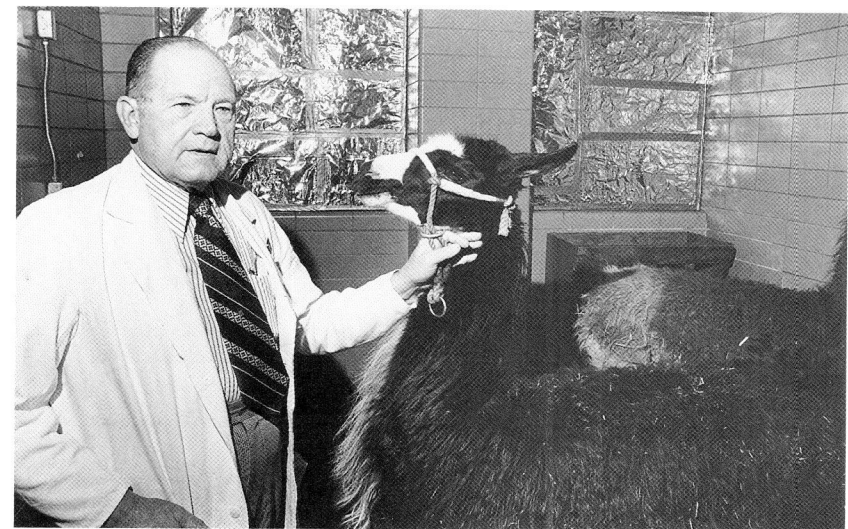

Murray Wardall, D.V.M., with llama.

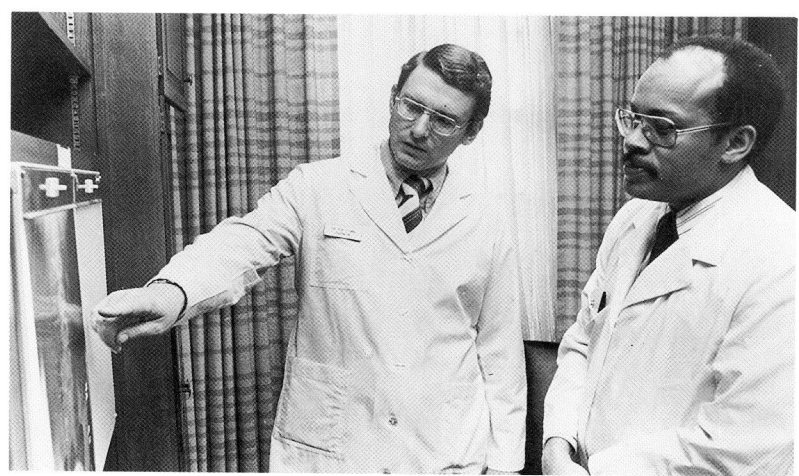

American Cancer Society Fellowship recipients James R.
Neff, M.D., and James H. Thomas, M.D., 1974.

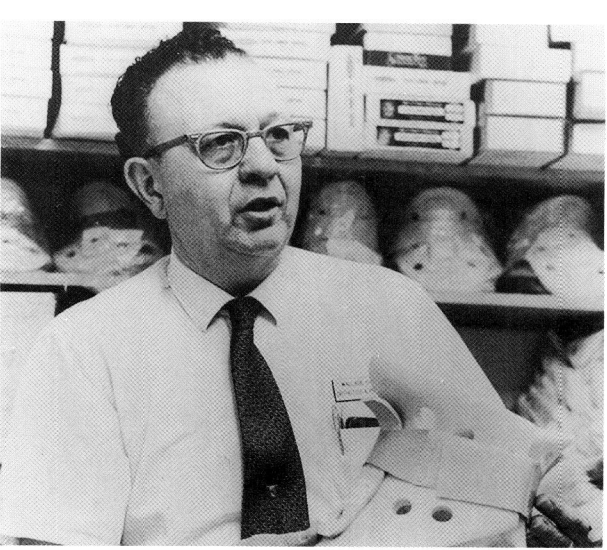

Wallace Whitney, head of the Department of Orthotics and
Prosthetics, October 1974.

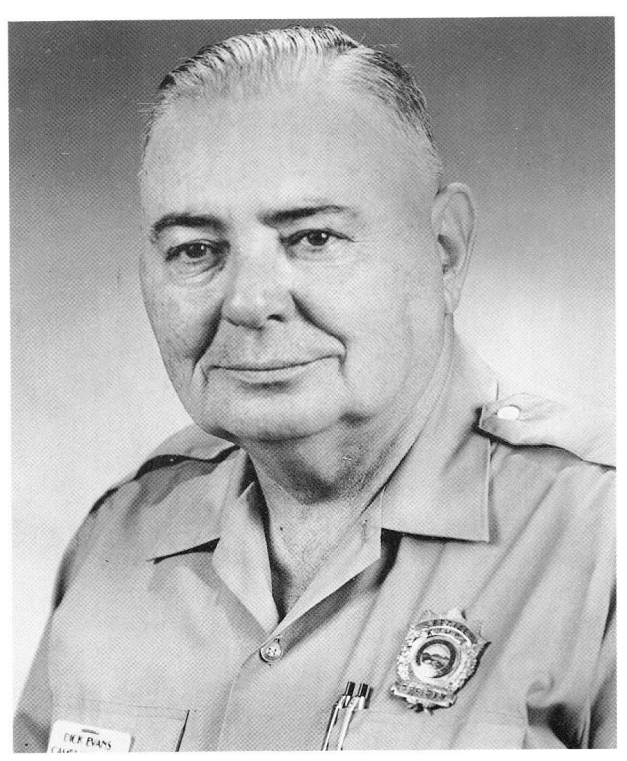

Richard Evans, campus patrol captain from 1967 to 1977.

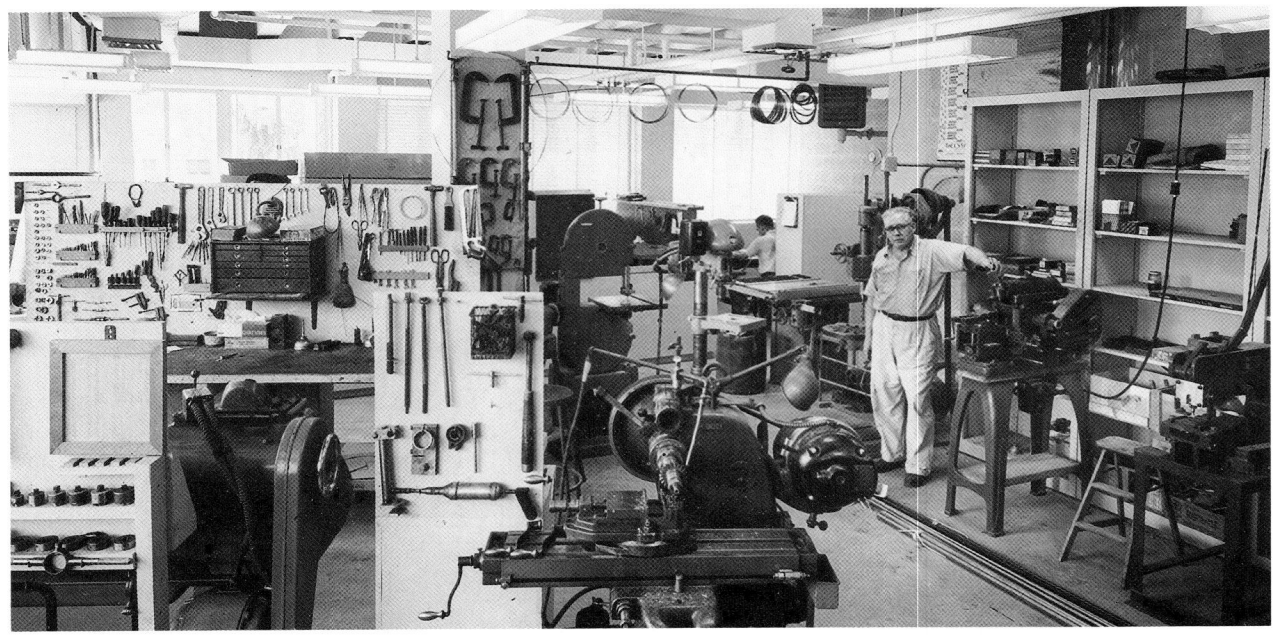

The instrument shop, 1961.

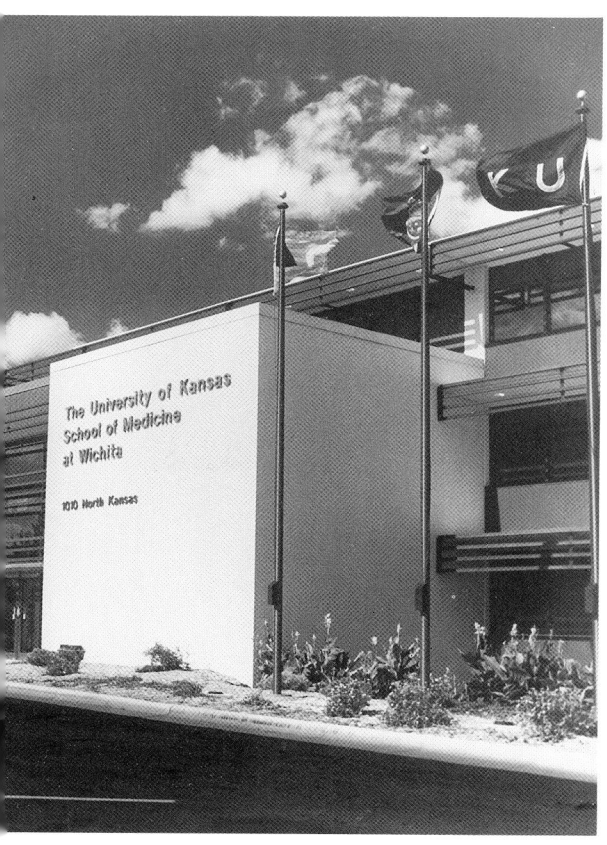

Eleven and one half years ago the State of Kansas opened a new facility for training physicians in Wichita. The official name of this institute is the University of Kansas School of Medicine at Wichita and it is located at the E. B. Allen Memorial Hospital building. Since this is a community based program, it does not have one teaching hospital but draws from the resources of four Wichita hospitals. St. Francis Regional Medical Center, St. Joseph Medical Center, and Wesley Medical Center are three of the four largest hospitals in Kansas. Also serving the School of Medicine is the Veterans Administration Center and Hospital.

But the Wichita program offers more than just the standard rotations between hospitals. They also provide a variety of outreach programs for the community. Other programs include rural health weekends, opportunities to rotate overseas, and a chance to be involved in several research projects.

The presence of the School of Medicine in Wichita has made possible more advanced techniques that fill a gap in the diagnostic and health care services. These include diagnosis of genetic disorders; diagnosis of vascular diseases; diagnosis, monitoring, and care of high risk neonates; diagnosis and treatment of infectious disease; and diabetes treatment.

The School of Medicine at Wichita offers a unique and varied experience to the student; utilizing hospitals, programs and research. But ultimately, the most valuable experience is the opportunity for the personal interaction necessary for personal growth.—*Jayhawker MD*, 1985–1986.

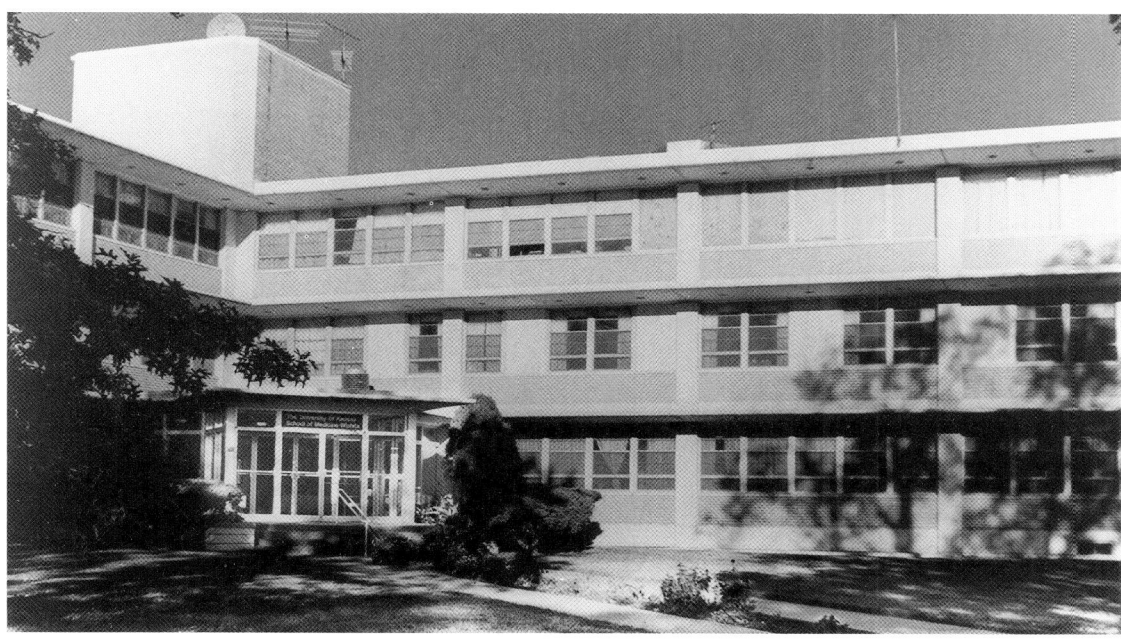

E. B. Allen Hospital, Wichita Campus, 1975.

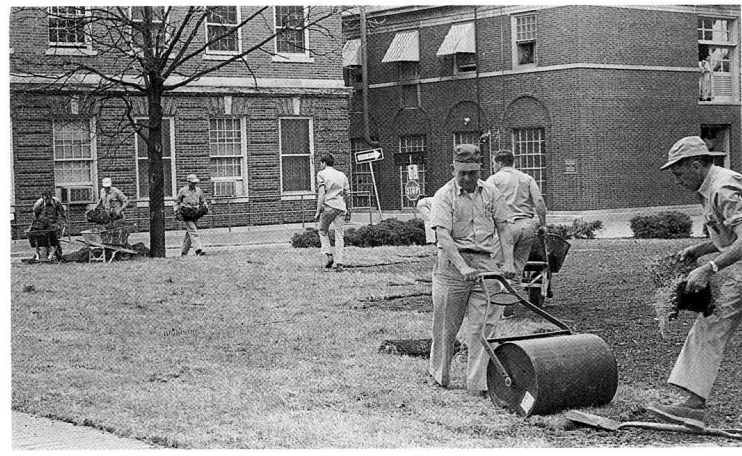

Buildings and Grounds employees laying sod, 1970s.

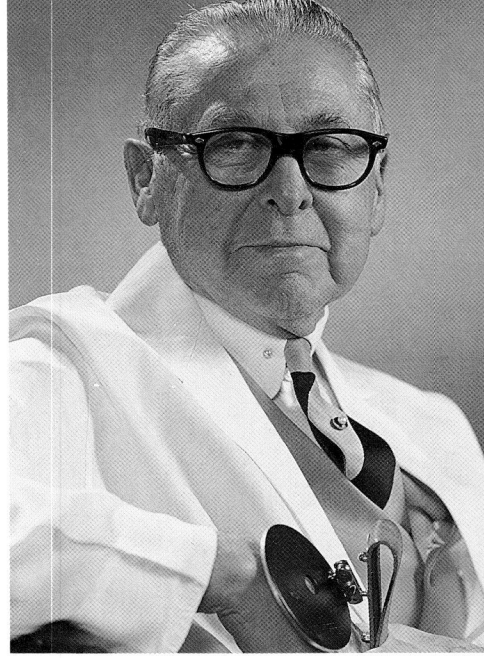

Sam E. Roberts, M.D., professor emeritus of Otorhinolaryngology, ca. 1960.

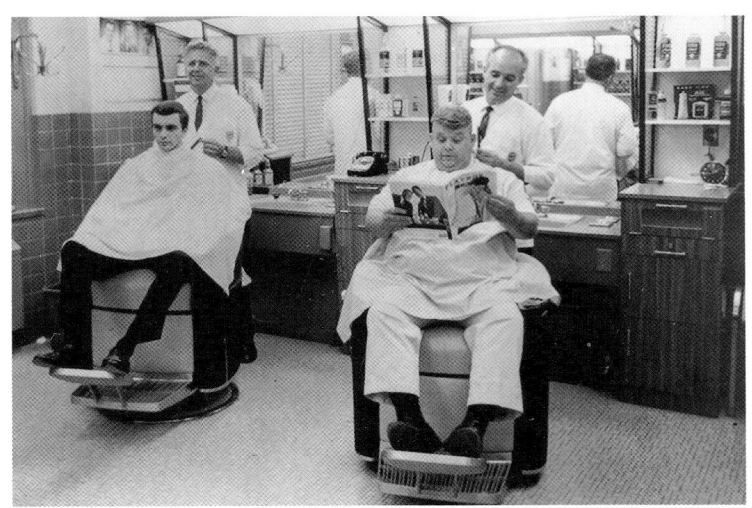

The barber shop in the Student Center with Jimmy Bowers (right) having his wig trimmed, 1970s.

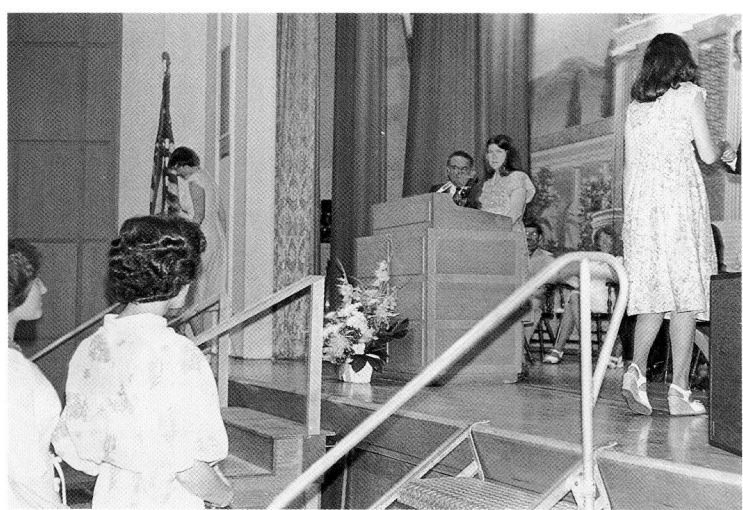

A 1970s School of Allied Health graduation ceremony.

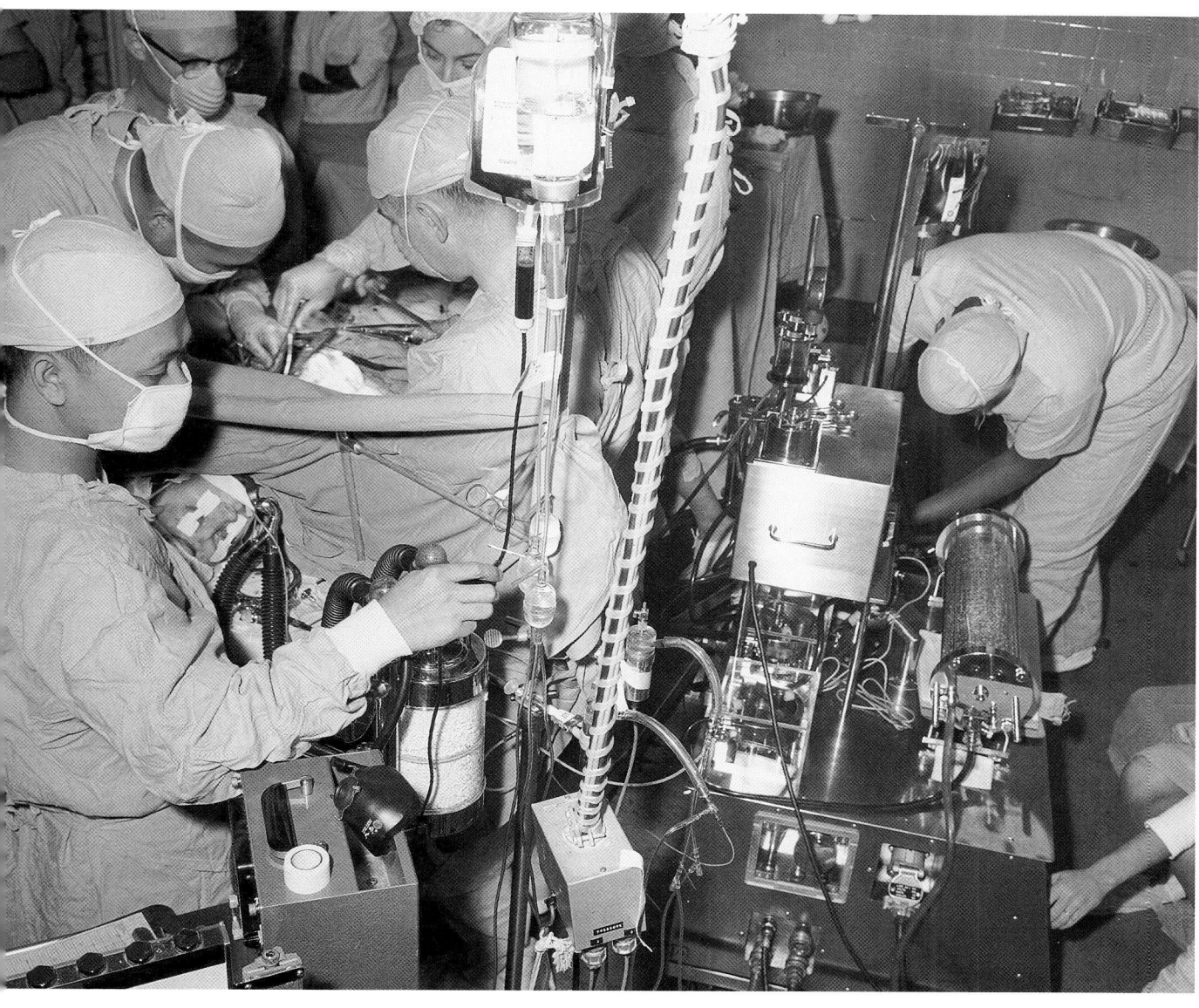

Anesthesiologists in surgery, 1960s.

The decline in our patient referral population may be attributed to a number of factors, one of the most important being our excellent resident training programs. Academic medicine, both here in Kansas and throughout the country, is doing an excellent job of putting itself out of business by training residents who are more skilled and capable of handling difficult problems. Many patients who in earlier times would have been referred to a medical center such as ours are now being cared for in physicians' offices and community hospitals by practicing physicians who are better equipped to handle complex problems and who are, in general, more highly skilled than their predecessors.—Burton A. Dudding, M.D., to David Waxman, M.D., September 27, 1977.

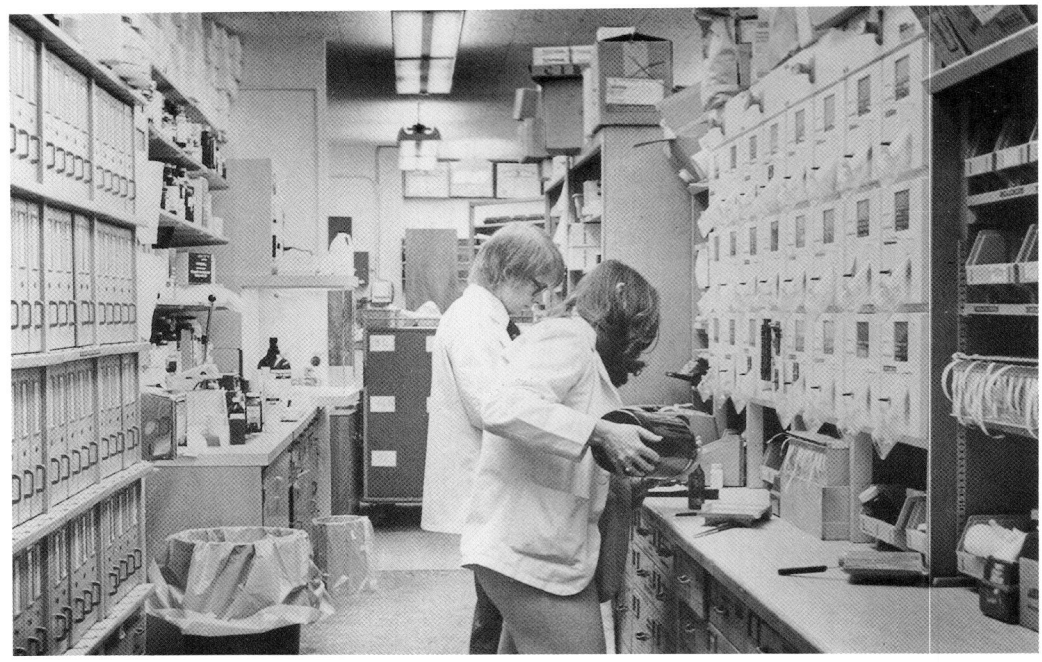

The pharmacy during the late 1970s.

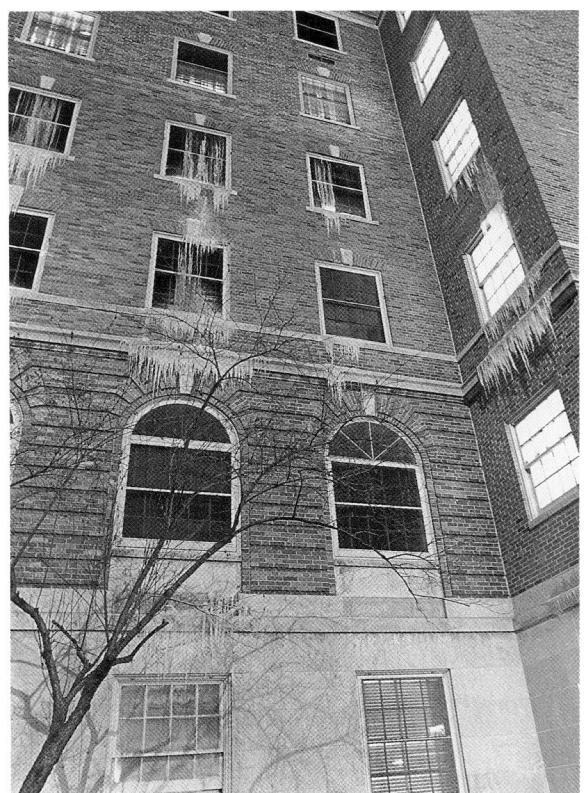

A winter flood in Sudler Hall, December 16, 1979.

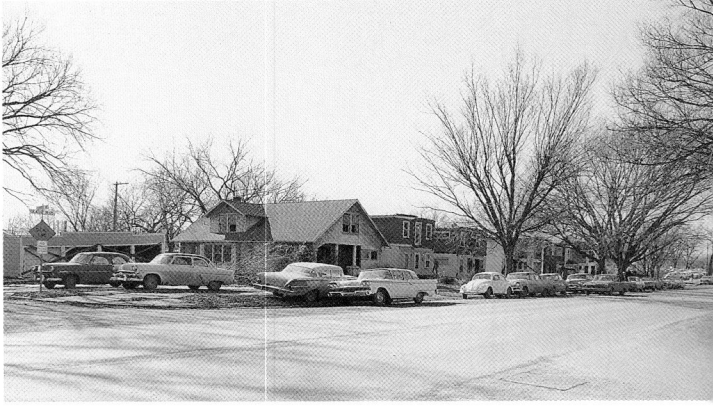

A view along Olathe Boulevard, January 1964.

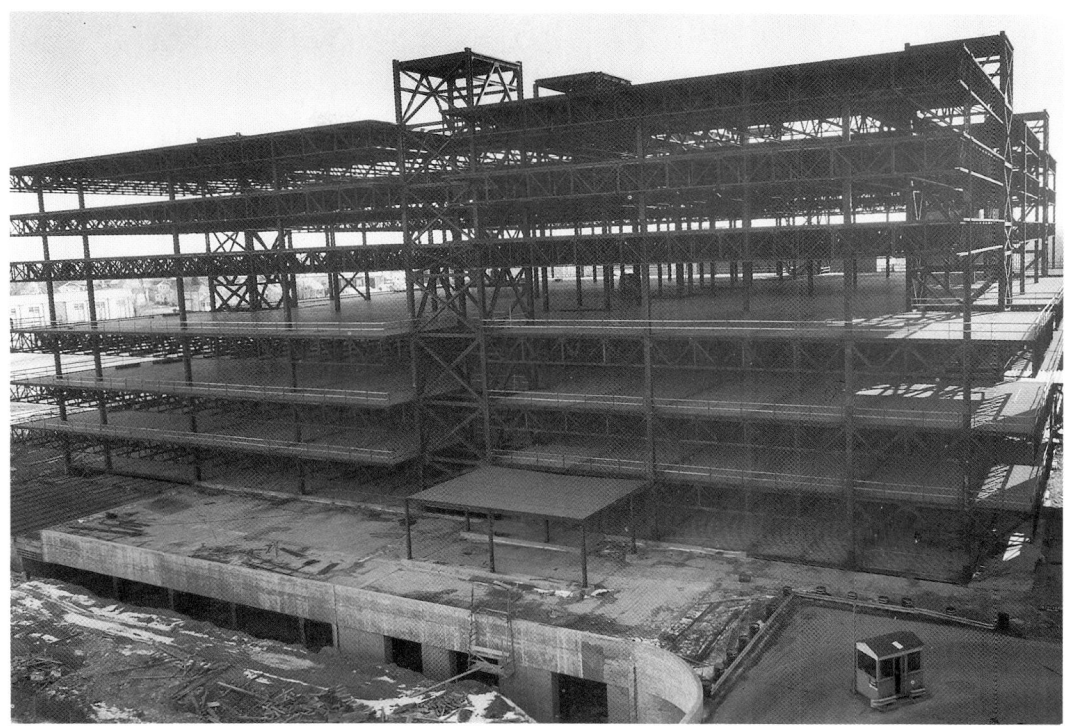

Early construction of the new University of Kansas Hospital, January 16, 1976.

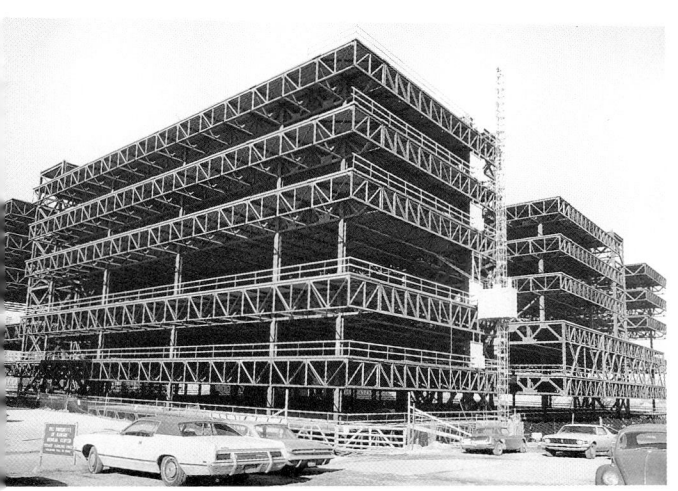

Friday the 13th of April was not at all an unlucky day! Governor Robert Docking invited the University of Kansas Medical Center's Central Administrative Planning Committee to formal ceremonies in his office in which he signed Senate bill 280 into law. This action represented the capstone to over three years of planning and discussion by members of the Medical Center staff, the Kansas Board of Regents, the Governor, and members of the Senate and House of Representatives.

The legislation passed by this year's session of the Senate and House and ultimately signed by the Governor provides nearly thirty-one million dollars for the expansion of Clinical and Basic Science facilities on this campus. In addition, this legislation authorizes the Board of Regents to sell up to 22 million dollars in revenue bonds. The Medical Center already had won approval for a federal grant of 5.1 million dollars for the Basic Sciences building. In total, our expansion program now has been approved and underwritten for nearly 60 million dollars. Never before in the history of the State of Kansas has any educational institution received direct support of such magnitude. This is a clear indication of the magnificent interest and help that we have received from our state legislature and from the executive branch of state government.
—KU Medical Center Expansion Program Memo, May 1, 1973.

The largest construction project in the history of the state of Kansas is currently underway, a project that will double the present Medical Center facilities. There will be nearly 800 beds and the 700,000 square-foot clinical facility will cost more than $50 million. Completion of this building is expected in the fall of 1977.

The main thrust of KUMC since its beginning has been teaching. During its history, 2,255 nurses have been graduated and 4,543 medical students have received their M.D.'s. That group of 75 students in two classes 50 years ago will increase to 200 in the freshman class alone when the new $6 million basic science building is completed in 1975.
—*Dodge City Daily Globe*, June 26, 1974.

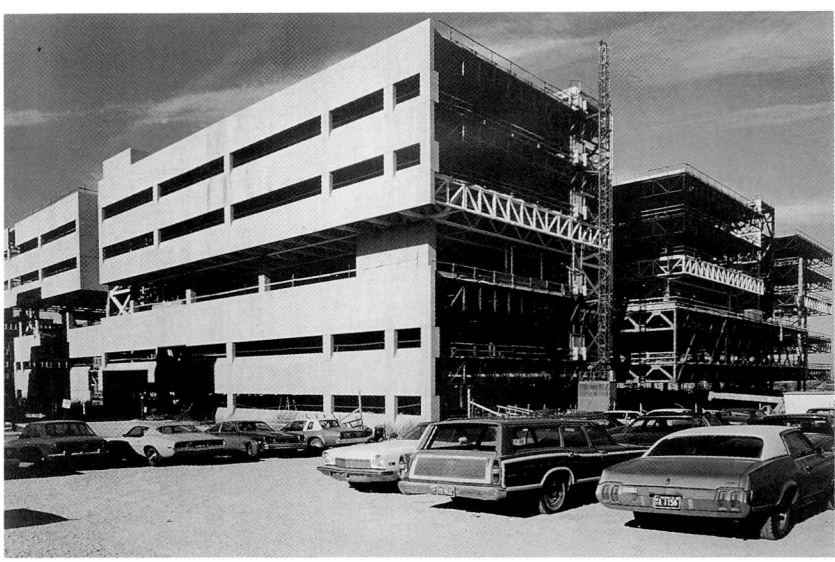

Two views of the hospital construction, late 1970s.

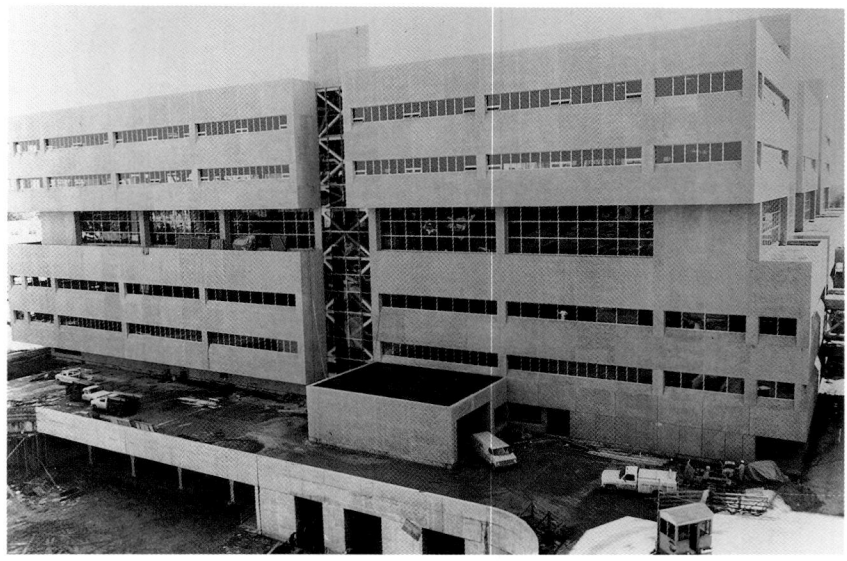

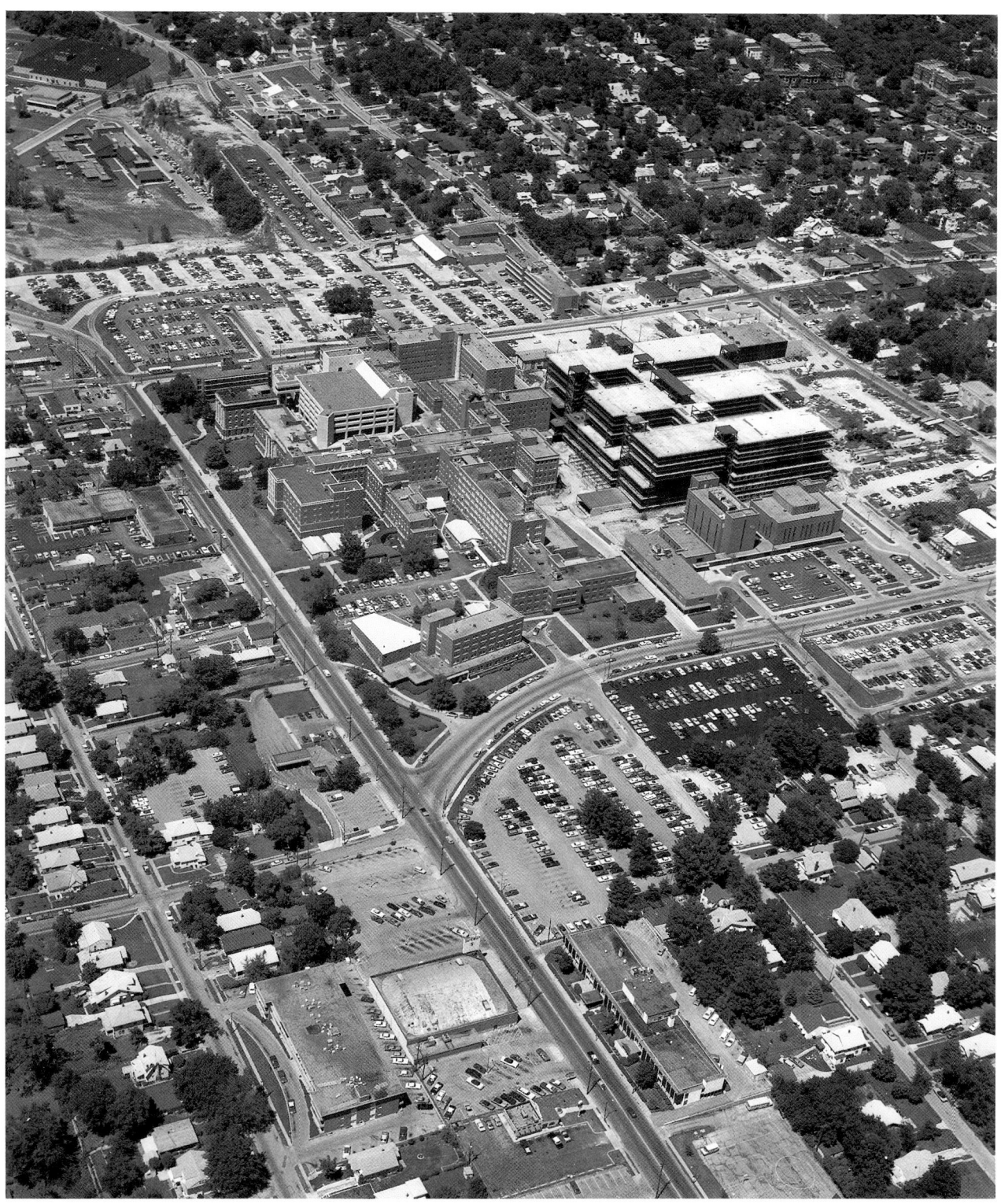

An aerial view of the Medical Center showing the new hospital under construction, ca. 1976.

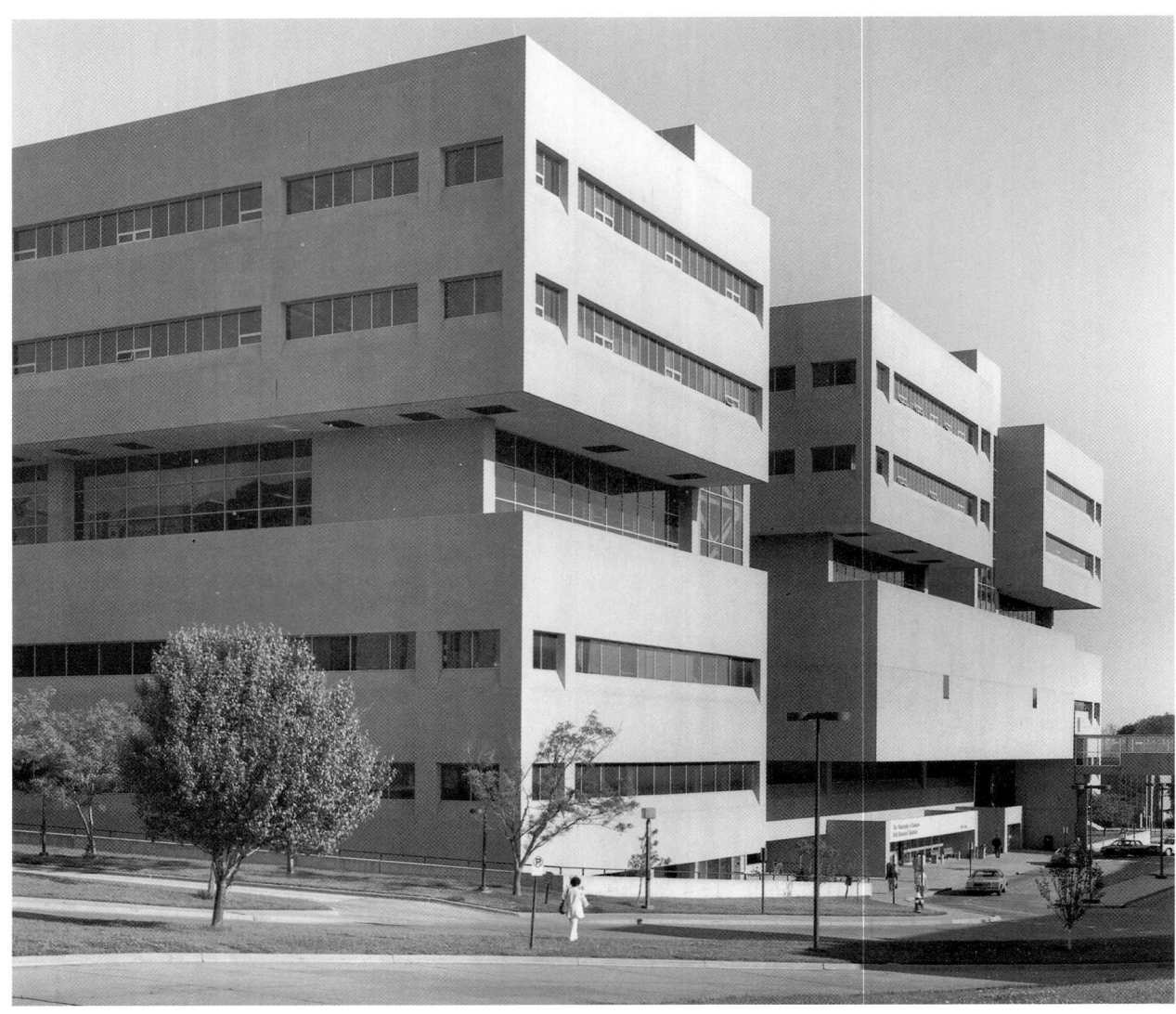

The University of Kansas Hospital, March 1990.

7

A Commitment to Excellence

On August 1, 1981, Gene A. Budig was appointed the fourteenth chancellor of the University of Kansas. The forty-two year old Budig, a native of McCook, Nebraska, brought impressive credentials to the position. Before entering higher education administration, he was a professional journalist and executive assistant to the governor of Nebraska. Long active in the Air National Guard, Budig rose to the rank of major general. He earned three degrees from the University of Nebraska, including a Doctorate of Education awarded in 1967. In 1972, Budig became an administrator at Illinois State University, assuming the presidency of that institution the following year. Four years later, in 1976, he was named president of West Virginia University, a post he held until his selection as chancellor by the University of Kansas Board of Regents.

The Kansas Regents viewed Budig as a skilled administrator with an outstanding record in operating both a major university and an accompanying medical center. In his new position, Chancellor Budig moved energetically to work closely with the Medical Center. Spending at least one day a week at 39th and Rainbow, he sought to broaden the scope of the Medical Center's research, while simultaneously continuing its commitment to teaching and clinical activities. Another important goal was upgrading the schools of Nursing and Allied Health. "I believe the Medical Center of the University of Kansas has the human resources to meet the most difficult of challenges," he said. "I also believe we have the will to succeed. I want and need a system that will foster the strongest possible Medical Center at the University of Kansas." Budig's prediction proved correct. During the 1980s, through a combination of his leadership and that provided by two executive vice chancellors, David Waxman,

M.D., and D. Kay Clawson, M.D., the University of Kansas Medical Center moved toward administrative and economic stabilization.

Dr. Waxman became executive vice chancellor in 1977, following Dr. Robert B. Kugel's abbreviated tenure. Since 1961, Waxman, a graduate of the Syracuse College of Medicine, had taught internal medicine and held several administrative positions at the Medical Center. A World War II Army Air Force officer, he retired from the United States Air Force Reserve in 1978 as a major general. The hallmarks of his tenure as executive vice chancellor, which began at a time of increasing competition for patients, were establishing high standards of patient care and eradicating the Medical Center's reputation for inefficiency. He directed a period of expansion and unprecedented growth that saw the opening of the new hospital, the establishment of a radiation therapy center, and the development of area health education centers in Hays, Garden City, and Chanute. Waxman resigned as executive vice chancellor in 1983, but continued his career at the Medical Center as director of Health Care Resources. In typical fashion, he told his successor, "Be patient and work hard. The reward is the work."

Dr. D. Kay Clawson, who became executive vice chancellor in the spring of 1983, had a national reputation in orthopaedics and medical education, and had been president of two major orthopaedic associations. A 1952 graduate of Harvard Medical School, Clawson came to the University of Kansas Medical Center from the University of Kentucky School of Medicine, where he had served for eight years as dean of the College of Medicine. Prior to his tenure in Kentucky, he was professor and chairman of the Orthopaedic Surgery Division/Department for sixteen years at the University of Washington in

Seattle. "We wanted someone with instant credibility," Chancellor Gene Budig stated in a May 5, 1983, interview in the *Kansas City Star*. "We also wanted someone who would relate well within the state."

During his first eight years at 39th and Rainbow, Clawson oversaw substantial improvements in financial conditions, presided over further expansion, enhanced the physical environment, and planned for an even larger institution by the twenty-first century. In an address that he delivered as chairman of the Association of American Medical Colleges in October 1989 in Washington, D.C., Clawson stressed the need for North American education to move in a direction better suited to the needs of individual students, emphasizing concepts rather than rote memorization. In addition to facility improvements, what he hoped to accomplish as executive vice chancellor was to change the course of health care education, placing the Medical Center in the forefront of international educational reform.

The new University of Kansas Hospital highlighted the revitalization of the Medical Center during the "Waxman-Clawson Era." The massive hospital facility, including a parking structure, virtually doubled the size of the 39th and Rainbow campus. At first, the hospital, which officially opened in 1979, fell short of projected revenues of $50 million a year. A terse assessment in an internal document, "Goals and Objectives," stated: "We must improve the efficiency of our services to patients and minimize the frustration they encounter; improve our relations with referring physicians; expand our range of specialized clinical services; improve our image as a health care and health educational resource; develop a more systematic approach to preventive medicine; expand our patient education programs; develop additional ambulatory care capabilities; and improve wages and working conditions for nursing and other hospital staff. In hand with all these, there must be constant improvement in our efforts to contain the cost of health care." A few critics, who had opposed building such a large hospital, suggested either selling it at a loss or leasing it to a private firm.

The financial condition of the new facility improved steadily following the appointment of Eugene L. Staples as hospital administrator in 1982, and vice chancellor of hospital administration in 1983. Staples, formerly the administrator of the 450-bed West Virginia University Hospital, intro-

duced systematic and intensive managerial methods which uniformly improved overall earnings. In 1988 the hospital had revenues in excess of $82 million and contributed over $15 million to the Medical Center budget. By 1990, as health costs skyrocketed, the University of Kansas Hospital's budget crossed the $110 million mark. With 18,000 inpatient and 360,000 outpatient visits at the expanded facility, Simeon Bell's vision of a great university medical complex had finally become a reality.

The new hospital underscored the Medical Center's commitment to modern technology and facilities. In an age of fierce competition, it was clear that a large health care center had to acquire and maintain the latest technological equipment at whatever cost. A modern medical center's faculty must also be leading practitioners of state-of-the-art life-saving techniques. In 1984, physicians at the University of Kansas Medical Center performed the first heart transplant in the Kansas City area, and in 1990, the area's first liver transplant program was initiated. The Medical Center's modern-day intensive care, radiology, pediatric, and experimental research facilities contrast sharply with their counterparts of the 1930s. The modern operating rooms are light-years away from those of pre–World War II. With this increased modernization, the "Wahl Years" fade into the distant past.

During the 1980s, the physical and learning atmosphere at the Medical Center continued to improve, characterized by continual building and refurbishing. The Archie R. Dykes Library, completed in 1983, provided students and faculty with a large, modern facility for study and research. This computerized learning center, housing nearly 150,000 volumes, contains more useable space than was available on the entire Goat Hill campus. Construction of the Research Support Facility and the Kirmayer Fitness Center and Sports Medicine Complex further enhanced the campus. The agenda at the Wichita Campus included obtaining additional land for expansion and bringing multiple residency programs under the university's umbrella.

Dr. Clawson's philosophy that "you never have a second chance at a first impression" led to vast improvements in the appearance of the buildings and grounds. A long series of improvement projects resulted in the remodeling of significant amounts of older space into modern office, classroom, and patient facilities and research laboratories, along with the construction of an expanded, modern bookstore in the Orr-Major building. Other physical improvements included the removal of all temporary structures, the re-landscaping of university property, and campus expansion through acquisition of adjacent residential and commercial properties.

A 586-space parking structure opened in 1989, but with over 12,000 people working at or visiting the Medical Center every business day, parking remains a pressing problem. The parking situation today is in sharp contrast to the photographs of thirty years earlier, when most people used public transportation and a few small, half-filled parking lots met the needs of faculty, staff, students, patients, and visitors.

During the decade of the 1980s, several important programmatic changes occurred. The already high quality of the instructional force steadily improved, and many faculty members achieved national prominence. The School of Medicine saw the rebuilding of the departments of Anatomy and Microbiology through more space, improved facilities, and the addition of many new faculty members. The School of Nursing reworked its curriculum and expanded its graduate degree offerings to include a Ph.D. The School of Allied Health, coming into its own under a full-time dean, expanded several programs, including physical therapy, occupational therapy, dietetics and nutrition, respiratory therapy, medical records, hearing and speech, and nurse anesthesia. The renovation of the Clendening Library and the Department of the History and Philosophy of Medicine enhanced the housing and programs of one of the finest collections of rare and classical medical books in North America. In 1988, largely due to Dr. Clawson's continuing support for preserving the history of the Medical Center, an institutional archives was added to this department.

Additionally, a new Center for Student Affairs and Educational Development consolidated and improved student support services, including psychological and education counseling. Finally, despite two budget recisions, new incentive plans allowed faculty members of most departments who excelled in research and patient care to increase their incomes to levels comparable to their peers at other institutions.

As an important part of the Medical Center's continual upgrading, research activities were in-creased significantly during the 1980s. This increase meant modifying the school's traditional emphasis on teaching. Research had the potential of both generating additional revenue and helping the Medical Center compete nationally. During this decade, public and private research at the Medical Center increased from just under $8 million to $26 million, but the shortage of suitable facilities still limits the growth of research activities. Although a planned $13 million research building now promises to alleviate some space shortages, this new facility will still leave the University of Kansas Medical Center behind comparable medical centers. Yet, the research controversy seems in keeping with the history of the Medical Center; every advance toward a higher level of performance leads directly to new challenges that require renewed action.

The visual images of the present-day Medical Center reflect progress toward the development of a modern facility. The highly technological and scientific environment conveys promise for resolving complex health care issues while providing an atmosphere conducive to resolving the many dilemmas facing modern medicine today. The very participation of the University of Kansas Medical Center in seeking solutions to contemporary medical problems is a further indication of its increasing national prominence. In 1990, the Medical Center had a budget of $219 million and a staff of 4,868. Official statistics for the fall of 1990 showed an enrollment of 737 in medicine, 578 in medical residencies spread through twenty-one subspecialties, 436 in nursing, 460 in allied health, and 99 in Ph.D. programs. The faculty totaled 788.

Large public institutions, when well-managed and supported, usually continue to expand, often very rapidly. By all accounts and signs, this maxim will define the decade of the 1990s for the Medical Center. The challenge, however, is not dealing either with growth or with policy questions. Rather, it is charting the best course to the pinnacle of medical education in the United States—one that emphasizes quality instruction and patient care along with innovative research. This course will mandate continued progress into the next century for the University of Kansas Medical Center.

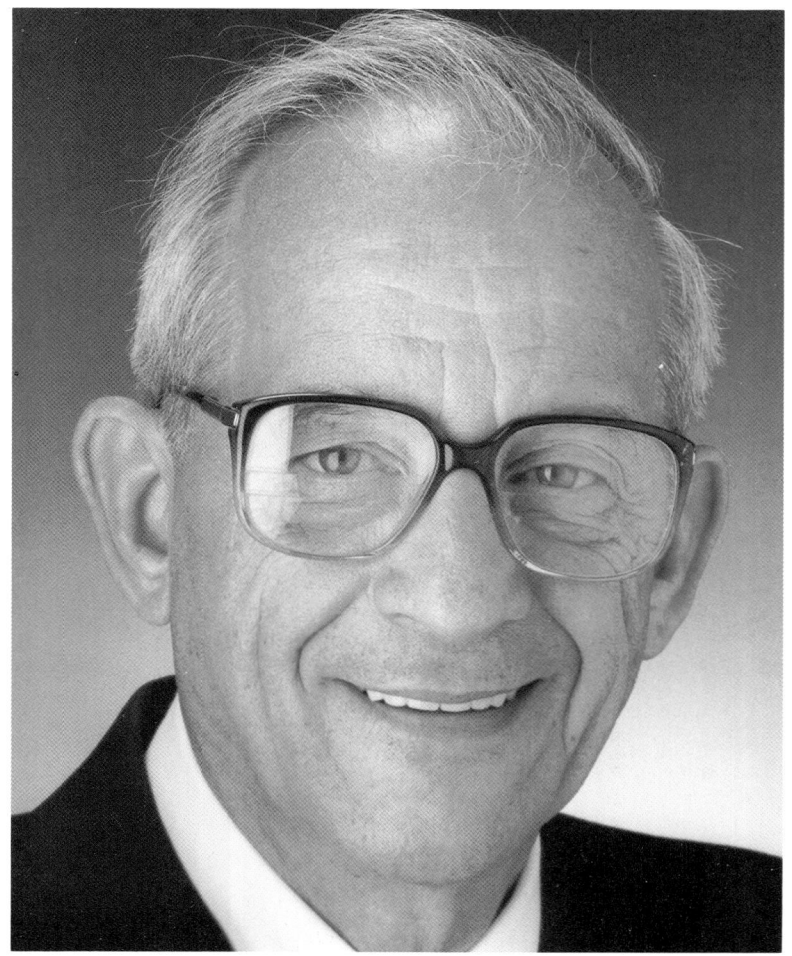

Eugene L. Staples, hospital administrator, 1982–1983; vice chancellor of hospital administration, 1983–1990.

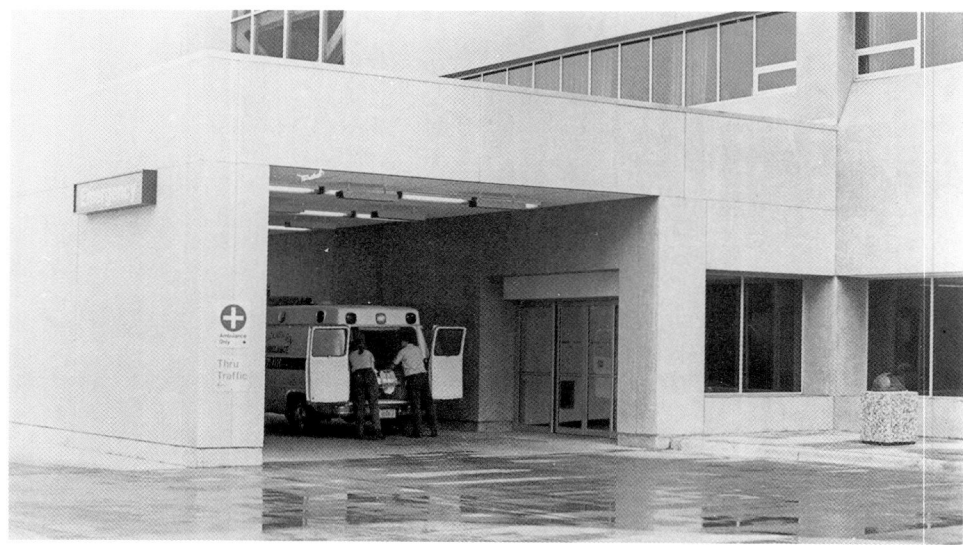

Hospital emergency entrance, 1980.

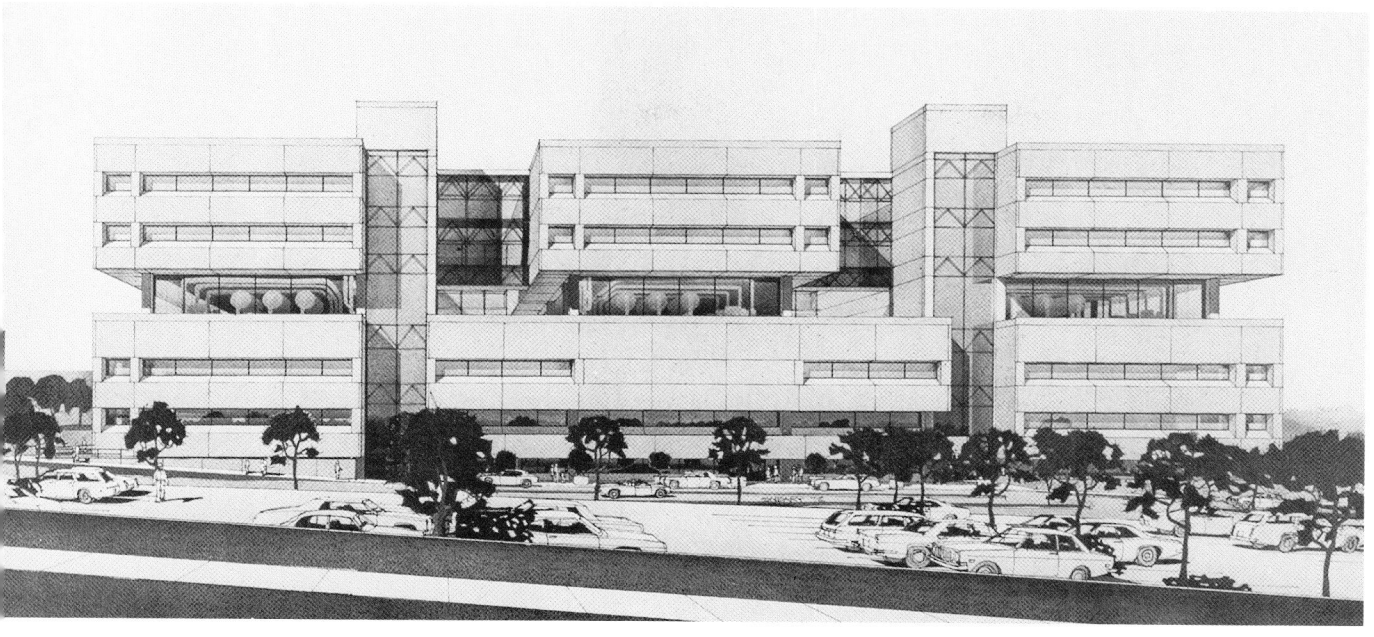

Architectural rendition of the new hospital, no date.

It appears that we could be facing a national crisis if the leading schools of medicine, such as ours, do not take decisive action. I want us to take a leading role in producing young scholars who will staff outstanding schools of medicine in the region and the nation.

In the years ahead, the school will need to place more emphasis on research and collaborative research with investigators from medicine, nursing and pharmacy. During the 1980s, the School of Allied Health deserves to be supported in its objectives to graduate students with high quality professional skills, to graduate students who are prepared for demanding clinical work, and to graduate students who have solid educational backgrounds.

I believe the Medical Center of the University of Kansas has the human resources to meet the most difficult of challenges. I also believe we have the will to succeed.
—Chancellor Gene A. Budig, University of Kansas Medical Center *Bulletin,* Winter 1982.

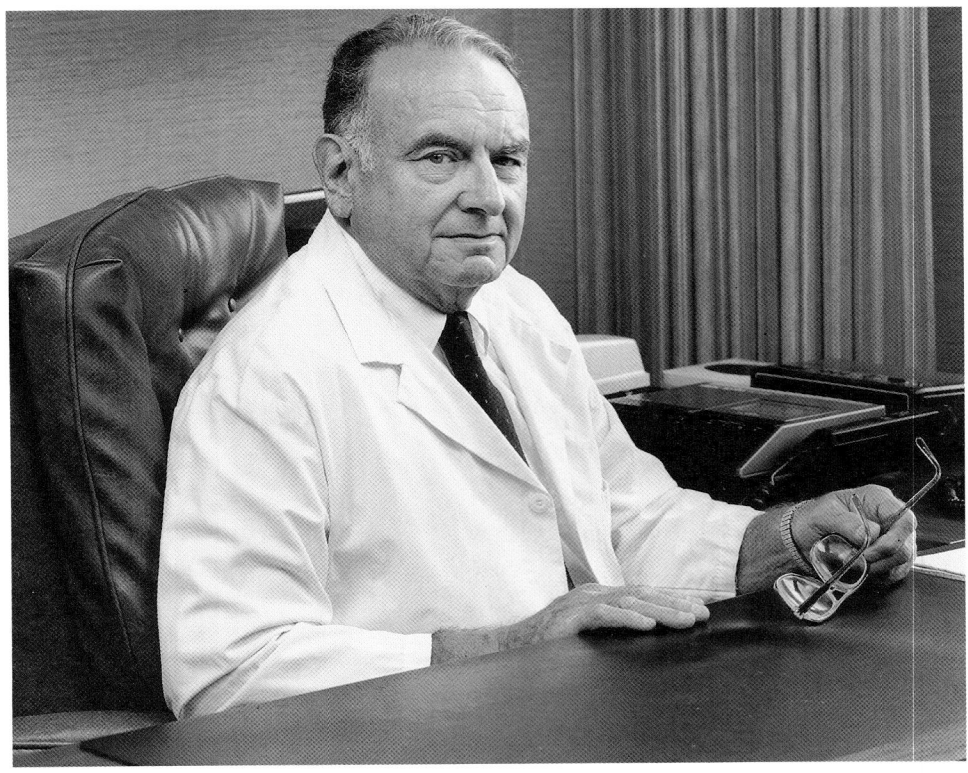

David Waxman, M.D., executive vice chancellor, 1977–1983.

The University of Kansas Bell Memorial Hospital is healthy and strong, and moving forward in the conduct of its very special mission for the state of Kansas. We have had budgetary problems, as have university hospitals across the nation. The proliferation of community hospitals and the ever-increasing commercialism and competition in health care have definitely had a negative impact upon teaching hospitals, especially, publicly-supported university hospitals. . . . Important changes have been made here within the last two years that place us in a very strong position to successfully cope with the pressures and challenges we are facing and will continue to face. We are in a position so that not only can we operate a financially sound hospital, but we can do it without adversely affecting our time-honored, traditional missions of *education, research,* and *public service.*
—The University of Kansas Medical Center/Bell Memorial Hospital Status Report, Dr. David Waxman, executive vice chancellor, to Legislative Budget Committee, July 20, 1983.

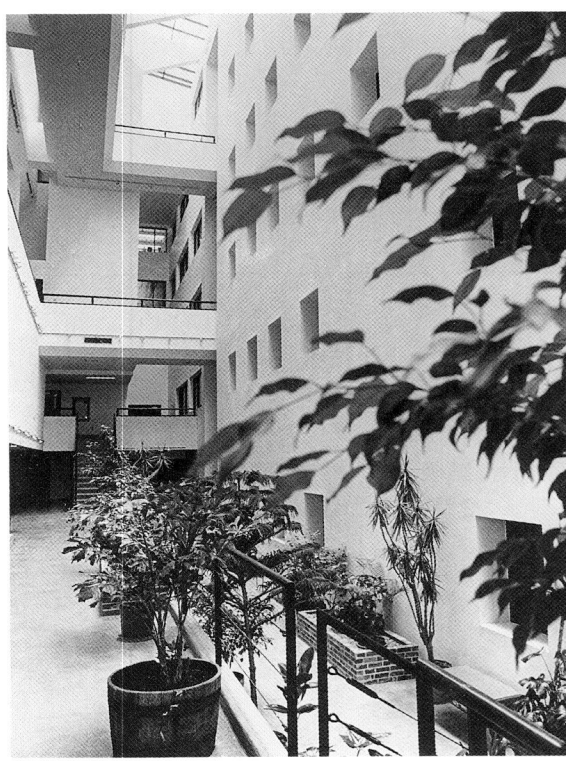

Interior of Orr-Major, 1979.

As one of the three foundations upon which academic health science centers are built, research activities at the College of Health Sciences contribute to making it the unique institution it is. The opportunities to conduct research and to teach future health professionals attract a special type of individual. Improvements in the research environment will ensure our continuing ability to recruit and retain the high quality of faculty expected of us.
—University of Kansas College of Health Sciences and Bell Memorial Hospital, "Goals and Objectives: Fiscal Years 1982–1983."

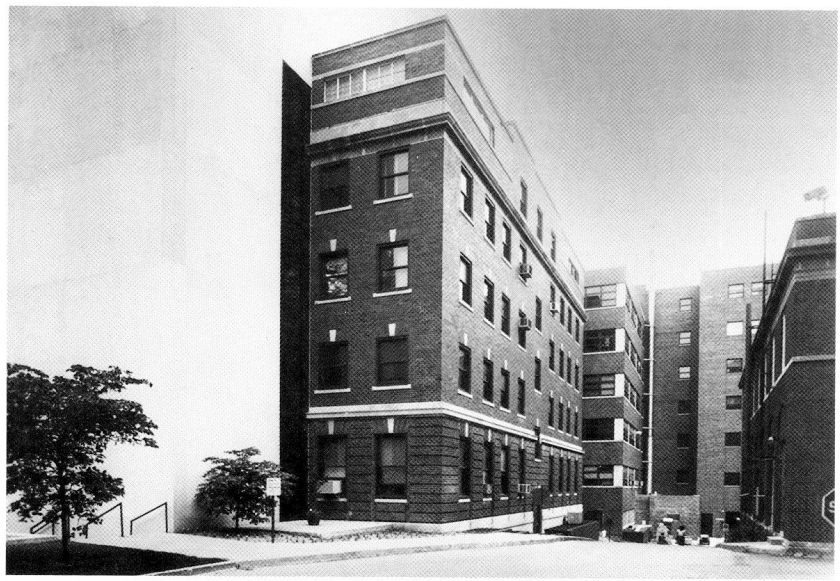

Hixon Laboratory and Orr-Major, 1980.

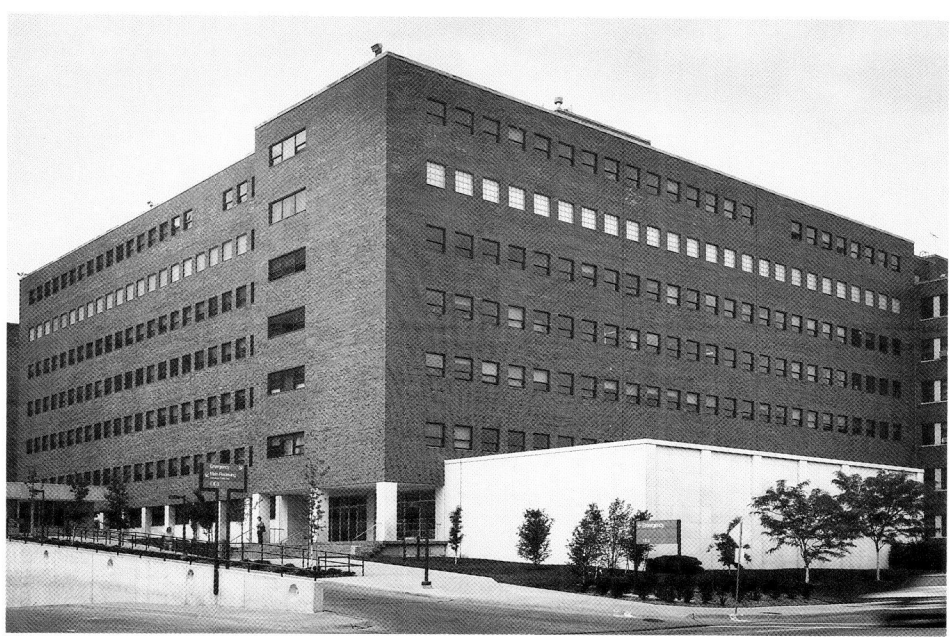

Wahl Hall East, May 1981.

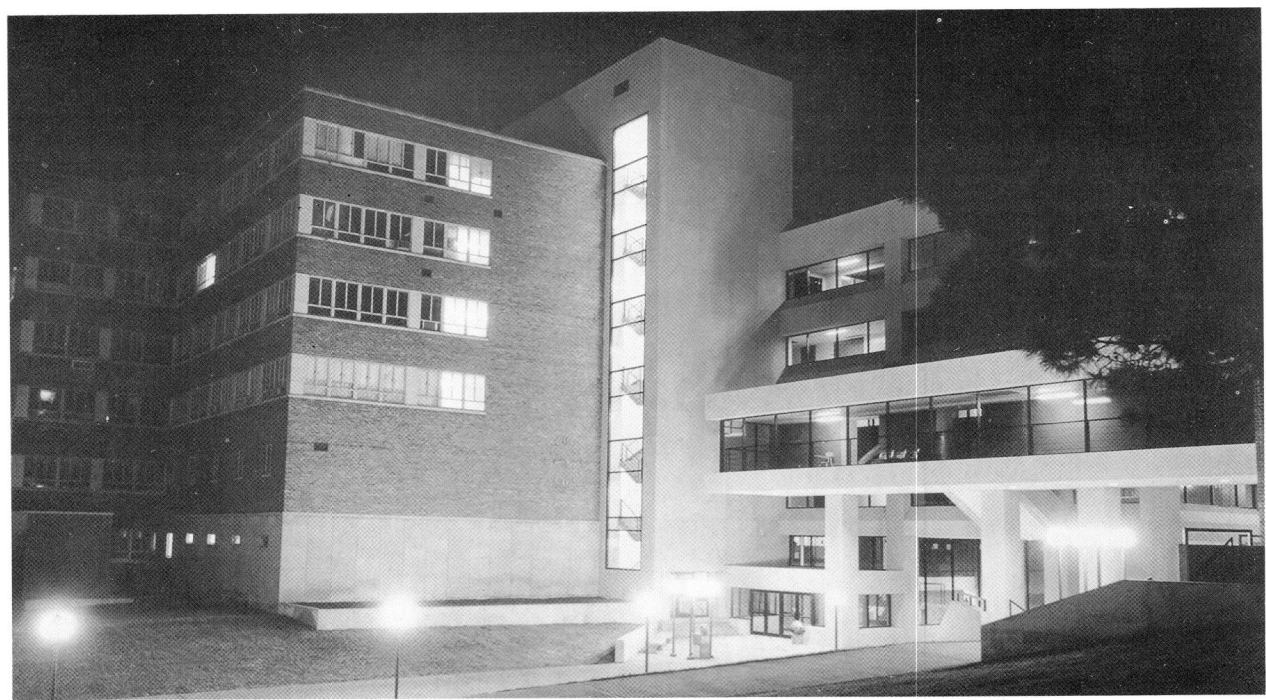

Wahl Hall West and Orr-Major, 1980.

The Kansas Board of Regents has approved plans for a new $5 million health sciences library at the Medical Center, to be built north of 39th Street across from Wahl Hall.

The new building will house all of the Medical Center's library except for the history of medicine and educational resources collections, which will remain in Robinson Hall (L).

The new library will include seating for more than 700 people in study carrels, small group study areas and reading lounges. It will be a two story, red brick building containing about 57,000 gross square feet and is designed to accommodate three additional floors for possible future expansion.—*Topics*, October 1980.

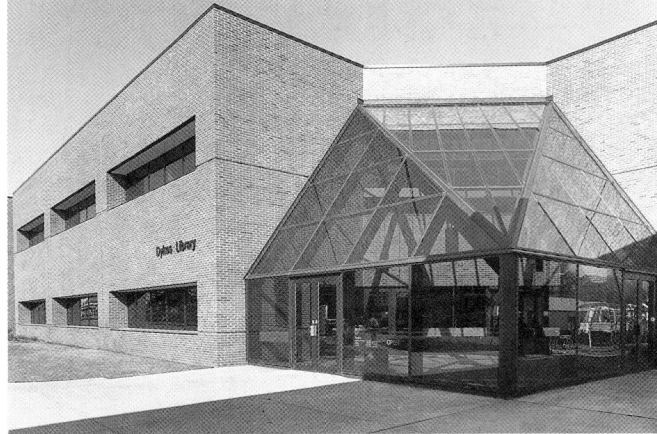

Archie R. Dykes Library, completed in 1983.

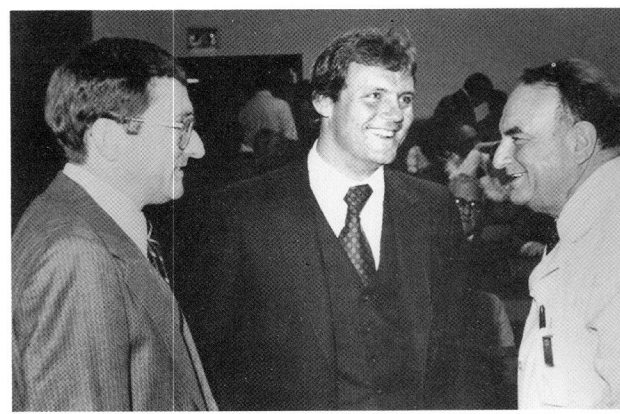

The dedication of the Amyotrophic Lateral Sclerosis (ALS) Regional Research Center with Chancellor Gene A. Budig, George Brett, and Executive Vice Chancellor David Waxman, M.D., 1982.

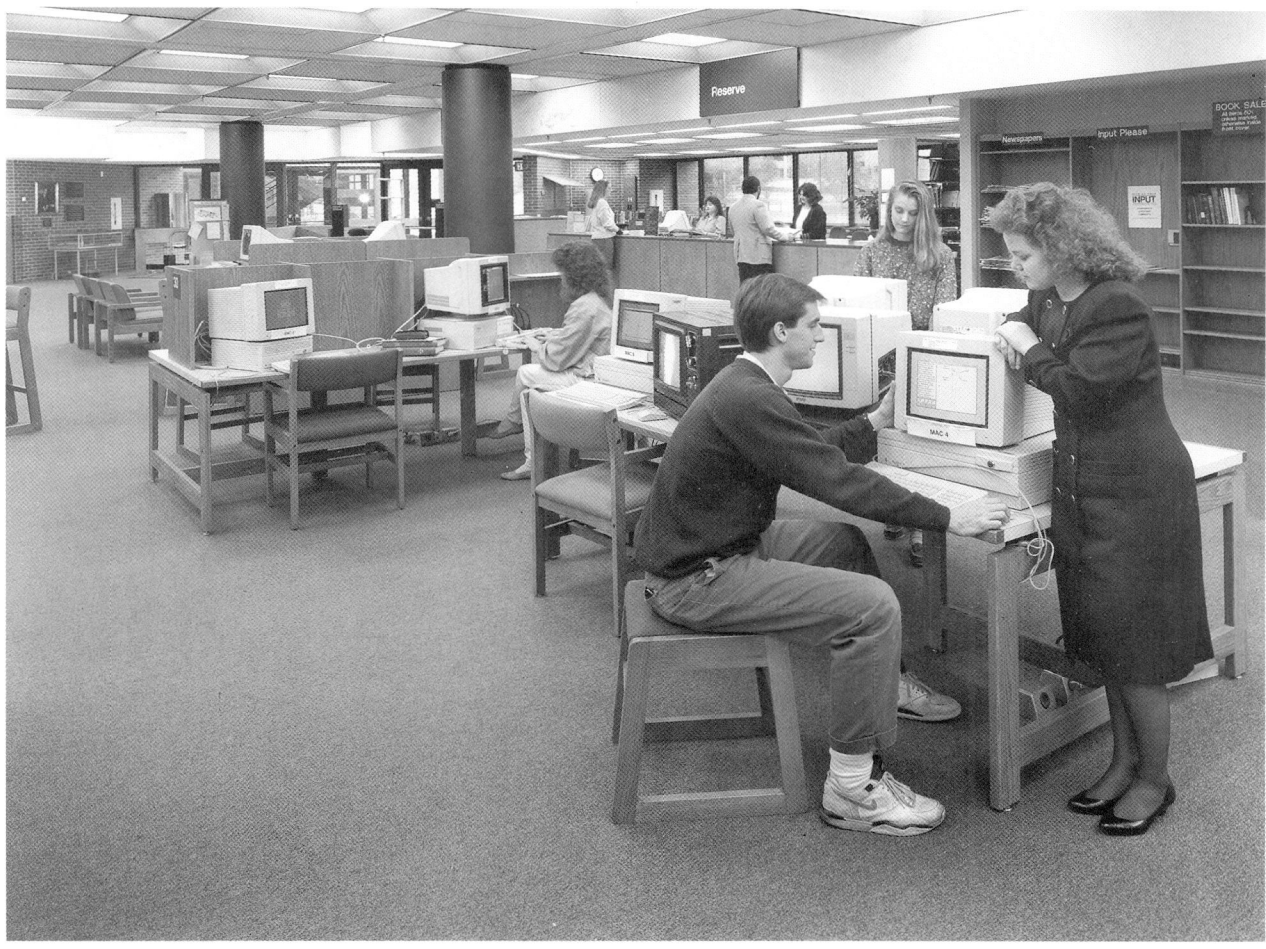

Students working at computers in Dykes Library, 1991.

In building a record of outstanding service and teaching, the center has developed corresponding strength in research. Investigators benefit from the resources of the university's libraries. In the Medical Center campus, the Archie R. Dykes Health Sciences Library, completed in 1983, contains more than 170,000 books, journals, and microforms. The Clendening History of Medicine Library houses 21,000 rare medical books.—University of Kansas *Bulletin*, 1989–1990.

The new Amyotrophic Lateral Sclerosis (ALS) Regional Research Center at the Medical Center will be formally dedicated . . . Wednesday, February 17, in Rieke Auditorium.

The dedication will recognize the commitment of funds from the ALS Society of America (ALSSOA) to establish the research center.

Guest speakers will include George Brett, Kansas City Royals, H. Eames Bishop, president of the ALS Society of America, and Keith Worthington, ALSSOA's area vice president.—*Topics*, February 1982.

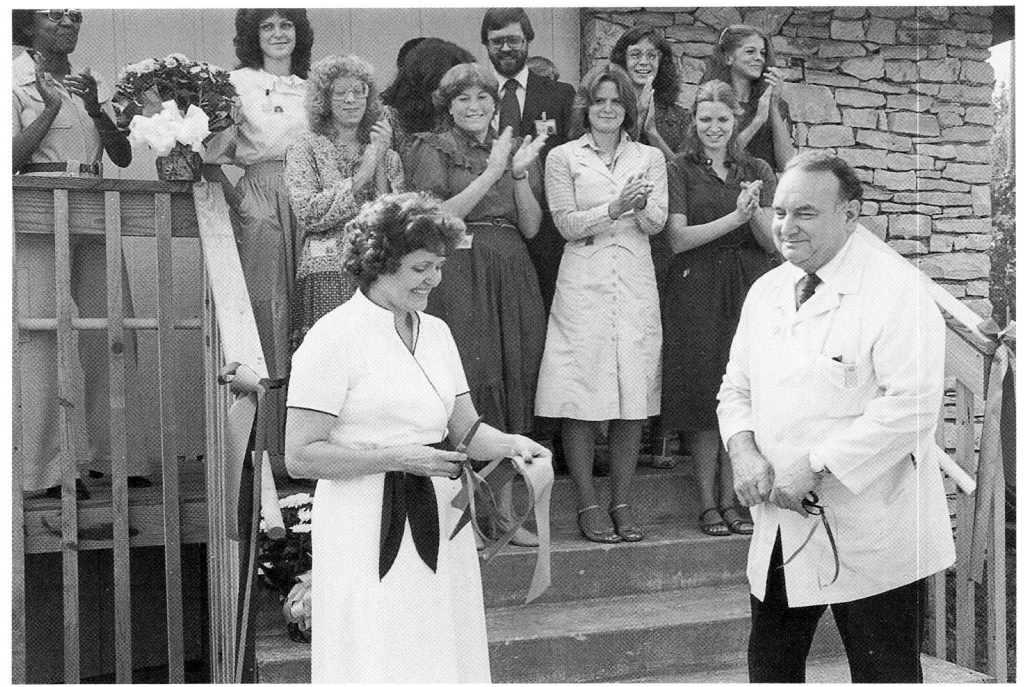

Dr. Waxman and Mrs. Pat Chapman at the ribbon-cutting ceremony for the Jay Care Learning Center, August 1982.

As an incentive to retain University of Kansas Medical Center staff, a new learning center has been established for the employees' children. . . .

The idea for the center originated one and a half years ago, because of complaints from medical students and nurses about the difficulty of finding child care services.

The auxiliary donated $38,000 and borrowed $64,000 from the Kansas University Endowment Association for equipment, general operating expenses and renovation of the former fraternity house and office building that houses the center.
—*University Daily Kansan*, August 31, 1982.

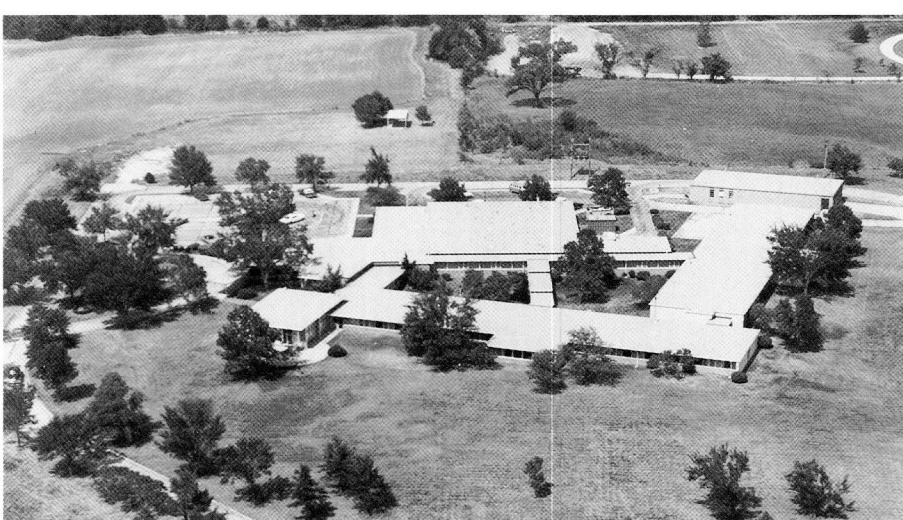

The Area Health Education Center in Chanute, Kansas.

The educational program of the University of Kansas School of Medicine is designed to assist the student in achieving his own goals for a professional career in medicine. The fundamentals provided should prepare the student for development of a career in family medicine as well as a specialty practice. The educational plan places importance on the student's ability to think for himself, to demonstrate initiative, imagination, intellectual curiosity, and scientific critique and resourcefulness; to face alternatives and make decisions; and to develop understanding of diseases and of persons rather than the knowledge of disease alone. Emphasis is placed upon performance, judgement, discrimination, and intellectual self-reliance. Although it is important that intellectual talents of the student should be developed to the fullest, it is equally vital that the qualities of temperament, human sympathy, and insight required for dealing with the many problems of the humanistic aspects of medical care be emphasized. The knowledge, skills, attitudes, and behavior essential to the practice of medicine are the goals of the educational program of this school.—University of Kansas Medical Center Report, 1981.

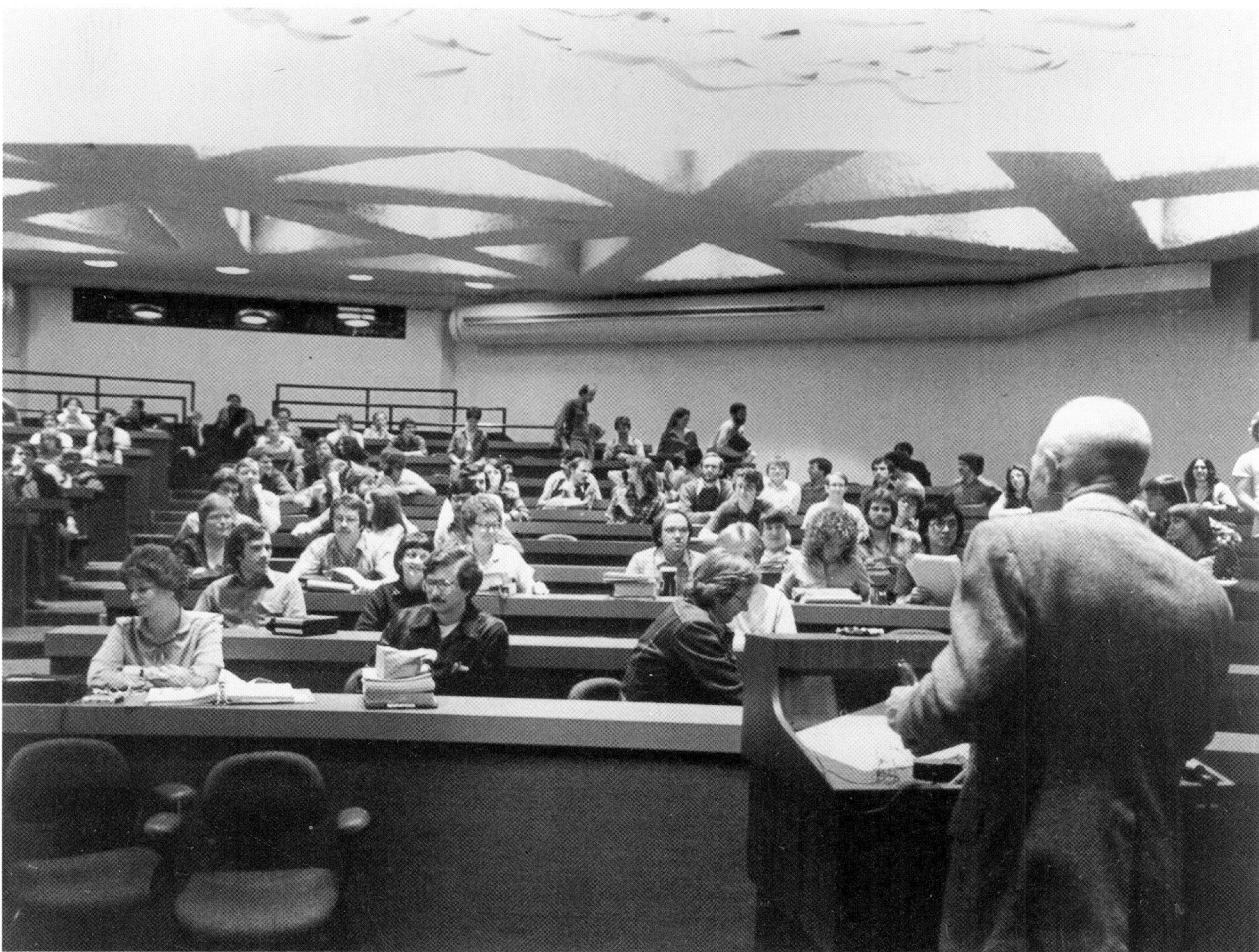

A class of medical students in Rieke Auditorium, December 1982.

You are an integral part of our College of Health Sciences and Hospital and must shoulder the responsibility in the years ahead to provide leadership in this your chosen profession. Your school has developed a faculty who are committed to excellence and are available to you from now on. Our Center which includes a beautiful new hospital is yours to work in and appreciate the best in modern equipment and technology. The Medical Center is here because you are here. Without you, there would be no Medical Center.

—David Waxman, M.D., School of Nursing Convocation, September 1, 1982.

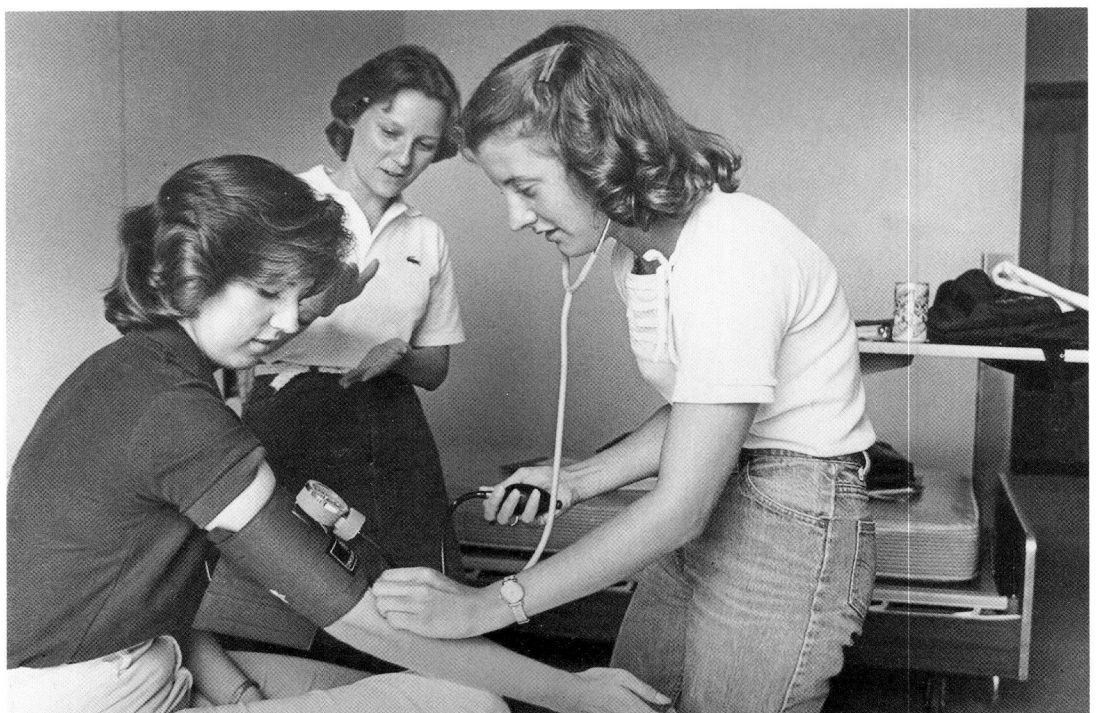

Nursing students practicing taking blood pressure.

A demonstration of the Jaystork, the Medical Center's Neonatal Intensive Care Unit, October 1980.

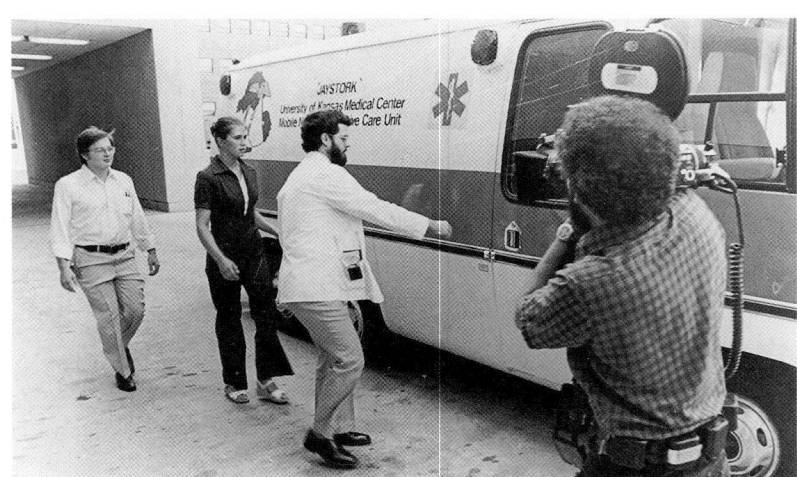

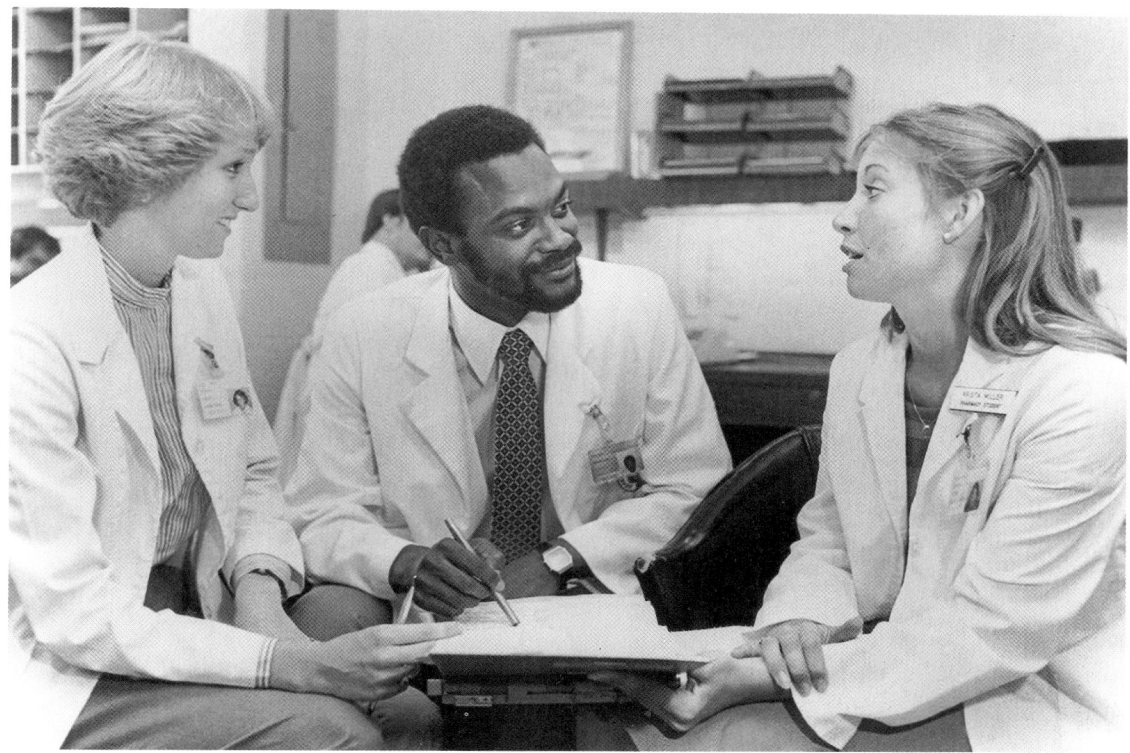

Students in pharmacy education, July 1982.

Students have an important responsibilty to acquire a vast array of information, concepts and skills. They also have a responsibility to adopt productive and efficient study regimes. They must constantly define priorities and budget their time and efforts accordingly. It is a responsibility of the faculty to communicate their expectations in as unambiguous and informative a manner as possible, so that the students can best meet the standards of achievement we have set for them.—University of Kansas College of Health Sciences and Bell Memorial Hospital, "Goals and Objectives: Fiscal Years 1982–1983."

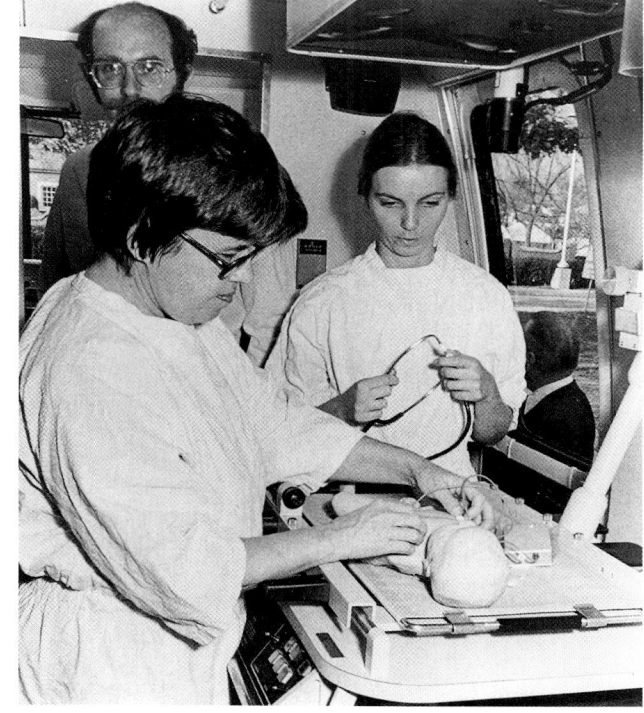

Warren Rosenthal, M.D., Mary McCue, R.N., and Jackie Moore, R.N., assist an infant in the Jaystork, ca. 1980.

The Gene and Barbara Burnett Burn Center (6th floor of B Building) celebrated its tenth anniversary of operation last month. Established in 1973 with the help of generous private donations, the burn center has served more than 1,000 severely burned patients.

Since opening 10 years ago, the burn center has been without a patient once and only once and that was for 11 hours. The number of patients being treated in the burn center increases each year. —*Topics*, July 1983.

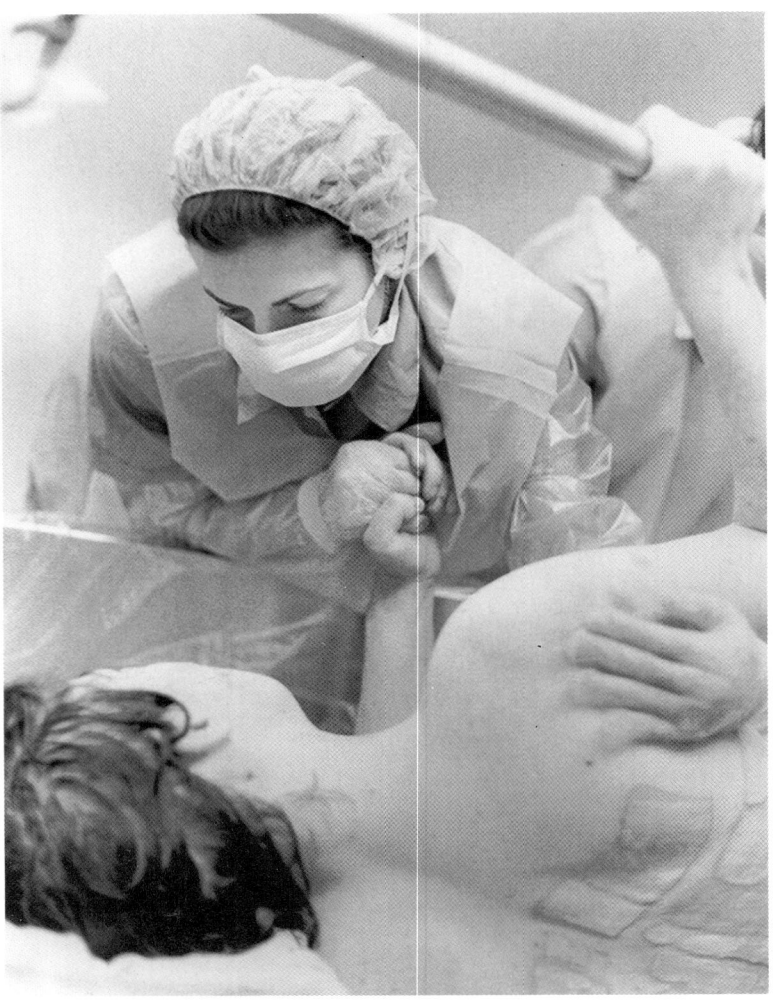

The Burnett Burn Center, ca. 1981.

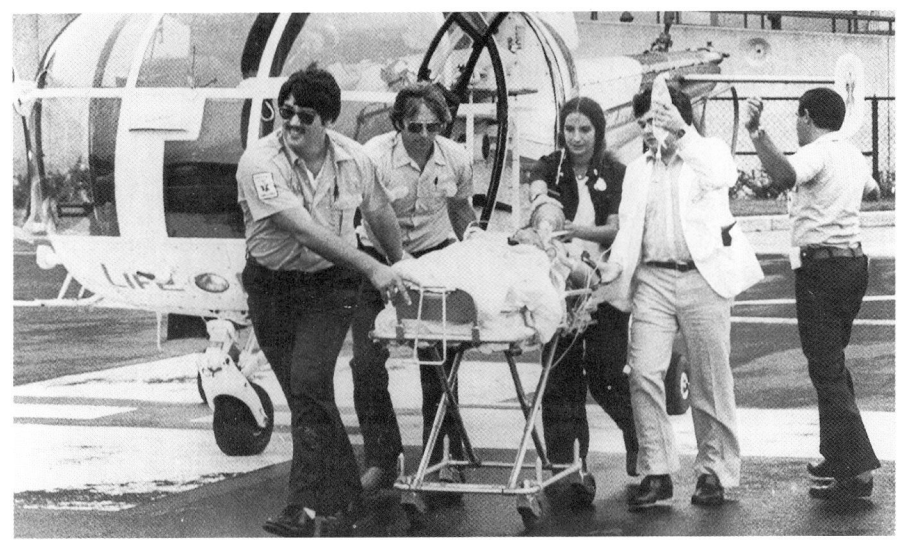

A patient brought to the Medical Center by Life Flight, 1981.

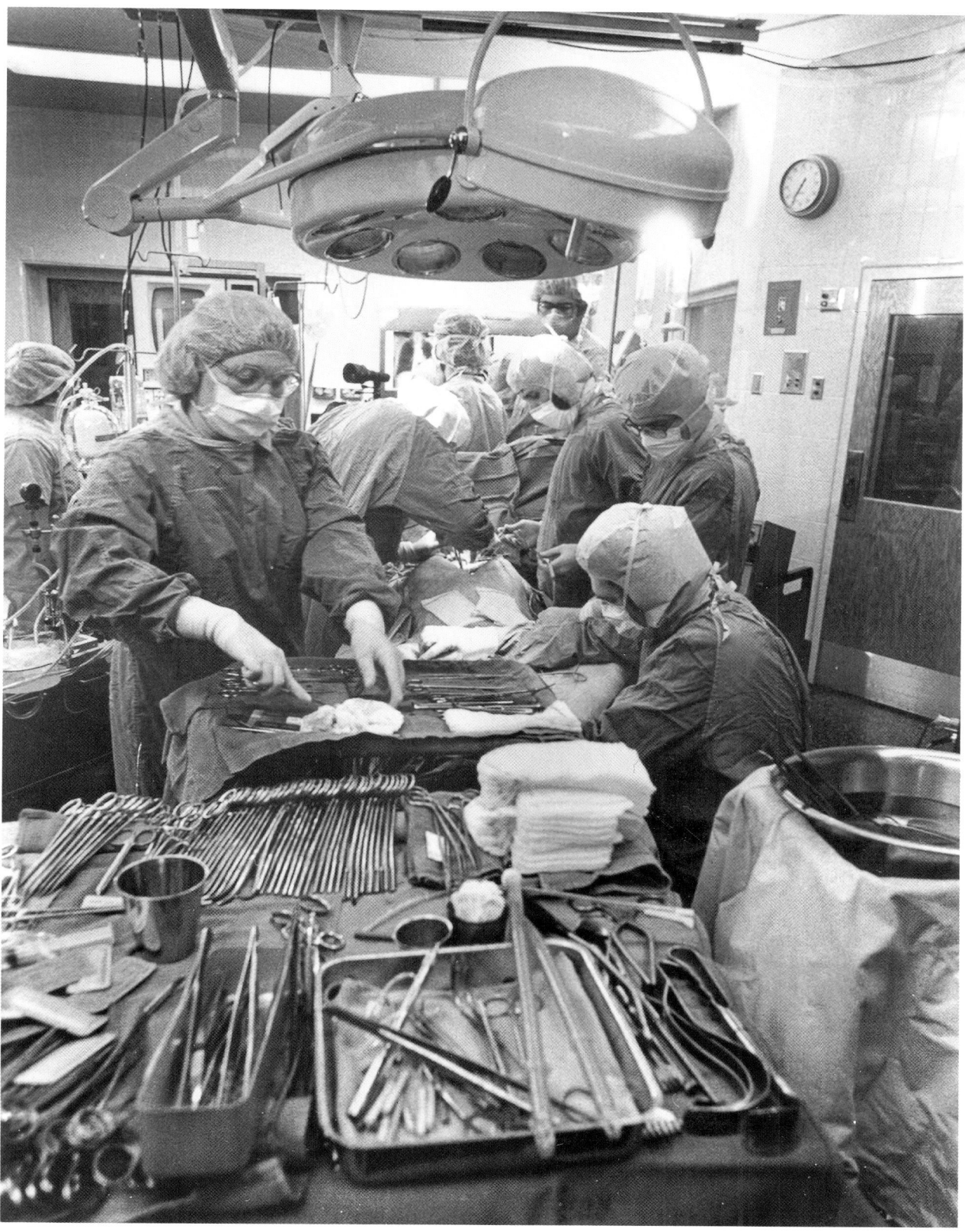

An operation in progress, fall 1980.

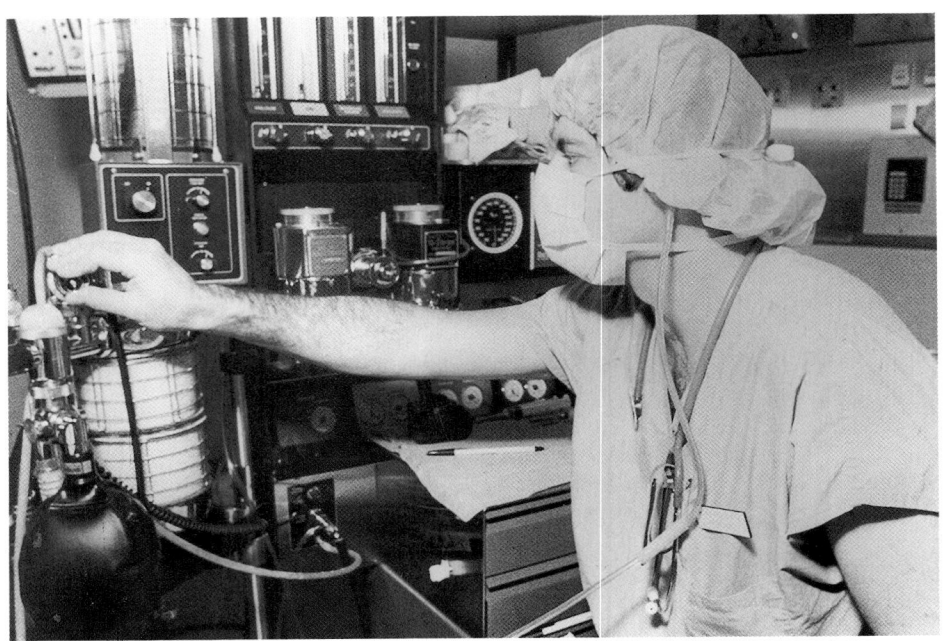

Nurse Anesthesia, 1981.

It is my belief that quality educational experiences are based on the findings from research. I also believe that research and scholarly endeavor are essential to upgrading or maintaining effective teaching. This view is held by many people in other disciplines and by most academicians. A major difference, however, is that few academic programs include a professional practice component. Research in nursing not only impacts the educational program but also, in the long run, the improvement of patient-care—our ultimate goal in nursing.
—Doris A. Geitgey, R.N., Ed.D., dean, *Janus*, Fall 1981.

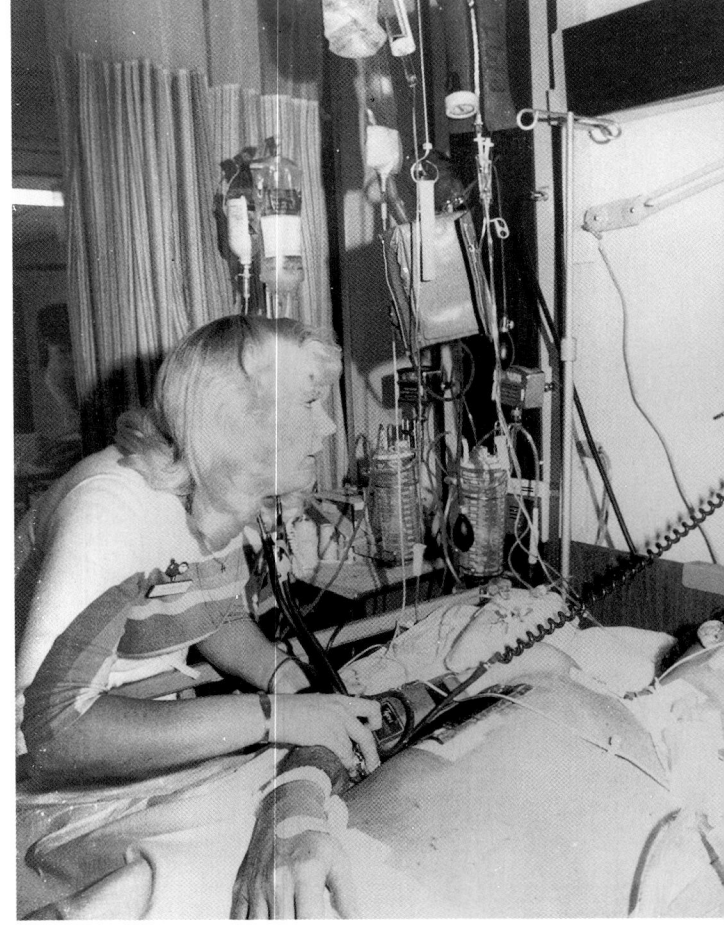

The Intensive Care Unit, October 1981.

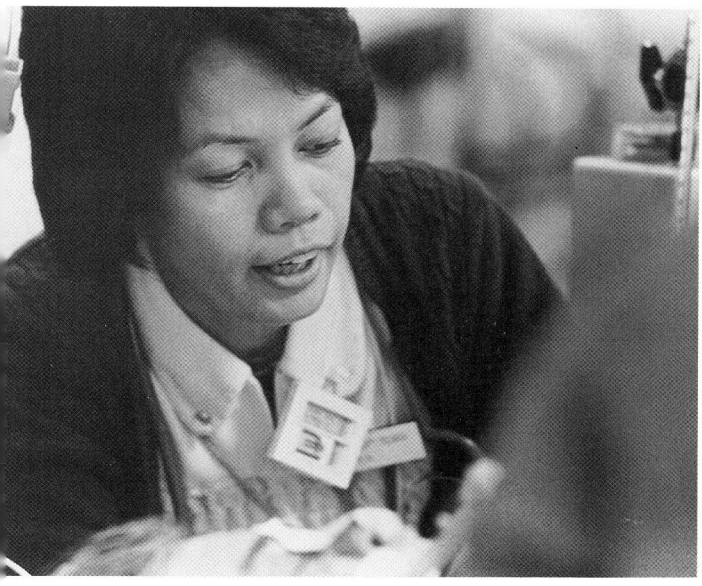

Nursing Services, February 1980.

Graduate education in nursing prepares the individual not only for advanced clinical practice but also clinical research. The increased emphasis on research in graduate programs in nursing is clearly an indicator of a growing interest both in expanding the knowledge base of nursing practice and in increasing sophistication of nurse faculty and students in research methodology. The launching of several successful new professional nursing journals dedicated to the reporting of nursing research is a clear indicator of the current zeal being demonstrated for pursuit of scholarly endeavors both in the classroom and in the practice setting.
—*Janus*, Fall 1981.

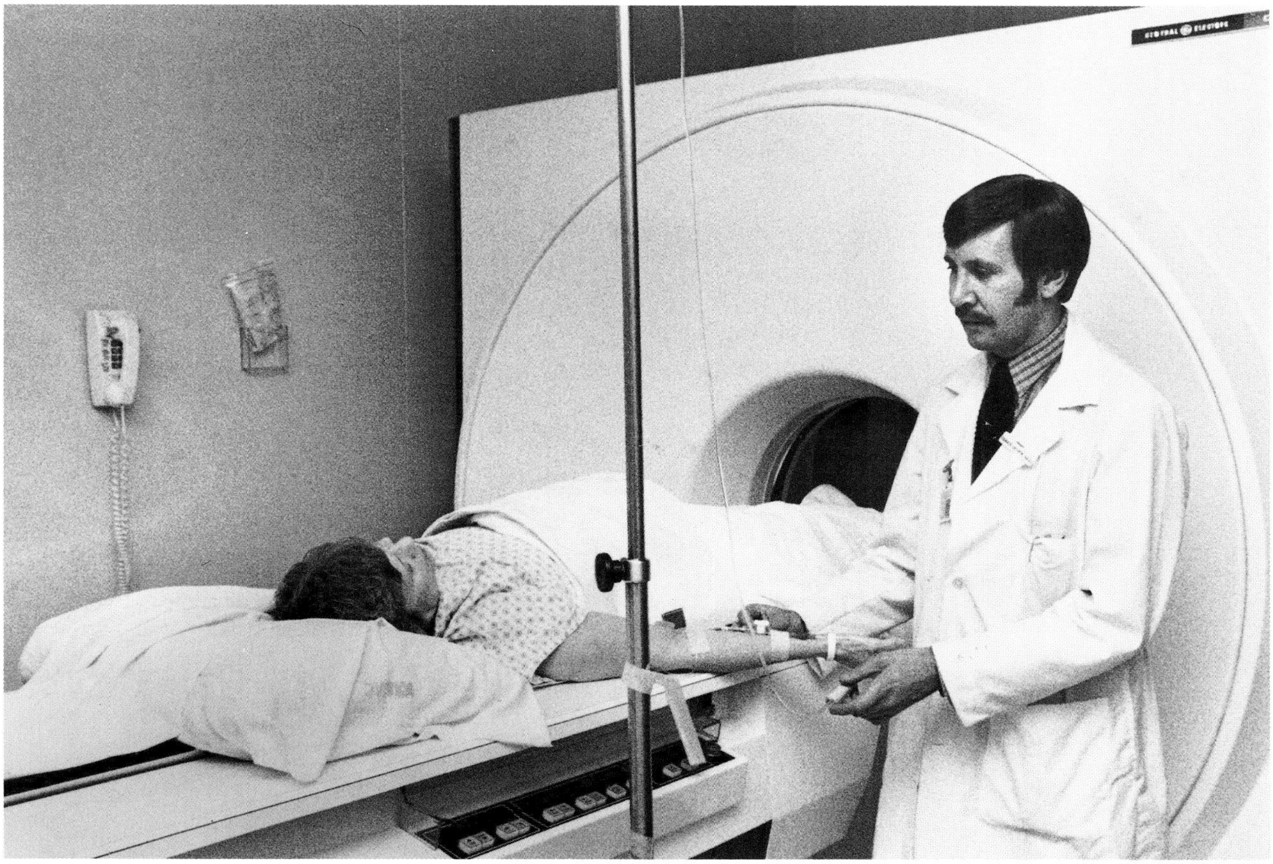

Errol Levine, M.D., with the CAT scanner, 1981.

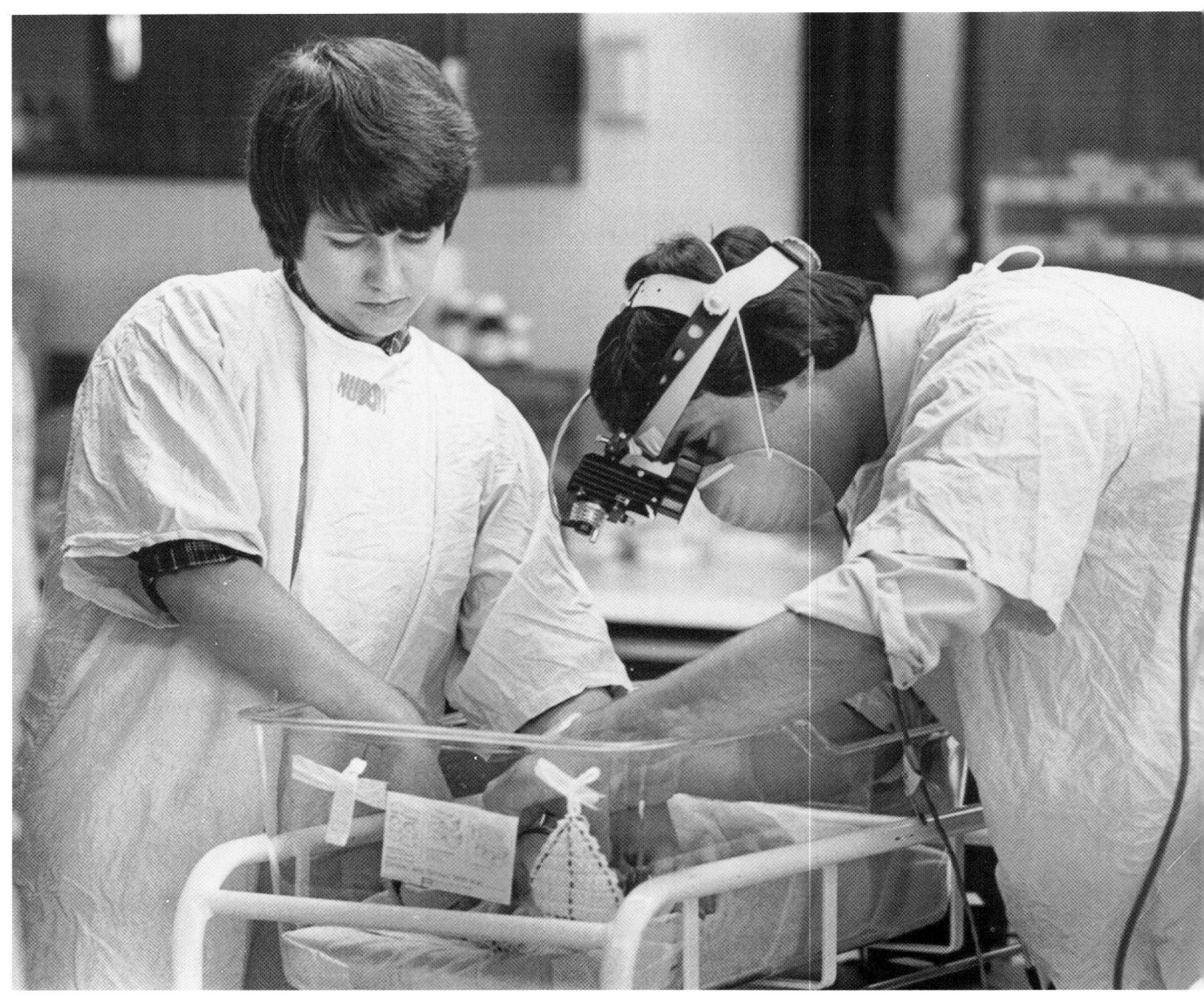

Ophthalmology care in the nursery, 1980.

I am extremely excited about this opportunity at the University of Kansas and its programs at the Medical Center, in Wichita and throughout the state. . . . This is a great school and I look forward to becoming a member of the excellent team at the University of Kansas. . . .

Kansas has excellent programs in health science teaching, research and service. I will strive for even greater levels of excellence.

—D. Kay Clawson, M.D., executive vice chancellor, *Topics*, May–June 1983.

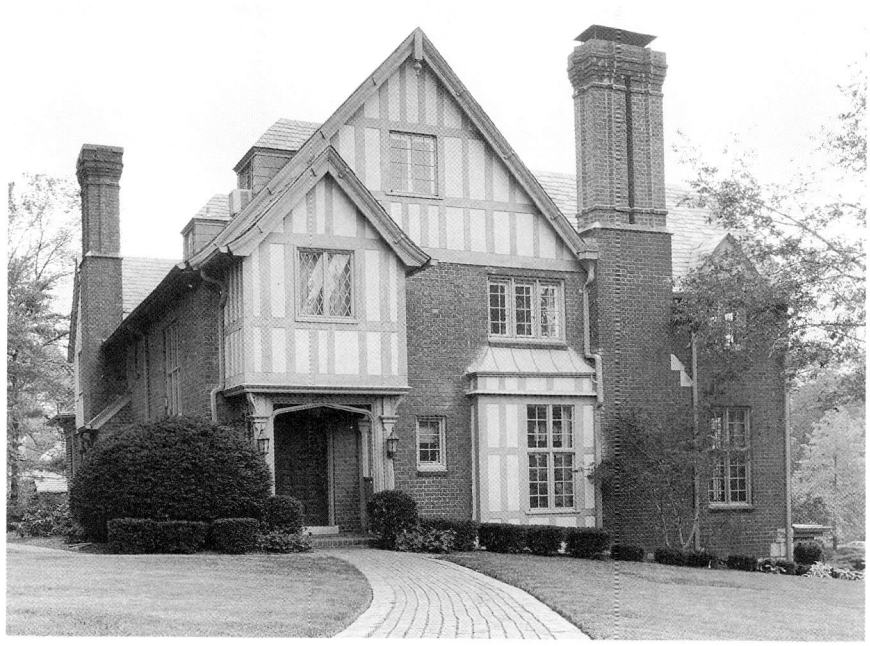

Spencer House, 1990.

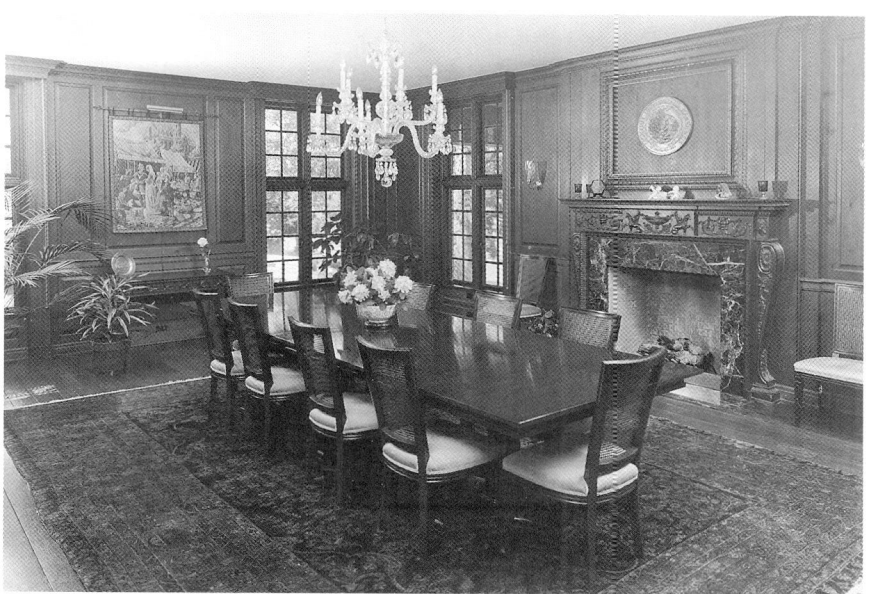

Spencer House interior, 1990.

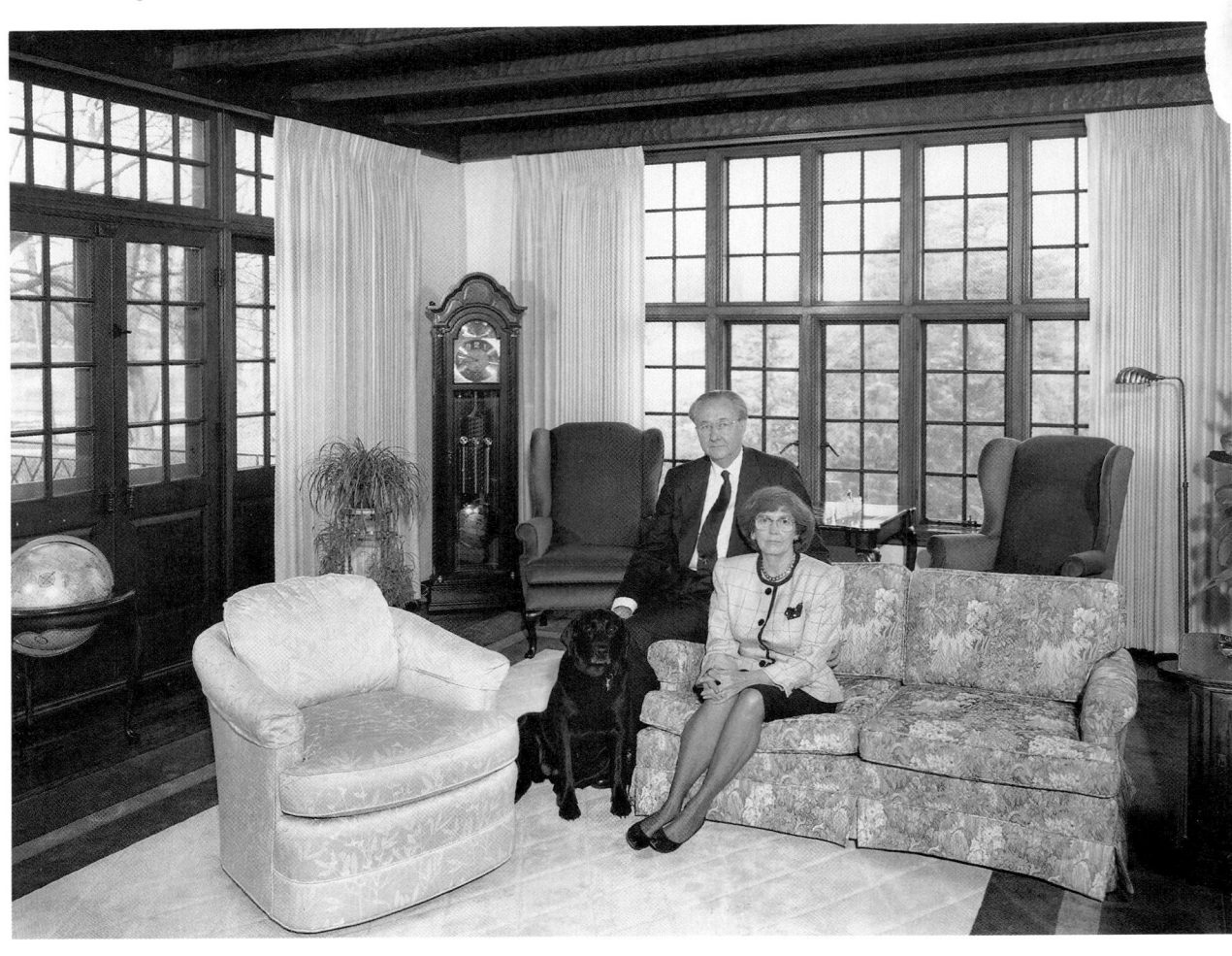

D. Kay Clawson, M.D., and Mrs. Clawson at Spencer House, the executive
vice chancellor's residence, April 20, 1990.

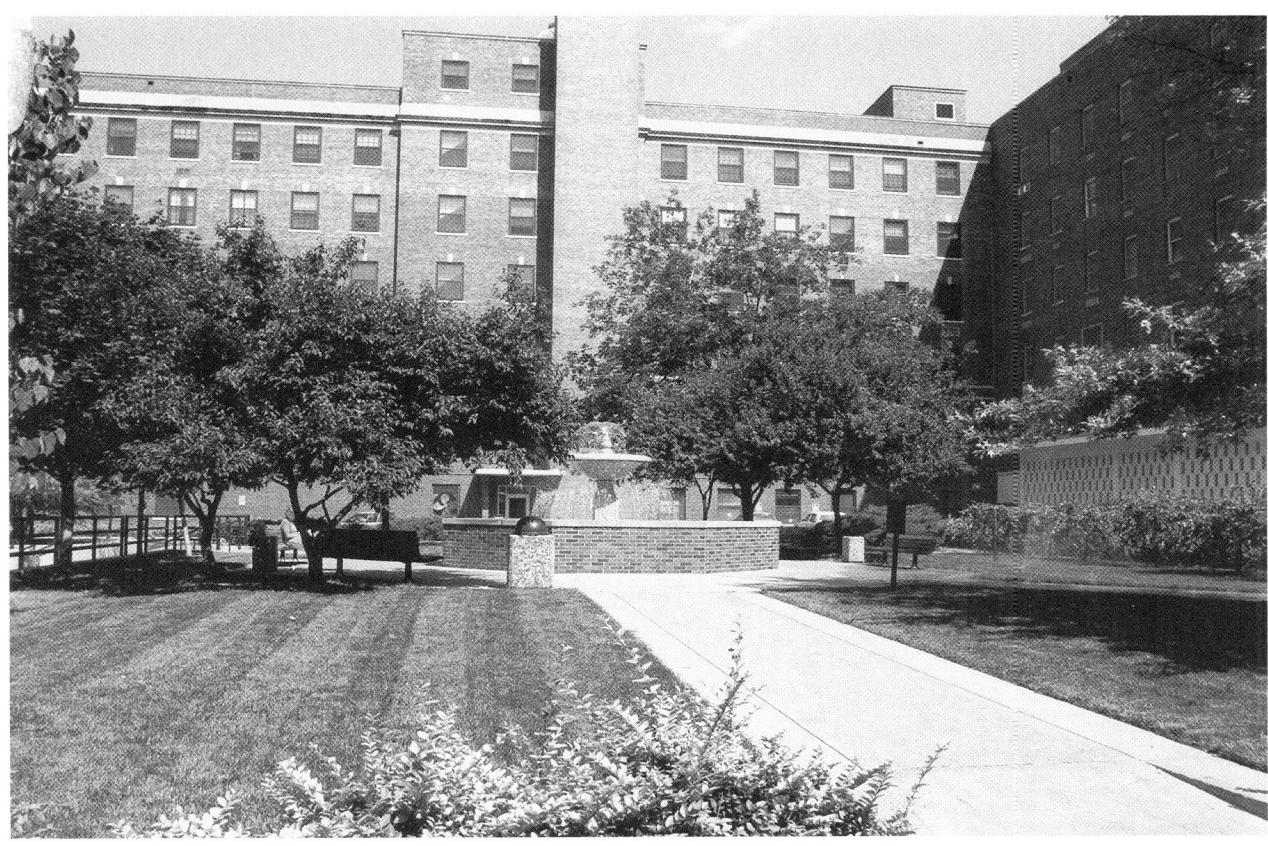

The Clendening fountain area on a summer day, by J. Tyler Motsinger, August 1989.

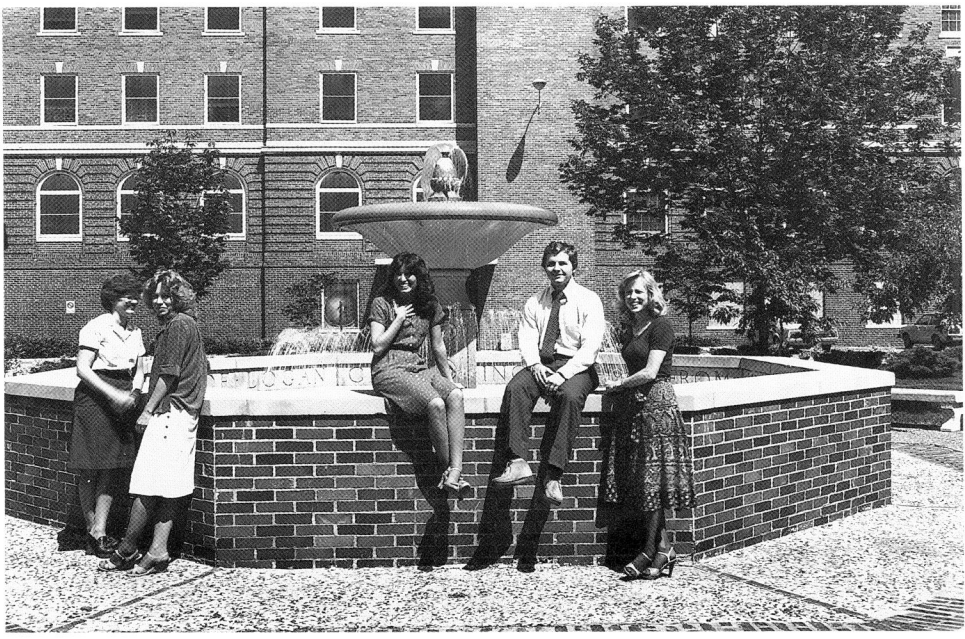

A group of students at the fountain, ca. 1989.

The University of Kansas School of Medicine is a very special institution. Our history is rich and our alumni accomplishments many. KU's contribution to the physician manpower of the state has steadily increased, and now 46.6% of all practicing Kansas physicians are K.U. graduates. Perhaps even more impressive is that 58% of the primary care physicians in the state are K.U. graduates and of physicians practicing in critically underserved areas, 71% represent our graduates, while in the underserved areas 92% of the physicians are K.U. graduates.—D. Kay Clawson, M.D., executive vice chancellor, speech at the Medical Alumni Banquet, May 1987.

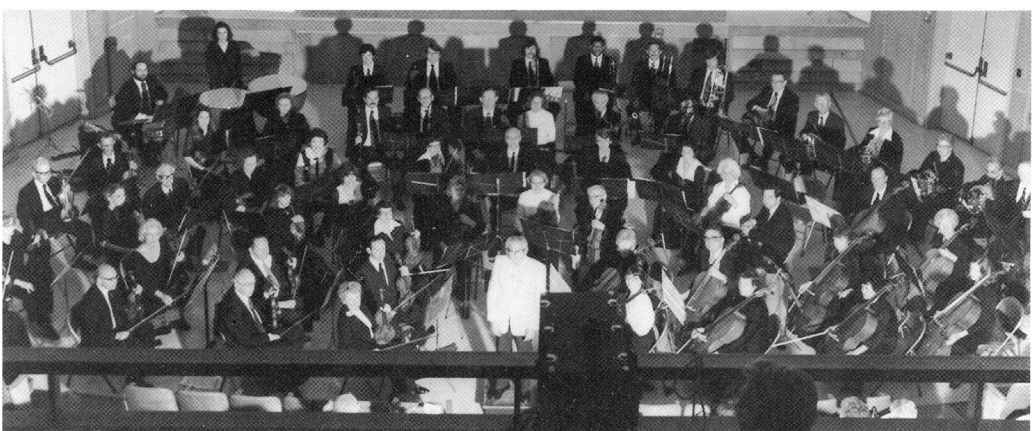

The Medical Arts Symphony, 1980s.

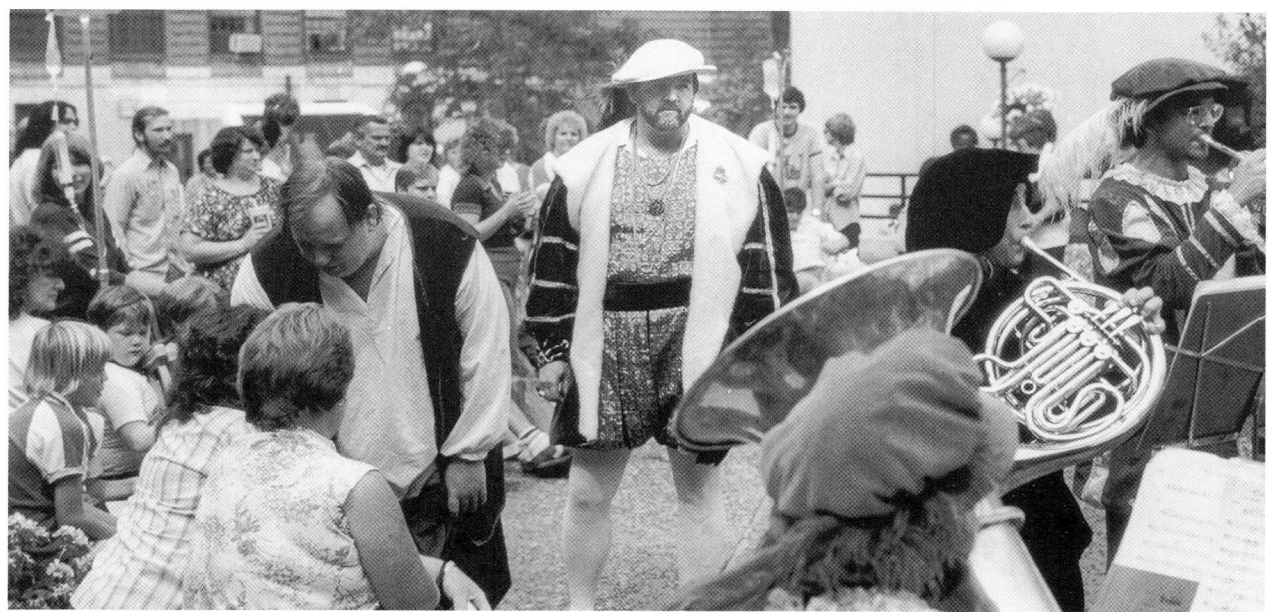

A Renaissance troupe entertaining near the Clendening fountain, ca. 1986.

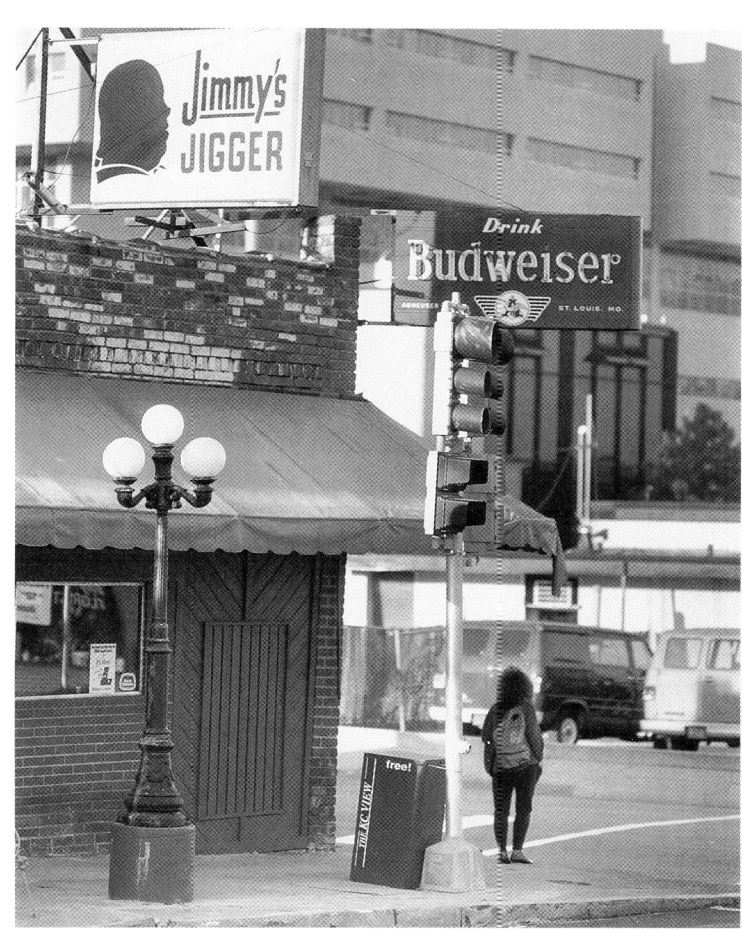

Jimmy's Jigger, a long-time favorite watering hole at 39th and State Line, September 1989.

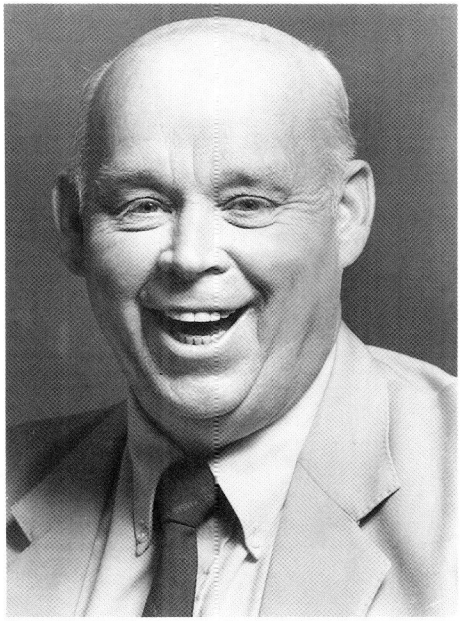

Jimmy Bowers of Jimmy's Jigger.

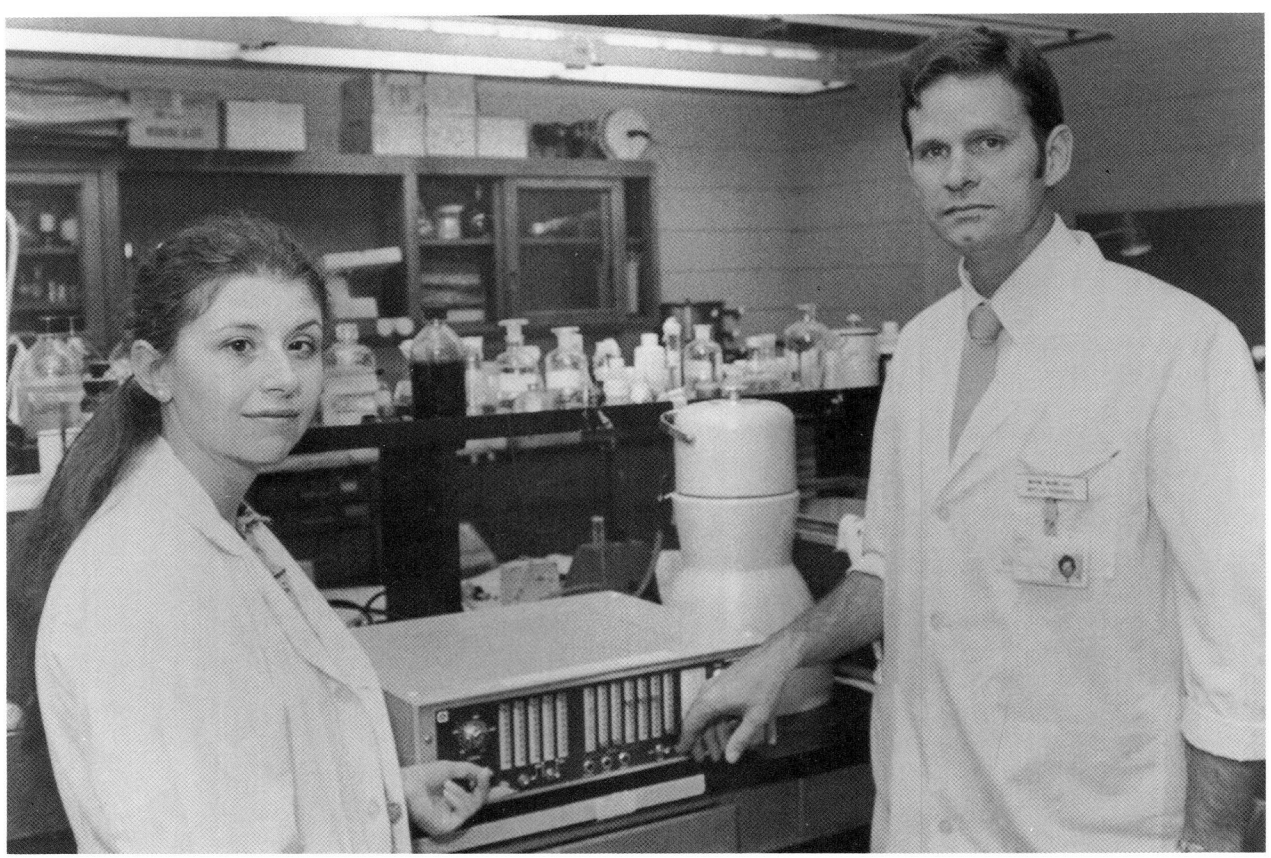

The Clinical Research Center, 1983.

Our research programs must be expanded and intensified. This emphasis need not be at the expense of our educational and clinical efforts. We are a "community of Scholars," but this does not refer to a sequestered, elite group of intellectuals removed from practical responsibilities; it refers to an environment within which new knowledge is generated, knowledge that maybe is translated into improved health—indirectly via education and directly via research. Therefore, we must reinforce this feature of our landscape.—University of Kansas College of Health Sciences and Bell Memorial Hospital, "Goals and Objectives: Fiscal Years 1982–1983."

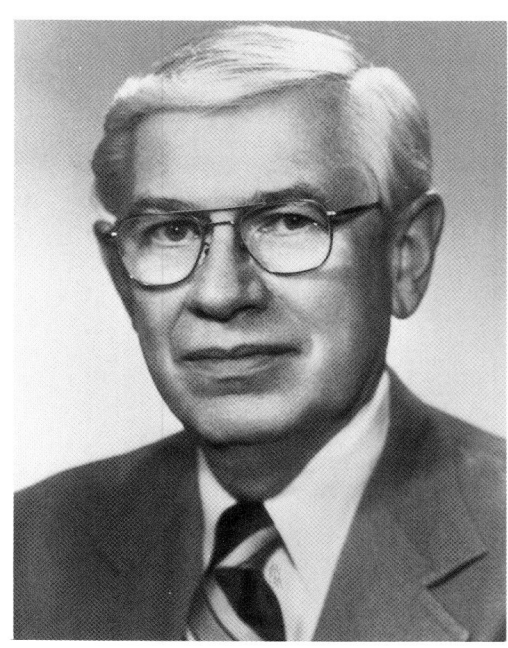

William J. Reals, M.D., vice chancellor and dean of the University of Kansas School of Medicine–Wichita.

The Department of Allied Health Sciences has two major functions: to provide advanced education to a wide variety of health care practitioners, and to develop core courses which are common to other programs in the School.

Those who enter the program may be certified in a variety of allied health occupations, including Radiologic Technology, Emergency Medical Training, Cytotechnology, Nuclear Medicine Technology, and Special Radiographic Procedures.

The second major function of the department is to develop common courses offered to all three Schools at the Med Center, presently exemplified by "Legal Aspects of Health Care" and "The Process of Patient Teaching". Future development of other courses is expected.—*Jayhawker MD*, 1984.

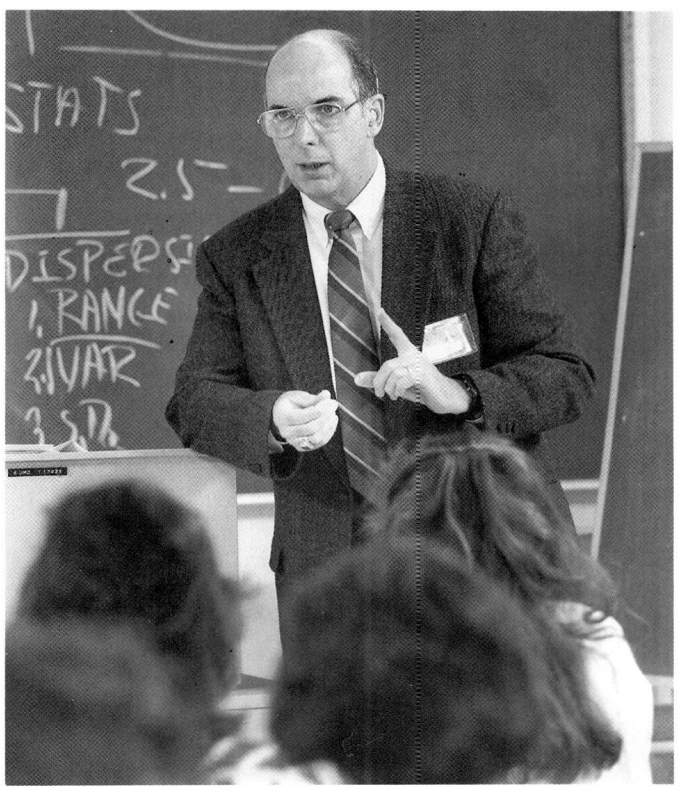

James P. Cooney, Ph.D., dean of the School of Allied Health.

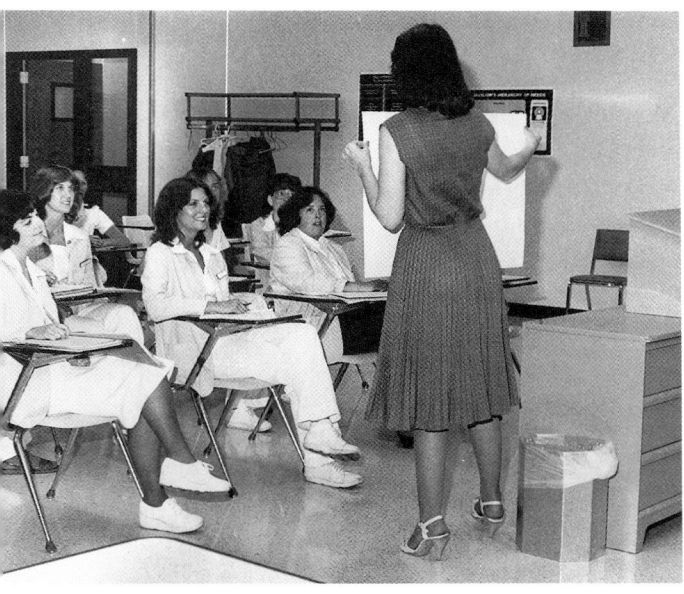

Medical Records Administration, 1981.

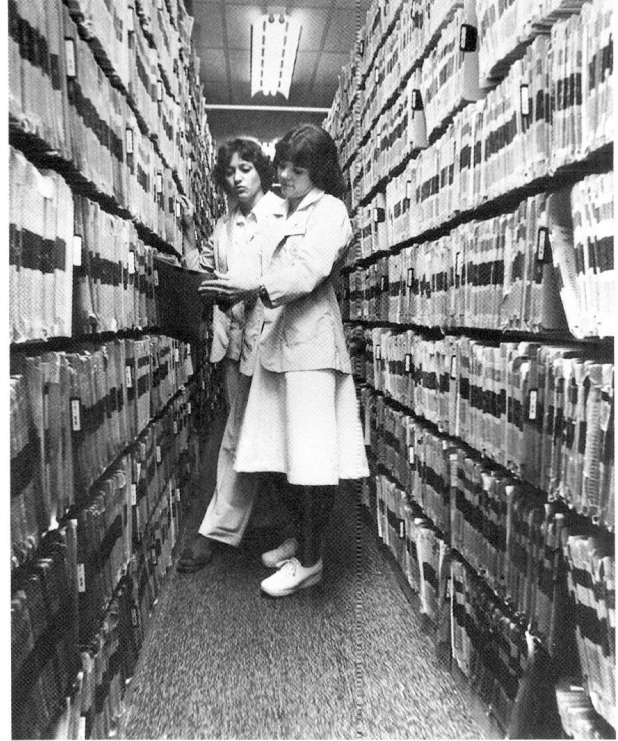

A medical records class, 1981.

Enrollment this year in the KU medical technology program is the highest in 10 years, and the increase may be attributable to increased recruiting in the face of a national shortage of medical technologists.

After years of meager enrollments, the School of Allied Health this year has drawn 25 students to the University of Kansas Medical Center for the final year of the four year med-tech program.—*University Daily Kansan*, August 28, 1989.

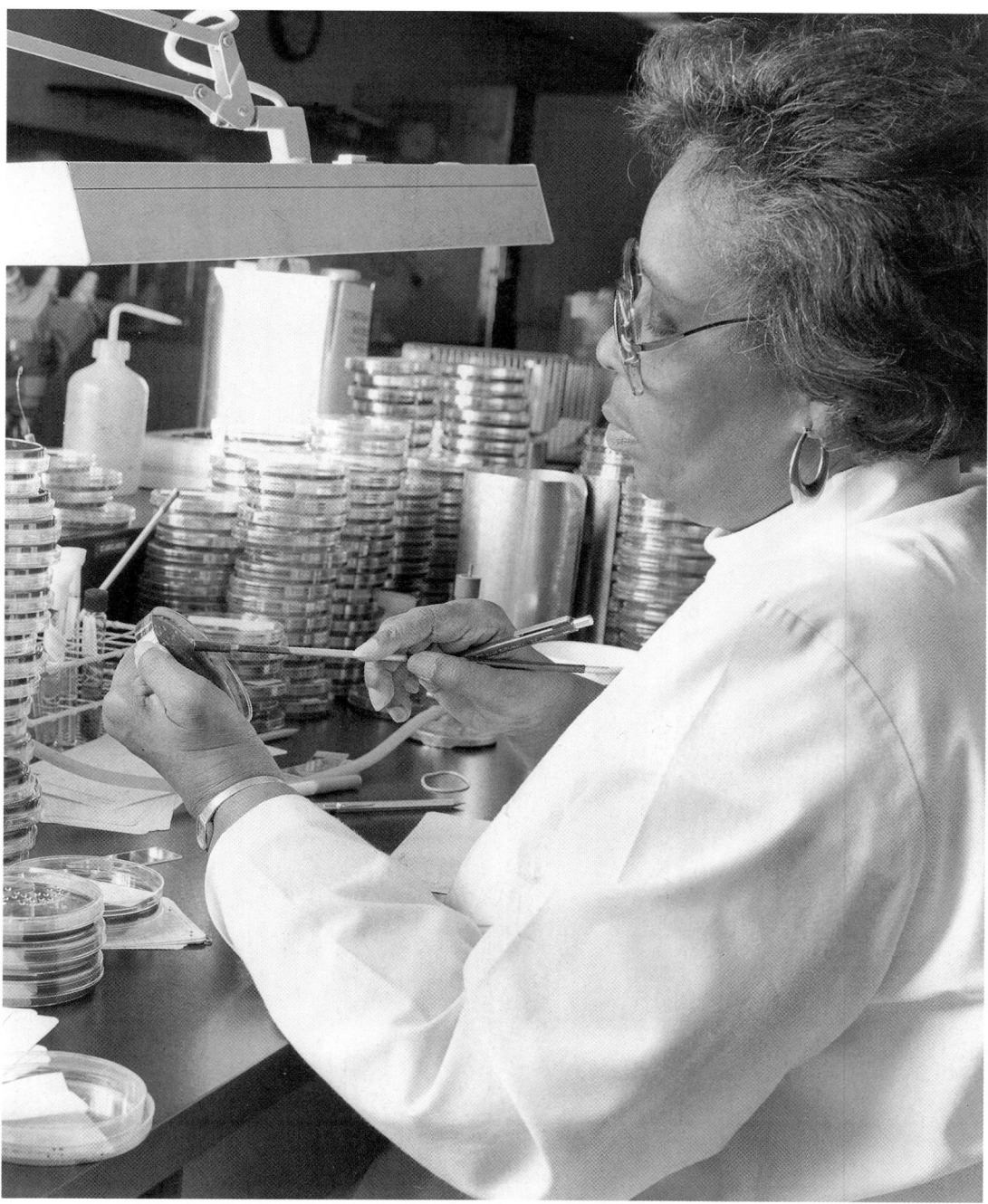

Medical technician Jaqueline Heath at work in the clinical lab, 1989.

You are entering into a career at a time in which your profession and what you can do is truly respected, at a time in which there is tremendous need for your services, at a time in which you are not only the compassionate caregiver that has been traditional for the nursing profession but the new technology and your skills to use it can truly mean the difference between life and death. The world into which you enter today, as far as it relates to health care, is one of tremendous opportunity in being able to make a living and at the same time enjoy the rewards of helping others when they can least help themselves. In this, you can find true happiness. As stated by James Berrie, "The secret of happiness is not in doing what one likes but in liking what one does."
—D. Kay Clawson, M.D., executive vice chancellor, speech at the School of Nursing Recognition Ceremony, May 1989.

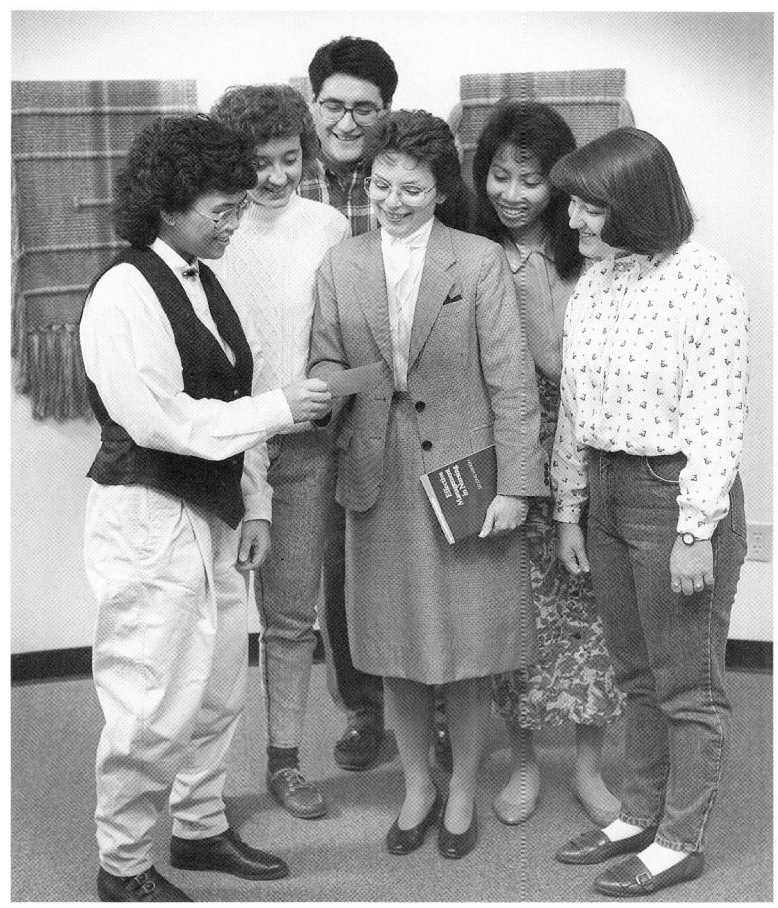

Eleanor Sullivan, R.N., Ed.D. (center), dean of the School of Nursing, with nursing students (left to right) Cecelia Labayan, Clarissa Haugsness, John Delgado, Thu Tran, and Amy Thomson, 1990.

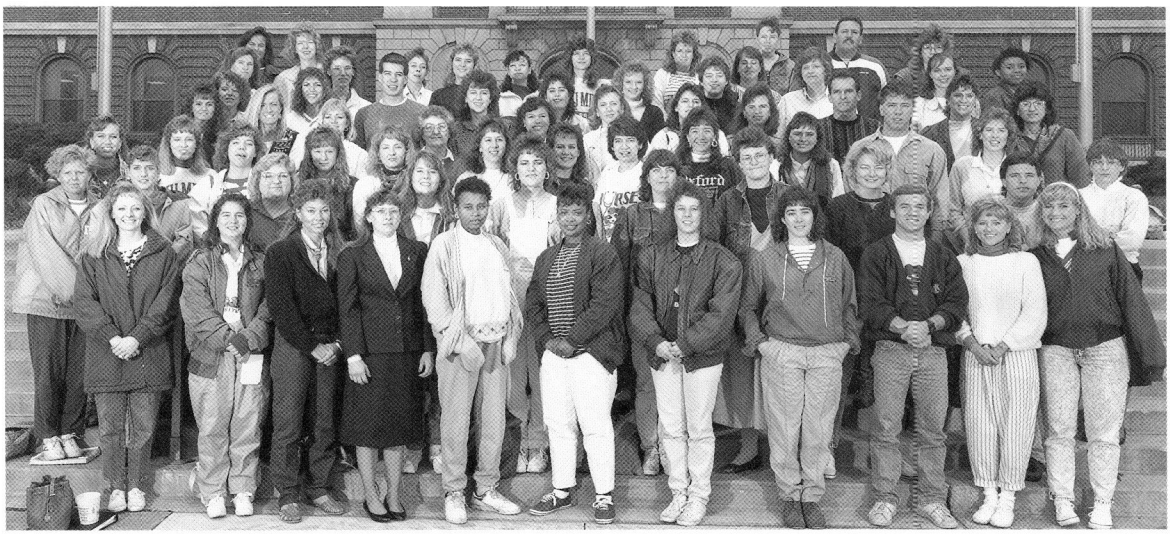

School of Nursing class of 1989.

This academic year the University of Kansas School of Nursing celebrates the 60th anniversary of its baccalaureate program. In 1929, one student enrolled in the newly created program. Today, students enrolled in the KU School of Nursing bachelor's program number 279. Since its inception, more than 2,000 students have received bachelor's degrees from the school.

Dean of the School of Nursing, Eleanor Sullivan, R.N., Ph.D., said, "The University of Kansas first offered nursing education in 1905 and has earned a reputation since that time for preparing outstanding nurses at the baccalaureate, master's and doctoral levels.

"Students in the School of Nursing have the opportunity to learn from some of the top people in the field. Our faculty members possess both clinical and academic expertise and are leaders in nursing research. Graduates of our programs are confident that they have received one of the best nursing educations in the country."—University of Kansas Medical Center *Bulletin*, Winter 1990.

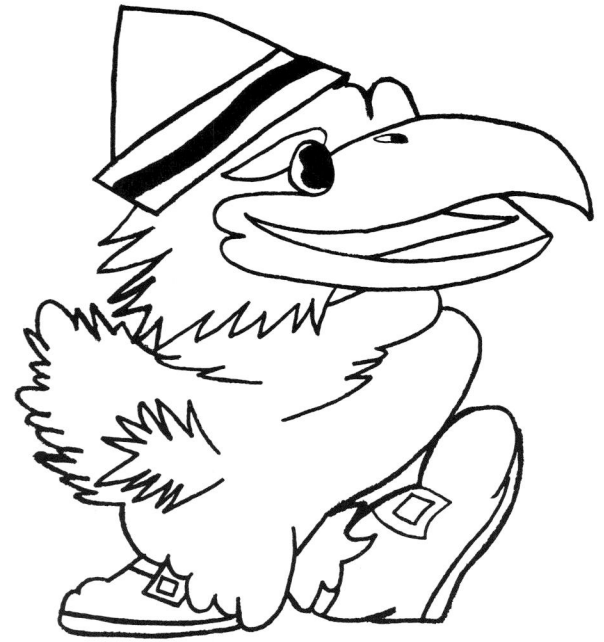

Jaynurse.

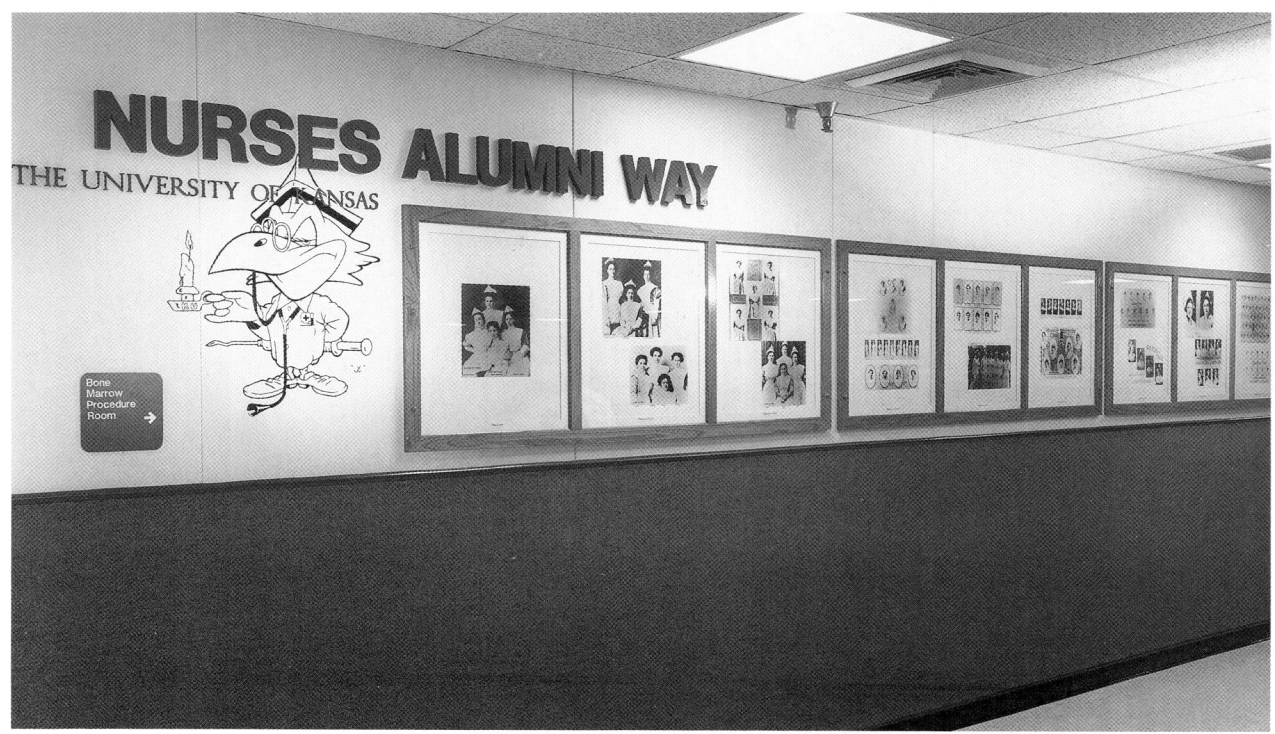

Jaynurse watches over Nurses Alumni Way, 1989.

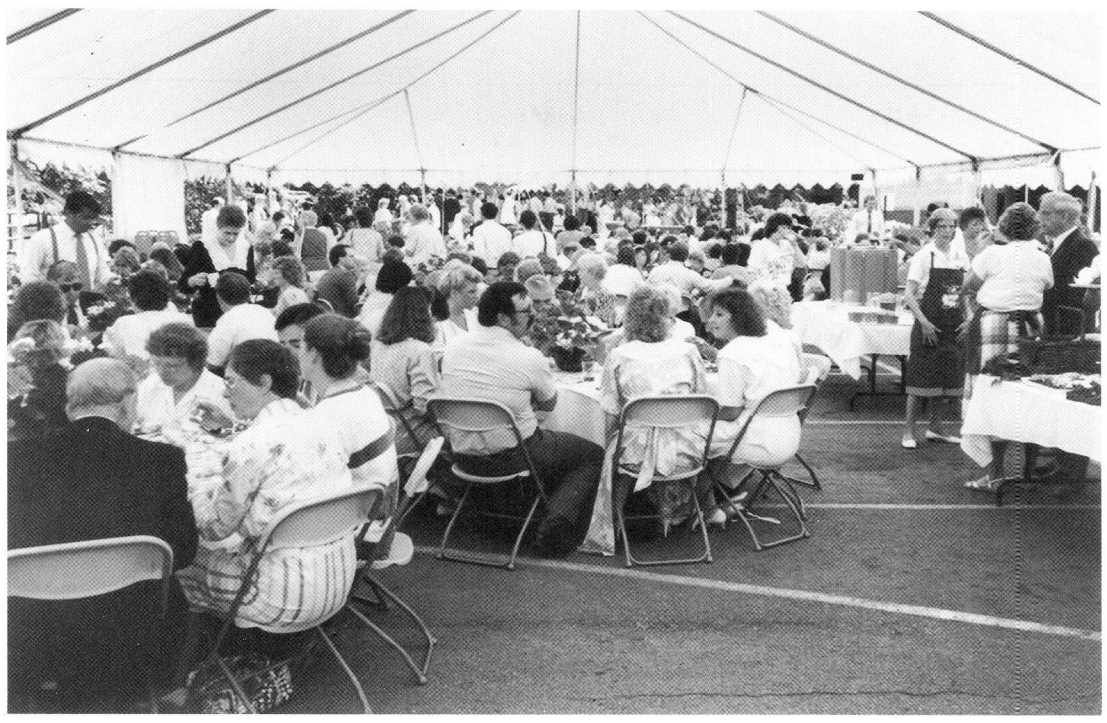

Graduating student brunch, spring 1989.

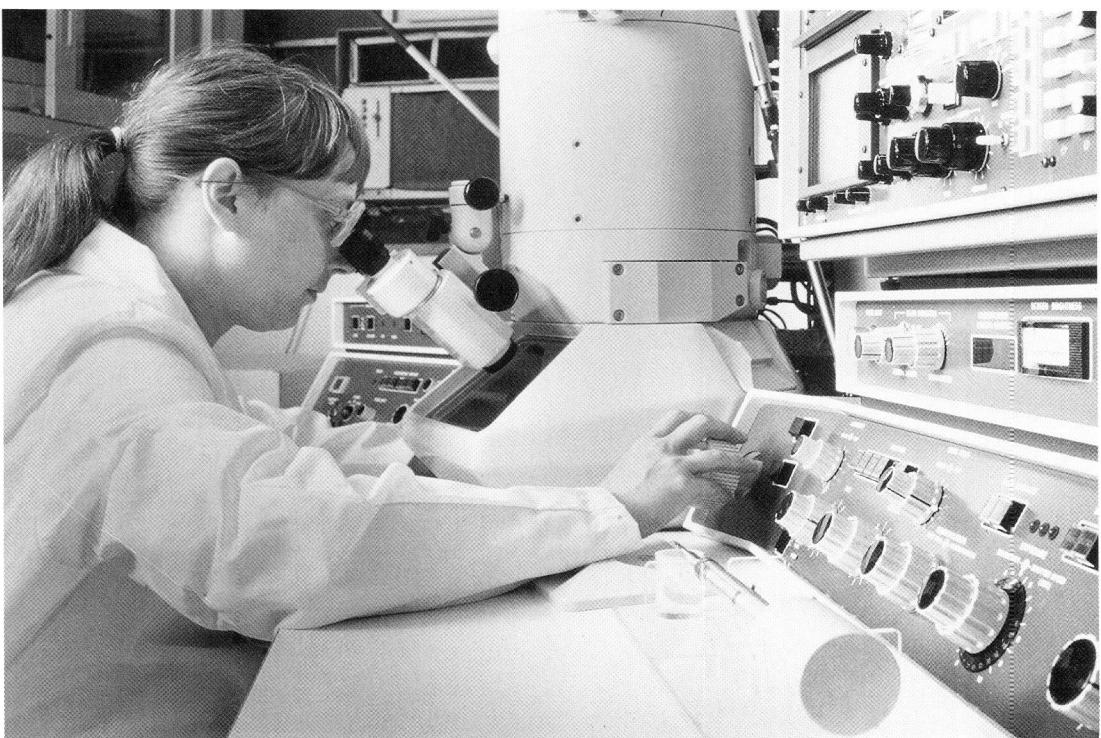

Electron microscopy with Barbara Fegley, Laboratory Manager, 1989.

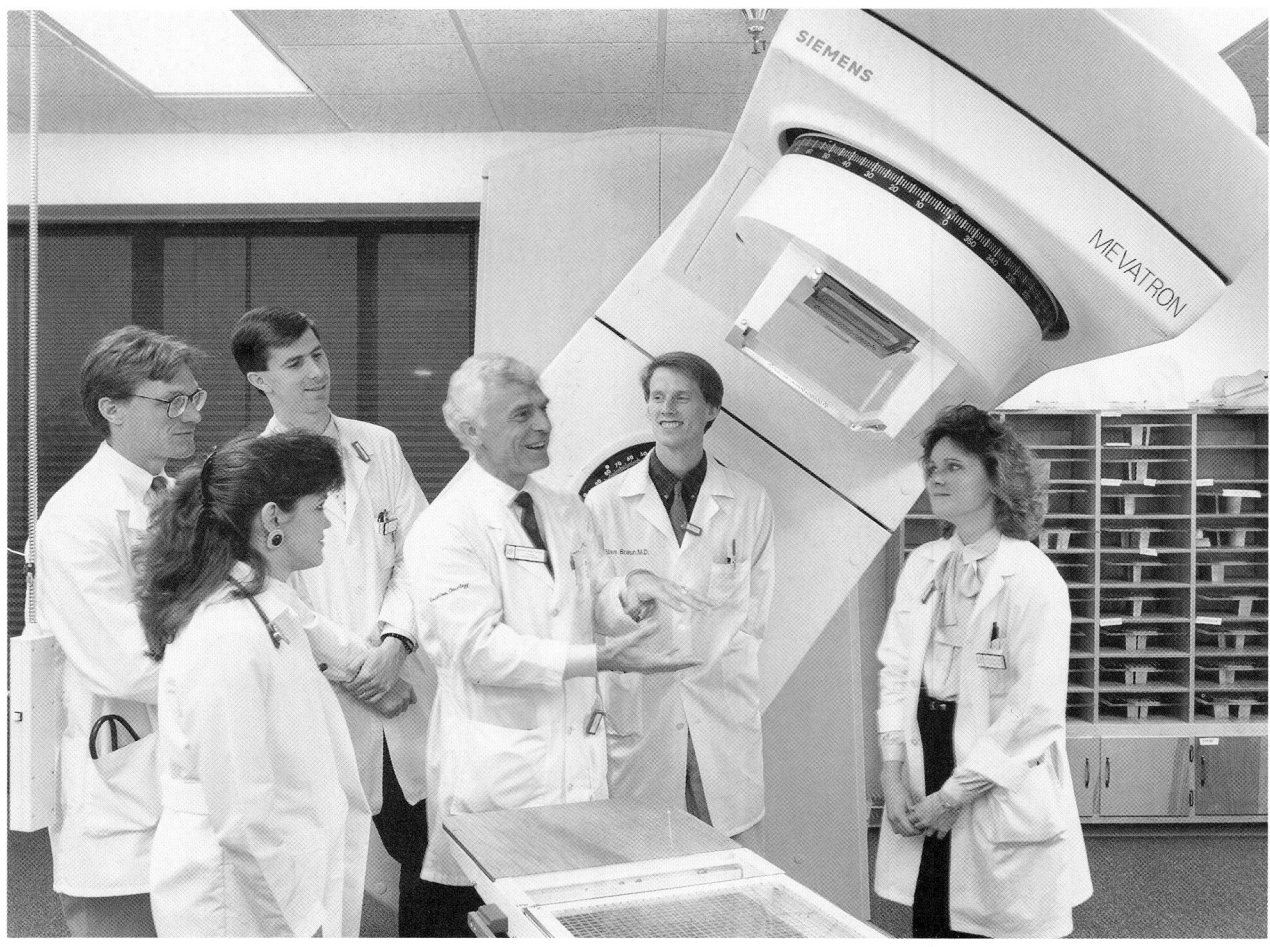

The linear accelerator in Radiation Oncology with Denise Trowbridge, M.D., Scott Cozad, M.D., Stephen Nigh, M.D., department chair Richard Evans, M.D., Ph.D., Steven Braun, M.D., and Barbara DeWitt, M.D., 1989.

Most diagnosis and treatment occurs at the University of Kansas Hospital, completed in 1979 at a cost of $61.5 million. As a teaching hospital, it supervises interns and residents from programs at KU and across the land.

In addition, a number of special units operate in conjunction with the schools and hospital: the KU Cancer Center, the Center on Aging, the Center on Environmental and Occupational Health, the Gene and Barbara Burnett Burn Center, the Children's Rehabilitation Unit, KU Care Flight, and Jaystork II. The hospital's Radiation Therapy Center is nationally known.

The Medical Center comprises a variety of academic and clinical units reflecting the complexity of health care today. Its fifty acres bustle with more than 5,000 employees, more than 2,300 students, and thousands of patients and visitors.
—University of Kansas *Bulletin*, 1989–1990.

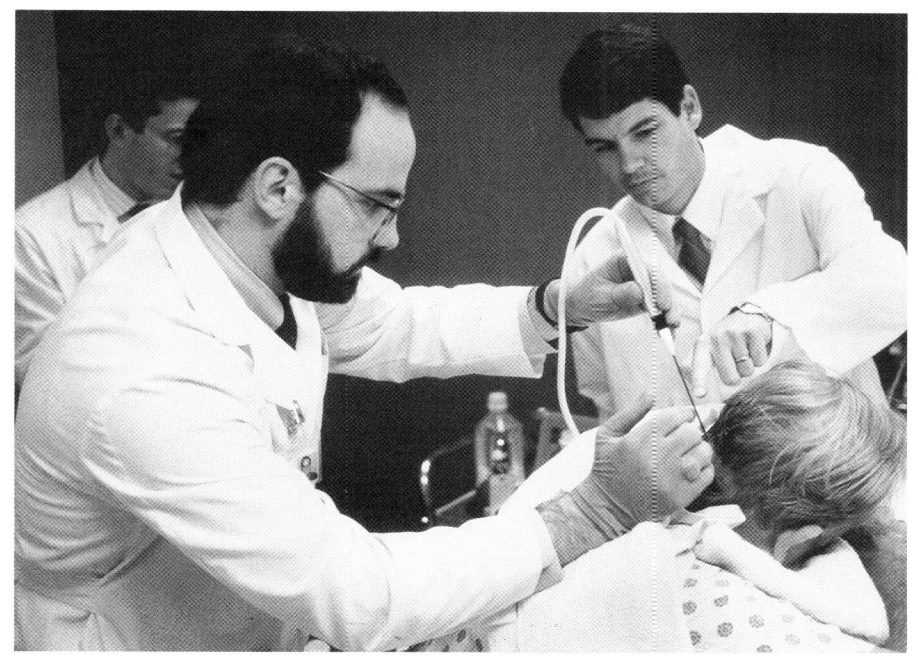

Craig Gilliland, M.D., and Brad Edmonds, M.D., in Diagnostic Radiology, 1989.

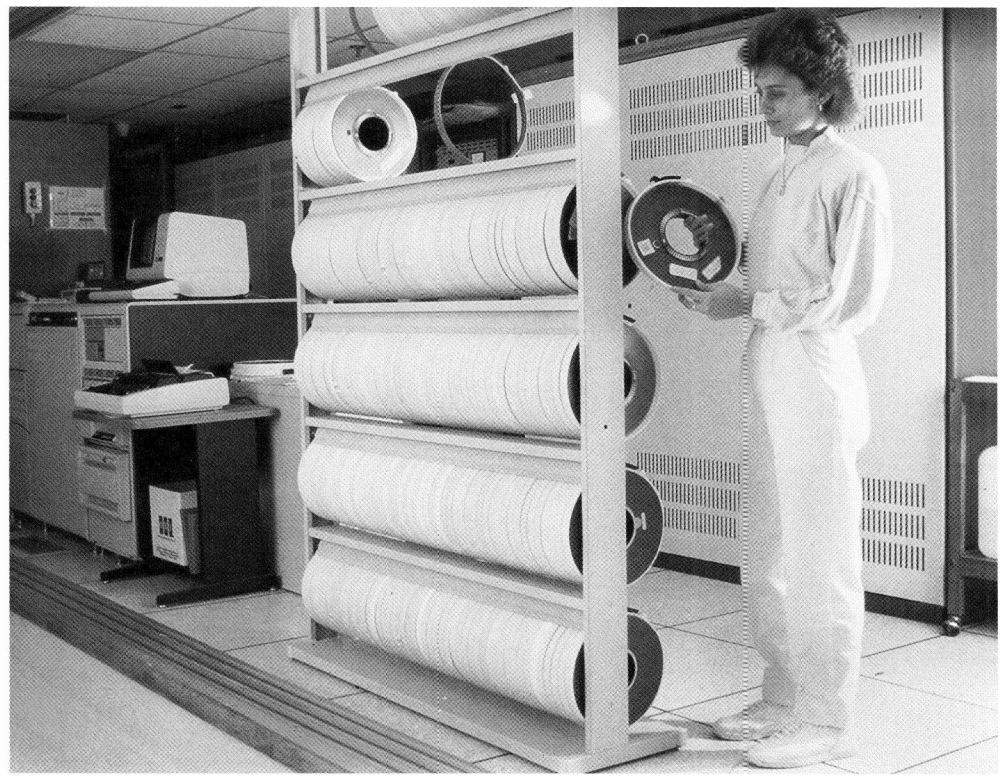

Stephanie Hoogasian in Diagnostic Radiology, 1989.

A new device at the University of Kansas Medical Center has reduced the need for surgery for some patients suffering from gallstones.

The process, called biliary lithotripsy, was first available in this country in 1988. The Med Center treated its first patient last February and since has treated about 30 patients.

The device is the only biliary lithotripsy unit in the state.
—*University Daily Kansan*, February 6, 1990.

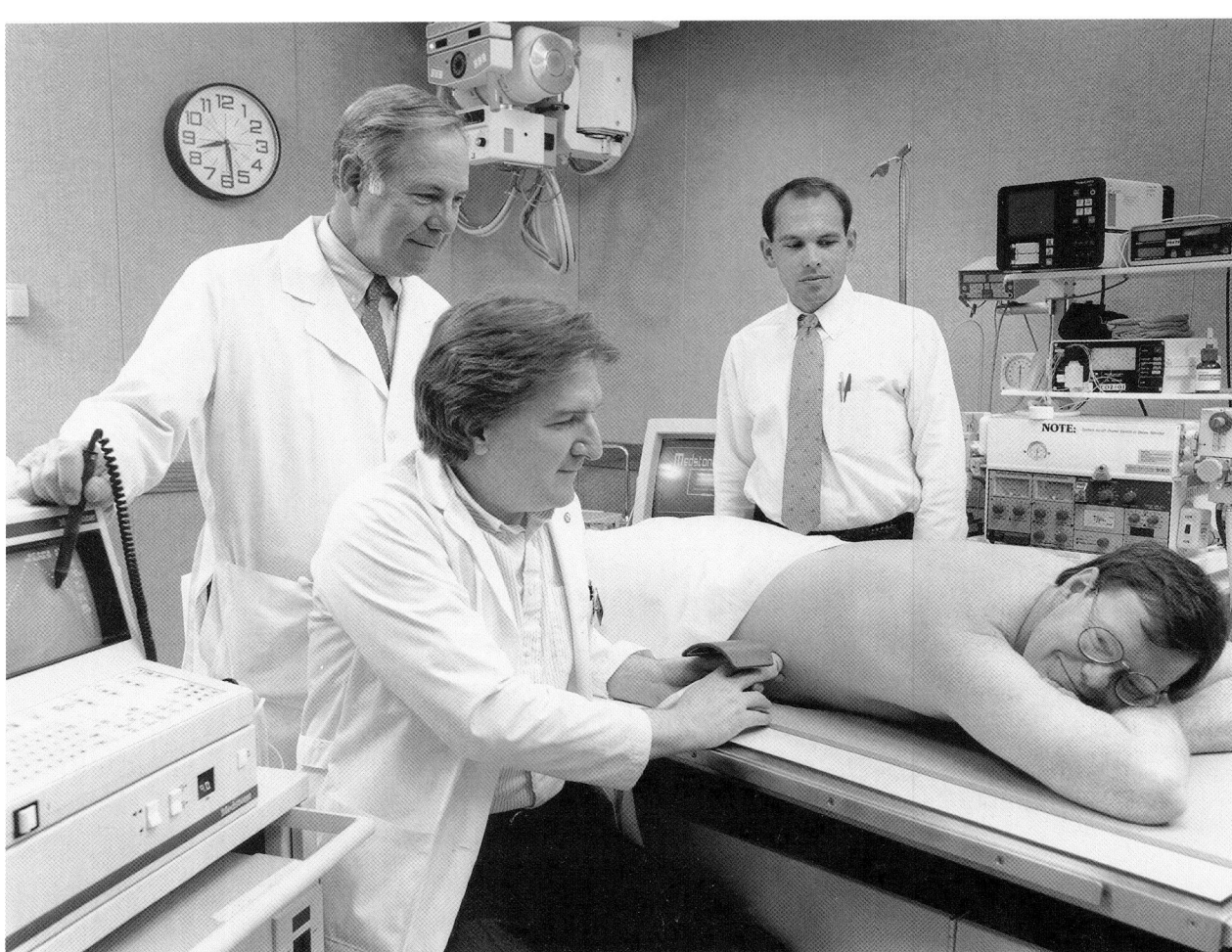

A demonstration of the gallstone lithotripter with Norton J. Greenburger, M.D., chairman of the Department of Medicine, Glendon Cox, M.D., associate professor of Diagnostic Radiology, Pete Nelson, M.D., resident, and on the table, Robert Sperry, M.D., chief resident, 1990.

KUMC's Dornier Kidney Lithotripter offers an alternative to surgery for approximately 80 percent of individuals suffering from kidney stones. The lithotripter . . . uses high-energy shock waves to shatter kidney stones, which are then passed harmlessly through the body's normal elimination process.

The $1.7 million machine is the only one of its kind in the region. Through an agreement made last year with the Medical Center and several area hospitals, KUMC established procedures for the referral and transfer of patients for lithotripter treatment.
—University of Kansas Medical Center *Bulletin*, Summer 1986.

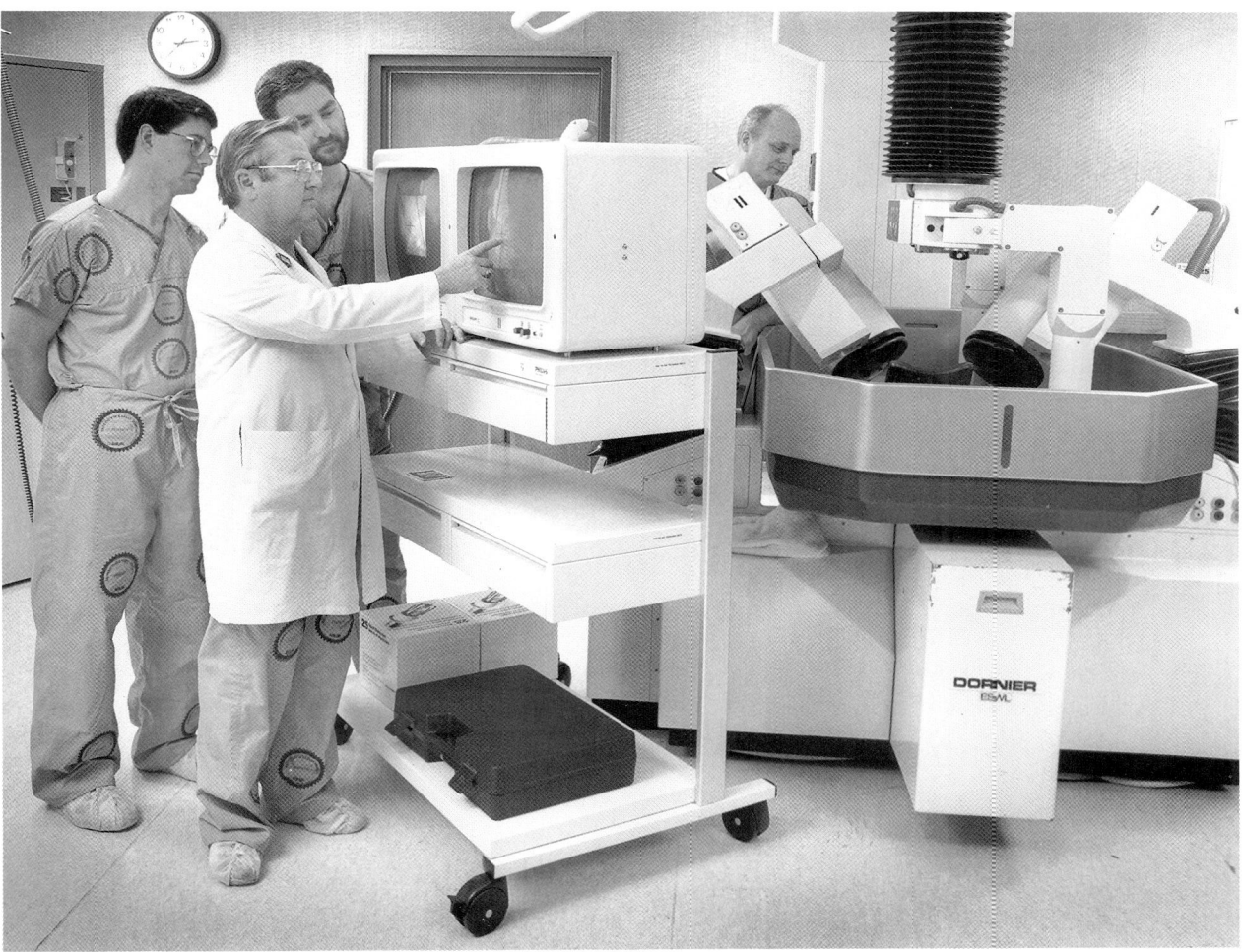

Winston K. Mebust, M.D., demonstrating the kidney stone lithotripter, 1990.

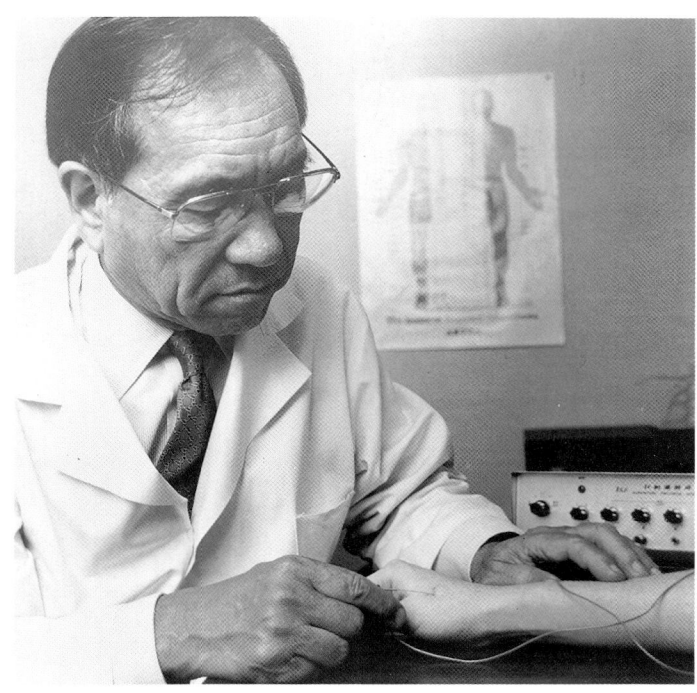

Chairman of the Department of
Anesthesiology Kasumi Arakawa, M.D.,
in the Pain Clinic, 1989.

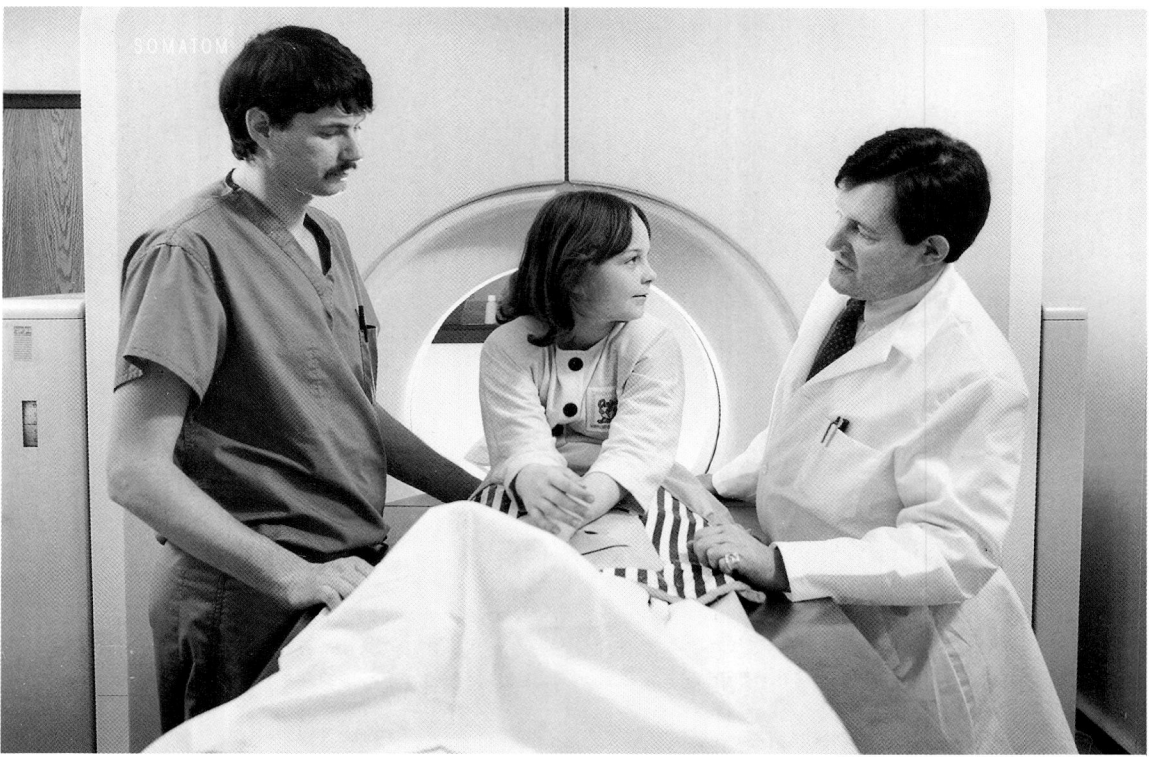

Solomon Batnitzky, M.D., professor of Diagnostic Radiology, demonstrating the CAT scan to
Don Siscoe and his daughter Angela, 1990.

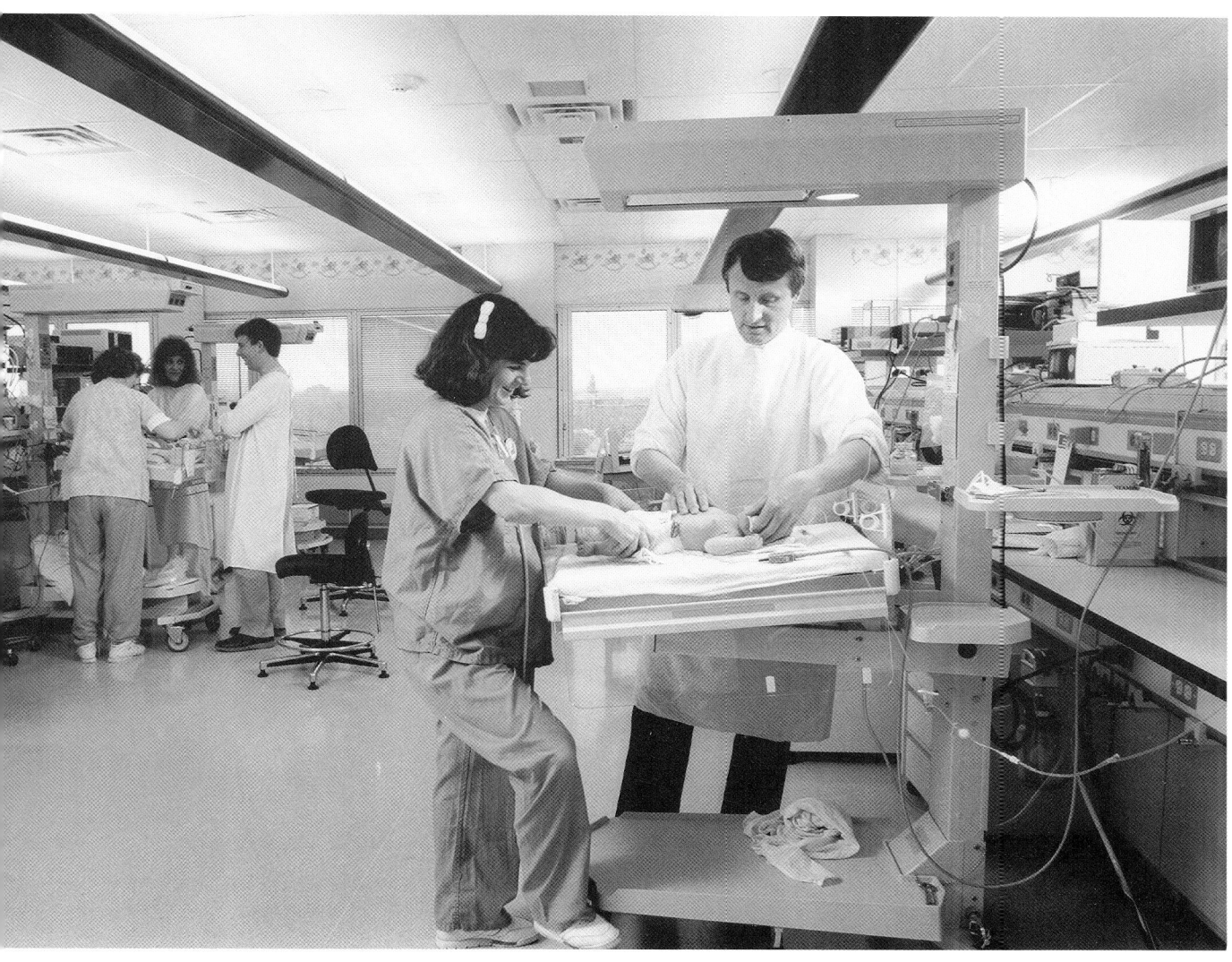

William Topper, M.D., associate professor of pediatrics, and Monica Grosdidier, R.N., 1990.

The Children's Unit, a state-of-the-art facility for pediatric inpatients, will serve ill children throughout the Midwest with a variety of services, facilities, clinics and programs for infants, toddlers, children and adolescents.

It features two nursing sections, a schoolroom that can be divided into two rooms, a play room, a consulting room for health care professionals, resident on-call rooms, a private office for the head nurse, office space for a clinical nurse specialist, a clinical social worker and a pediatric dietician.
—*Kansas City Kansan*, July 11, 1989.

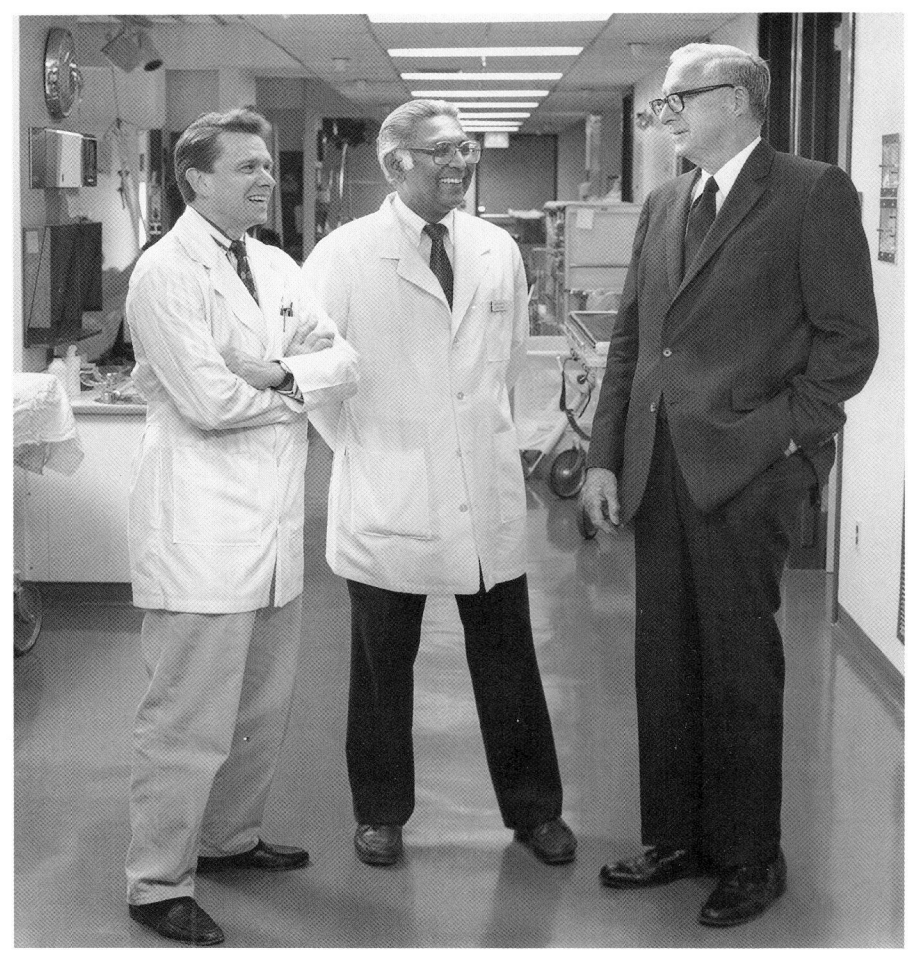

John Hiebert, M.D.,
Mani Mani, M.D., and
David Robinson, M.D.,
in the Burnett Burn
Center, 1990.

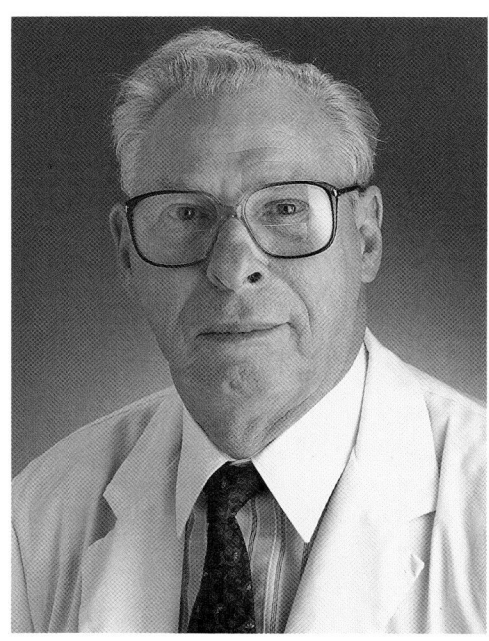

Kermit Krantz, M.D., University Distinguished Professor,
professor of obstetrics and gynecology, and professor of
anatomy, 1990.

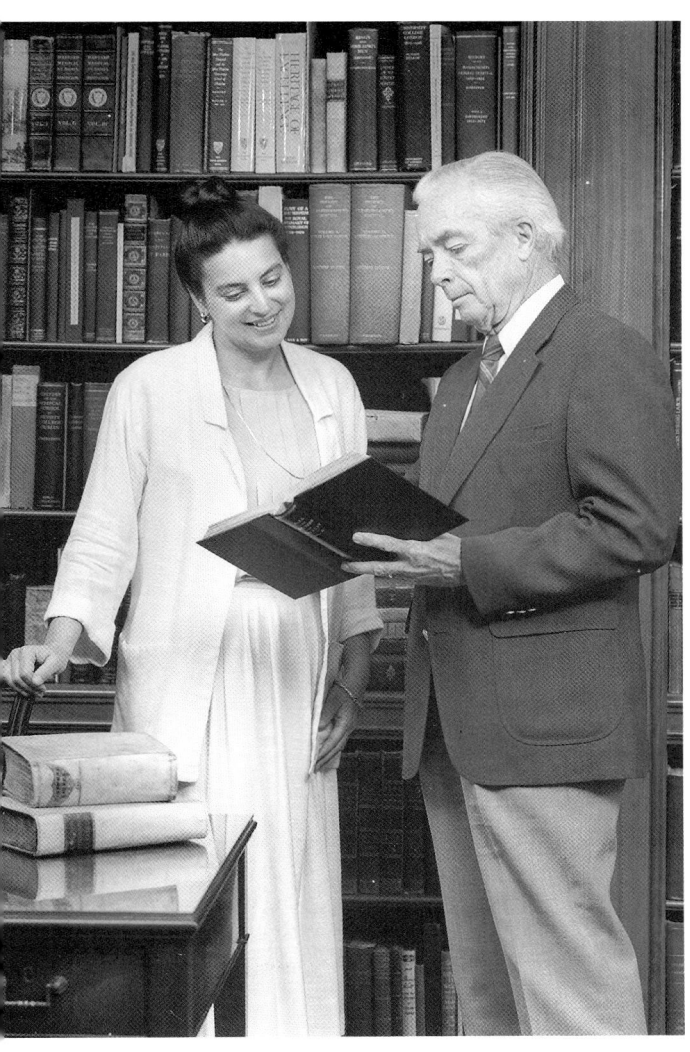

Robert P. Hudson, M.D., chairman of the Department of the History and Philosophy of Medicine, with Susan B. Case, rare books librarian, in the Clendening Reading Room, 1990.

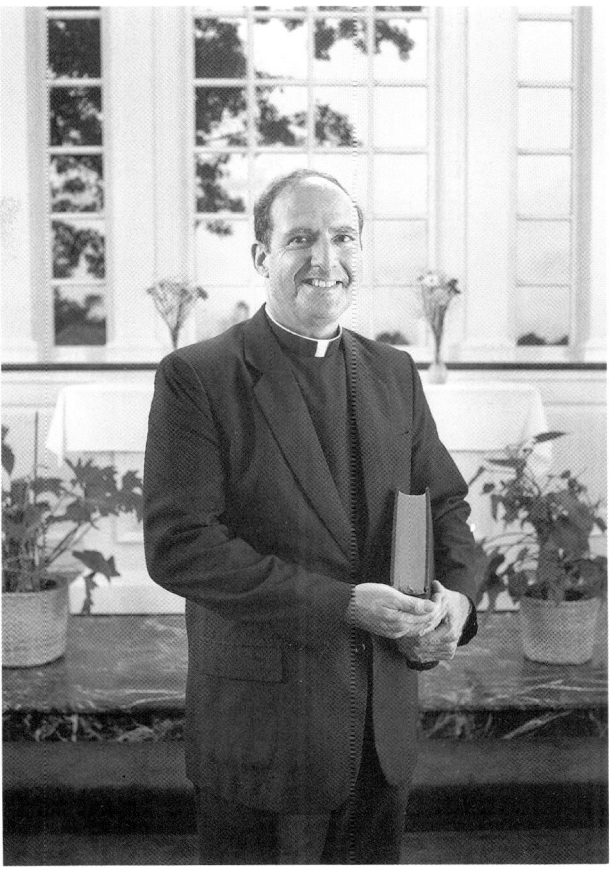

Father Jerry L. Spencer, 1991. Father Spencer has served as Catholic chaplain at the Medical Center since September 12, 1967. He is also an associate in the Department of the History and Philosophy of Medicine.

The Logan Clendening History of Medicine Library is one of the most notable libraries of its type. The priceless nucleus of the present library collection was bequeathed in 1945 by Dr. Logan Clendening to the University of Kansas School of Medicine. . . . Further endowments from distinguished physicians, alumni and faculty of the University, friends of the library and the late Dorothy Hixon Clendening Clark have provided significant bibliographic contributions and funds for collection development.
—*Dusty Shelf*, January 1988.

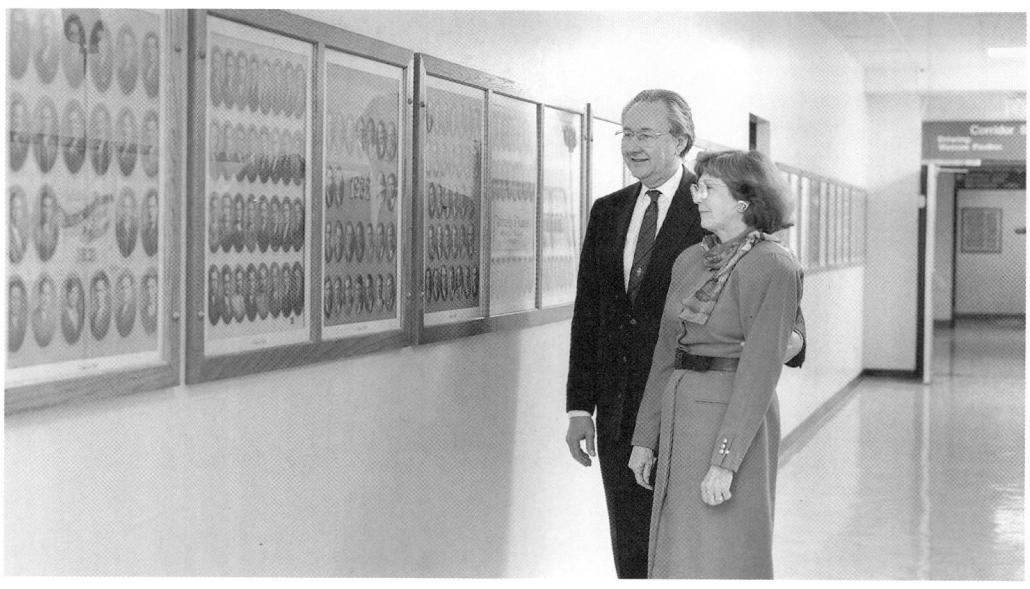

D. Kay Clawson, M.D., and Mrs. Clawson view Alumni Way, 1990.

The past few years have been exciting because they are times of great stress in the health care system and particularly in medical education. They are times of rapid change and everyone finds change difficult. This is particularly true for our faculty who are pressured from all sides. They are expected to improve the quality of the educational experience for students, to adapt to new teaching technologies, and at the same time to be intensely competitive for research funding while increasing their patient care activities. While some have found this most difficult, most have adjusted well. At the present time, our institution is as strong as it has been at any time in its history.—D. Kay Clawson, M.D., executive vice chancellor, speech to the Medical Alumni Banquet, May 1987.

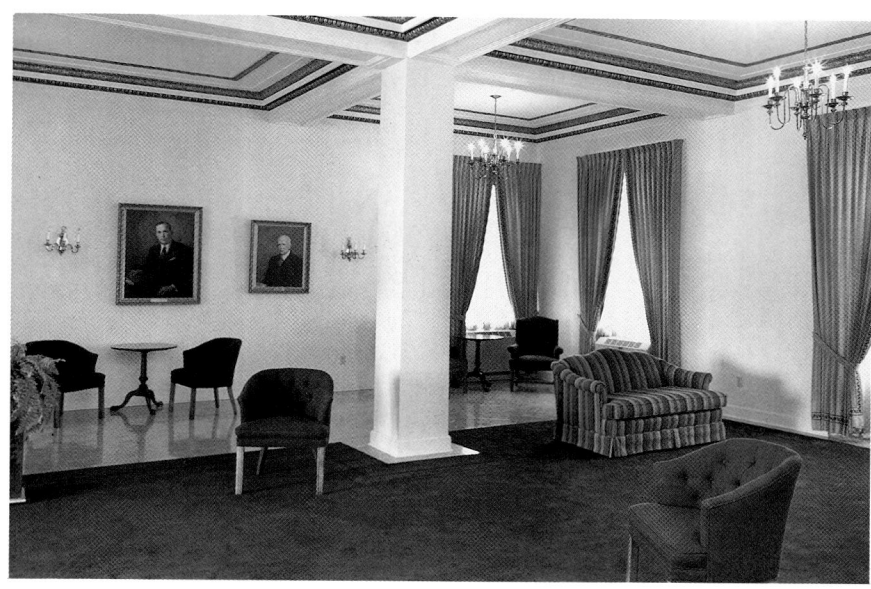

The reception area of the Murphy Administration Building, 1990. Both the remodeling of this area and the development of Alumni Way were among the many improvements initiated by Dr. and Mrs. Clawson.

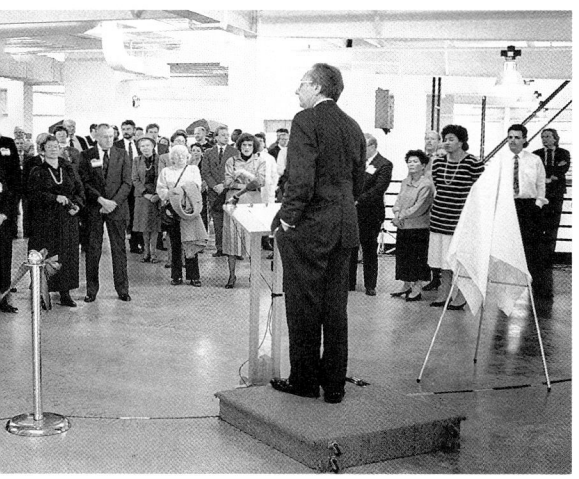

D. Kay Clawson, M.D., executive vice chancellor, speaking at the opening of the Fitness Center, February 1, 1990.

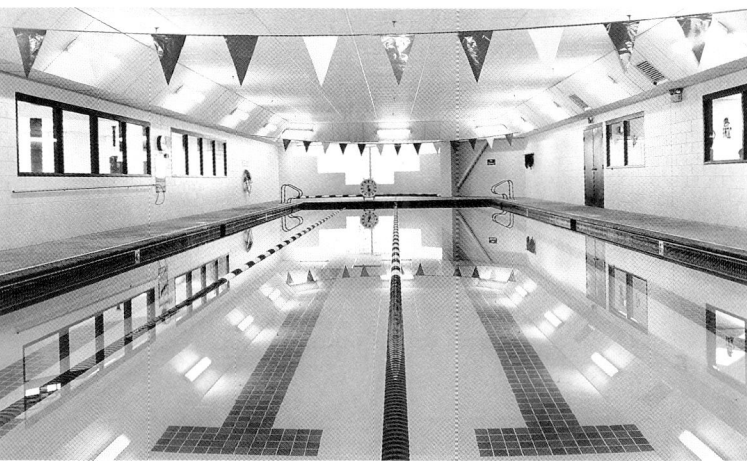

Fitness Center swimming pool, 1991.

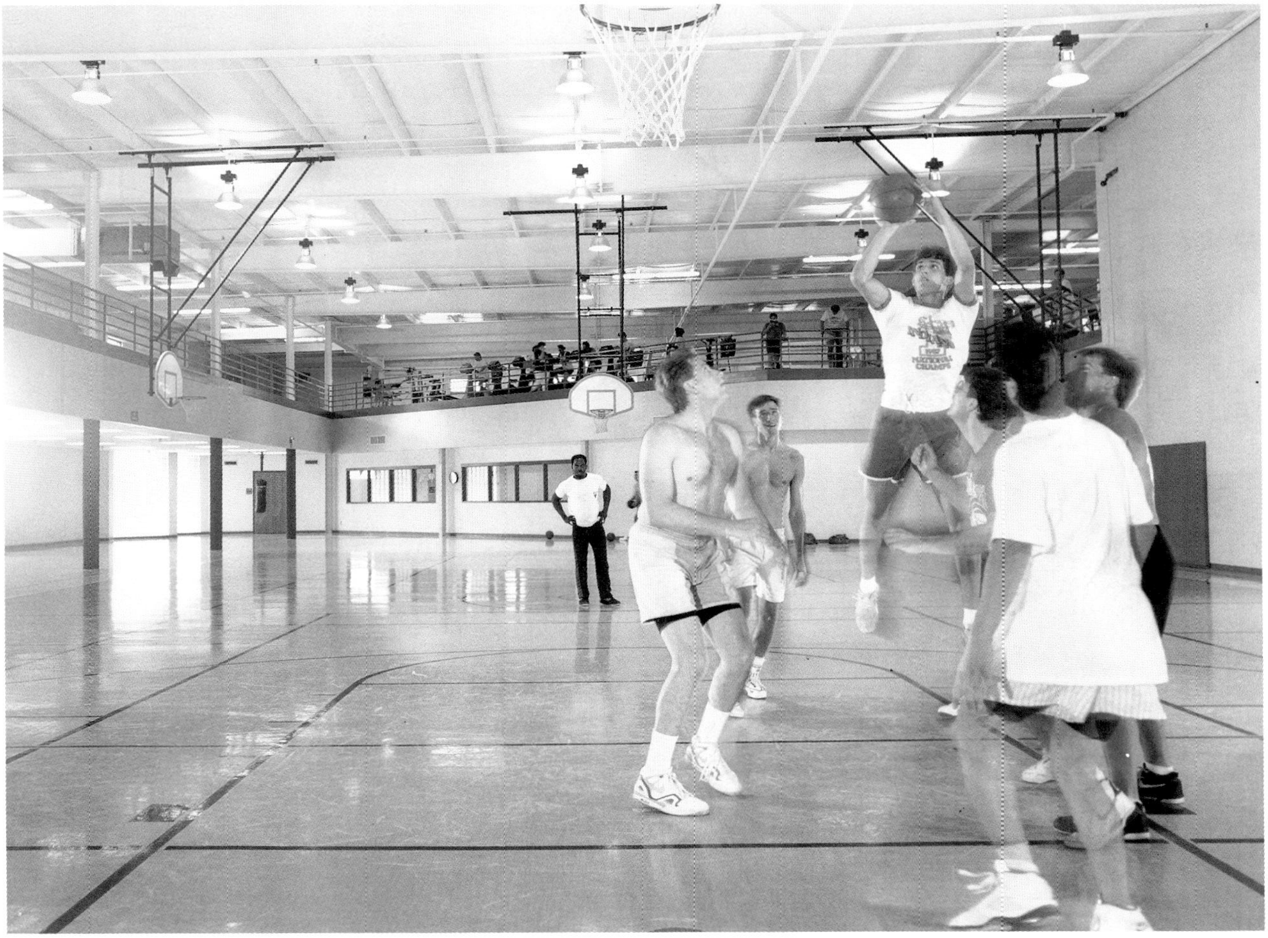

![Fitness Center basketball court](basketball court image)

Fitness Center basketball court, 1991.

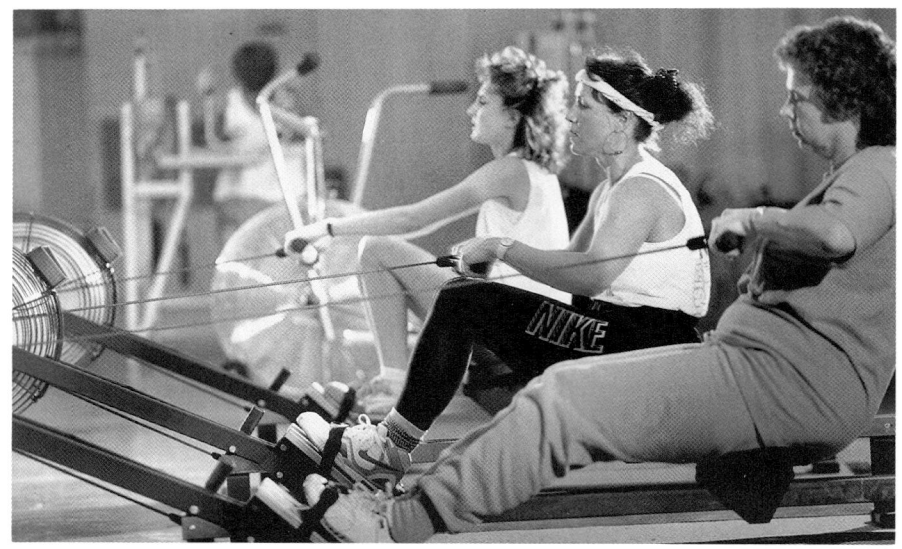

Susan Hein, Sharon Hall, and Janice Van Natta making use of the Fitness Center, 1990.

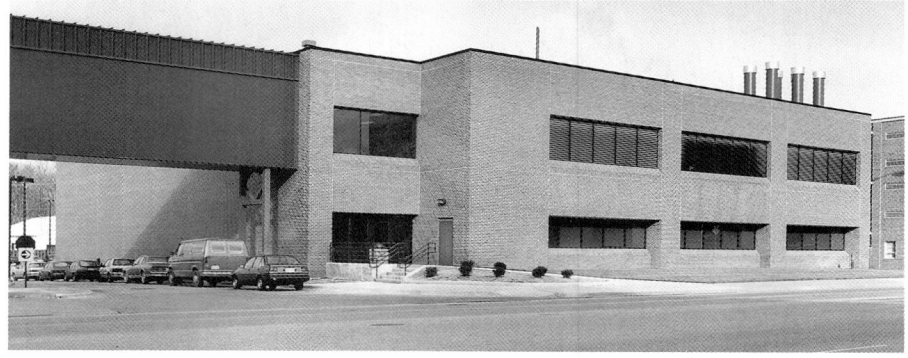

Research Support Facility, 1991.

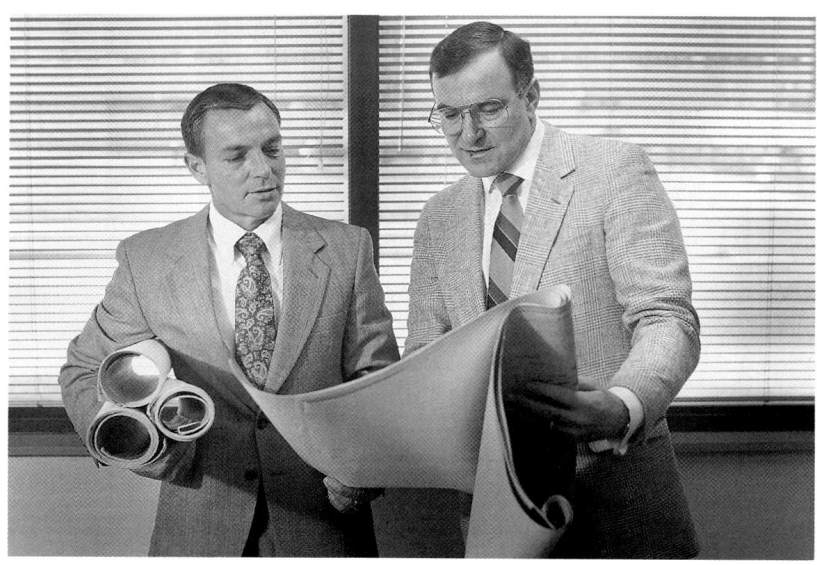

Roger Lambson, Ph.D., vice chancellor for administration, and Tony David, D.V.M., director of laboratory animal resources, 1990.

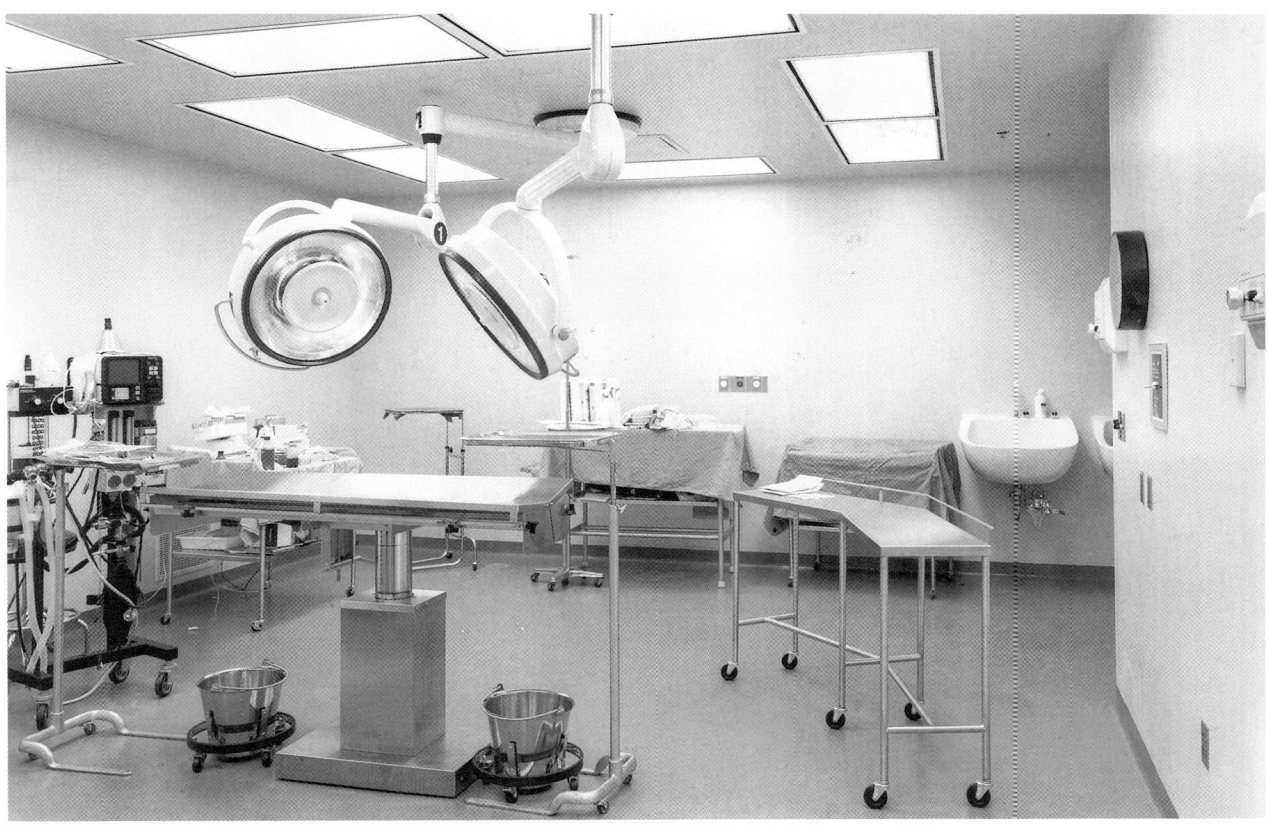

Interior, Research Support Facility, 1990.

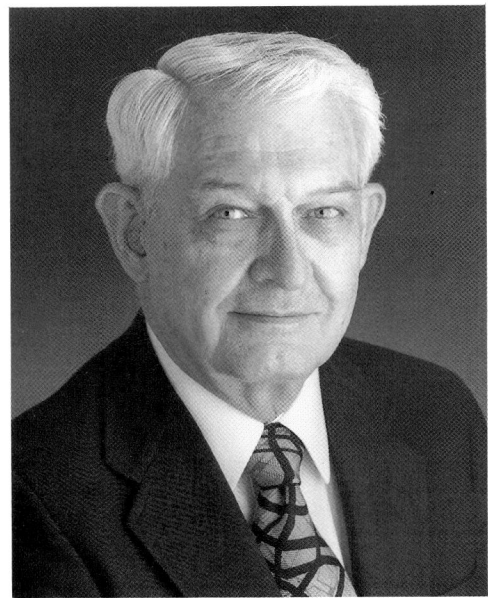

James Price, M.D., executive dean, School of
Medicine, and professor of family practice.

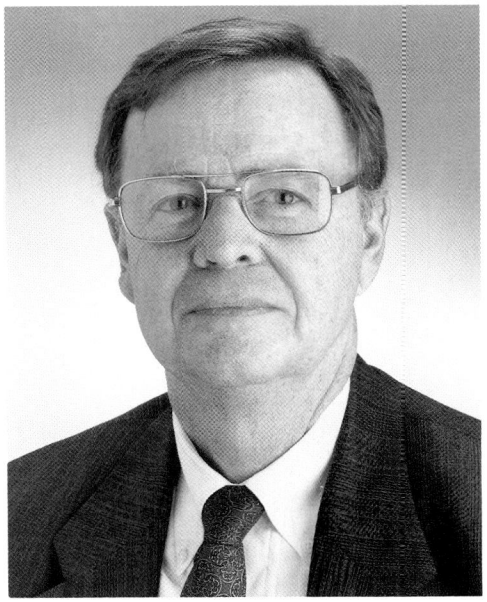

A. L. Chapman, Ph.D., dean of Graduate
Studies and Research, and professor of
anatomy and cell biology.

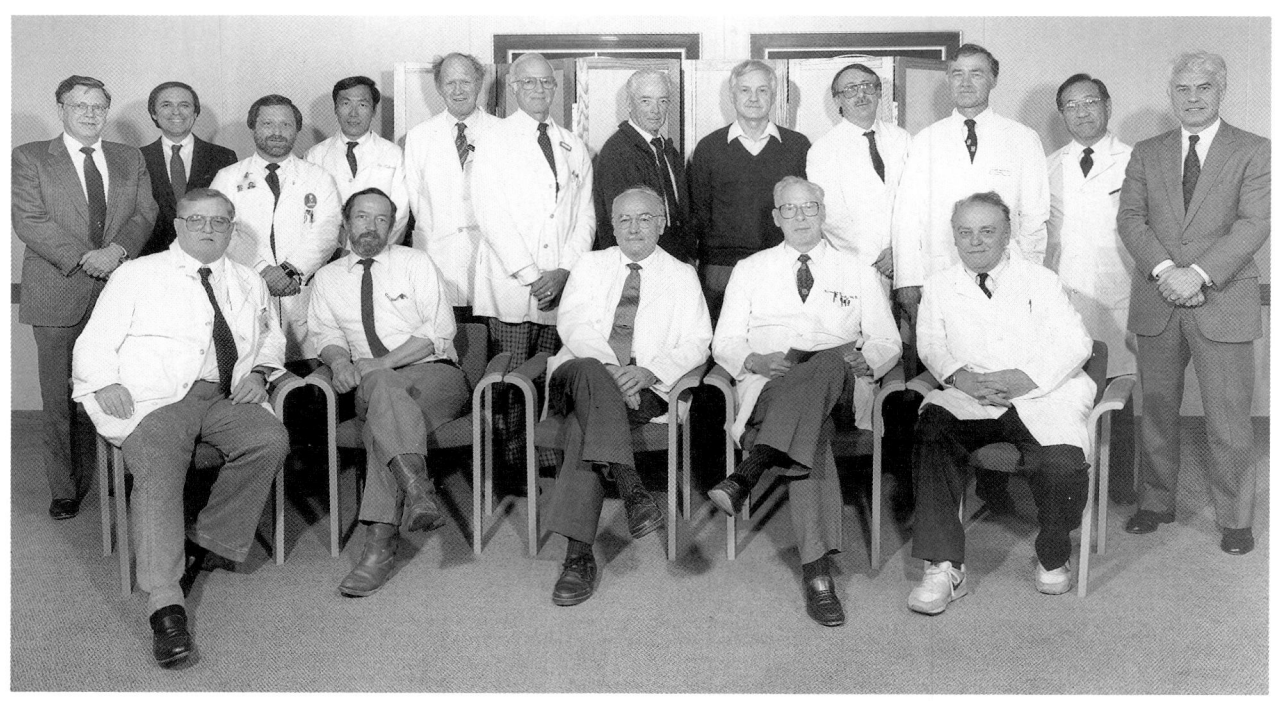

Department chairs, 1990. Front, left to right: Don W. Goodwin, M.D., professor and chair, psychiatry; David C. Morrison, Ph.D., professor and chair, microbiology; Charles W. Norris, M.D., chief of staff, hospital administration; Kermit Krantz, M.D., professor and chair, obstetrics and gynecology; and Edward J. Walaszek, Ph.D., professor and chair, pharmacology, toxicology, and therapeutics.
Back, left to right: Theodore Lawwill, M.D., professor and chair, ophthalmology; Martin Pernoll, M.D., executive dean, School of Medicine; Allen P. Erenberg, M.D., professor and chair, pediatrics; Laurence Y. Cheung, M.D., professor and chair, surgery; John Redford, M.D., professor and chair, rehabilitation medicine; Arch Templeton, M.D., professor and chair, diagnostic radiology; Robert P. Hudson, M.D., chairman, history and philosophy of medicine; Kurt Ebner, Ph.D., professor, biochemistry; William C. Koller, M.D., Ph.D., professor and chair, neurology; H. C. Anderson, M.D., professor and chair, pathology; Kasumi Arakawa, M.D., professor and chair, anesthesiology; and Richard G. Evans, M.D., Ph.D., chairman, radiation oncology.

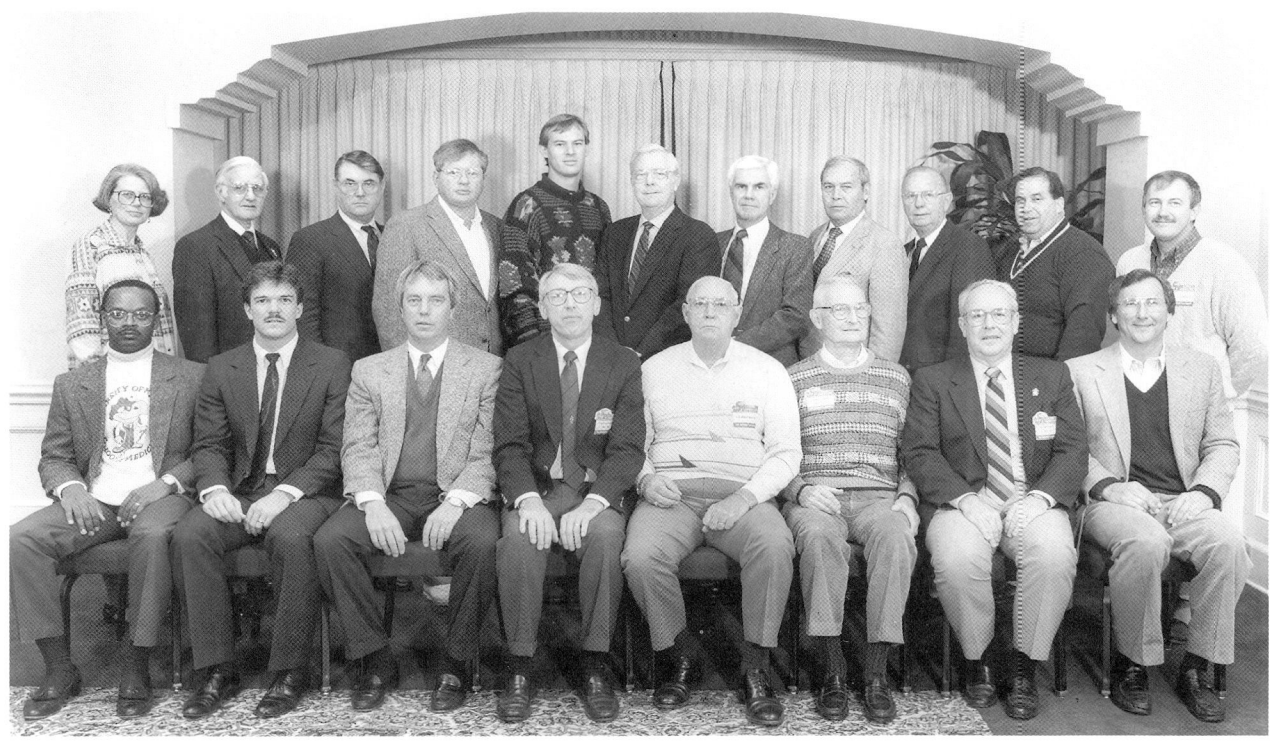

KU Medical Alumni Association, 1990–1991, Board of Directors. Standing, left to right: Donna Daily, M.D., president-elect; William E. Larsen, M.D., chairman, 45-year reunion; George F. Sheldon, M.D., national member-at-large; Ralph G. Robinson, M.D., chairman, membership and elections; Cris D. Barnthouse, M.D., co-chairman, 10-year reunion; John S. Trombold, M.D., national member-at-large; Joseph L. Kyner, M.D., treasurer; Don C. McIlrath, M.D., national member-at-large; Jack D. Walker, M.D., lieutenant governor, state of Kansas, chairman, fund-raising committee; G. Charles Loveland, M.D., statewide member-at-large; Ray Lash, M.D., metropolitan member-at-large.

Seated, left to right: Walter Rayford, senior medical student, Kansas City campus; Wade Gaeddert, senior medical student, Wichita campus; Tom G. Sullivan, M.D., president; Frederic M. Gilhousen, M.D., chairman, 25-year reunion; L. G. Agee, M.D., chairman, 40-year reunion; John F. McDonnell, M.D., chairman, 50-year reunion; Joseph C. Meek, Jr., M.D., chairman, Department of Internal Medicine, and dean, University of Kansas School of Medicine–Wichita; Cranston J. Cederlind, M.D., chairman, 20-year reunion. Board members not present in picture: John R. Goheen, M.D., immediate past president; Gerald R. Kirby, M.D., membership and elections committee; Ann Allegre, M.D., metropolitan member-at-large; Richard E. Davis, M.D., metropolitan member-at-large; Jimmie Gleason, M.D., statewide member-at-large; Carol Connor, M.D., co-chairman, 10-year reunion; Perri Ginder, M.D., chairman, 15-year reunion; Robert H. Durie, M.D., chairman, 30-year reunion; Richard M. Childs, M.D., chairman, 35-year reunion; Franklin G. Bilchmeier, M.D., chairman, Distinguished Medical Teaching Fund Trustees.

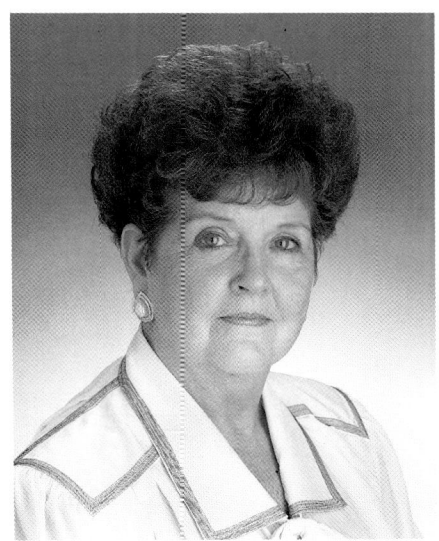

Patricia Head, director, Alumni Center.

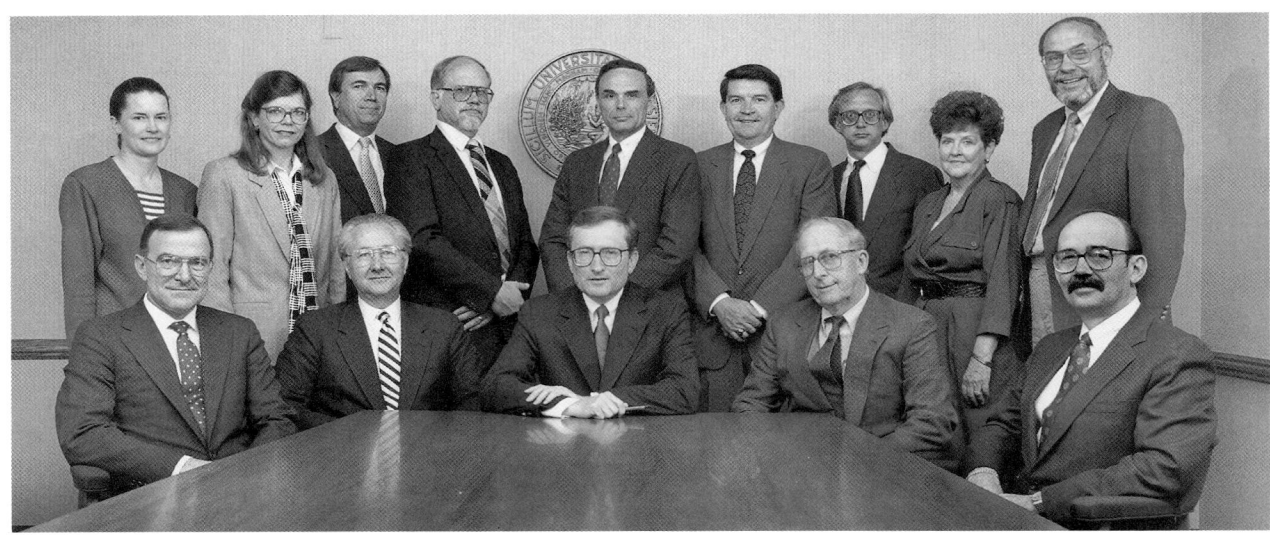

Chancellor's management team, 1990. Seated, left to right: Roger O. Lambson, vice chancellor for administration; D. Kay Clawson, M.D., executive vice chancellor; Gene A. Budig, chancellor; Keith L. Nitcher, university director of business and fiscal affairs; Glenn Potter, vice chancellor for hospital administration.
Standing, left to right: Jane Henney, M.D., vice chancellor for health policy and programs; Ann Victoria Thomas, general counsel of the university; R. Mike Keeble, director, business affairs; Allen Wiechert, university director of facilities planning; Richard L. Mann, university director of information resources; Rodger Oroke, university director of support services; Randy Attwood, director of university relations, Medical Center; Patricia Head, director, alumni association, Medical Center; Marlin Rein, associate university director, business and fiscal affairs.

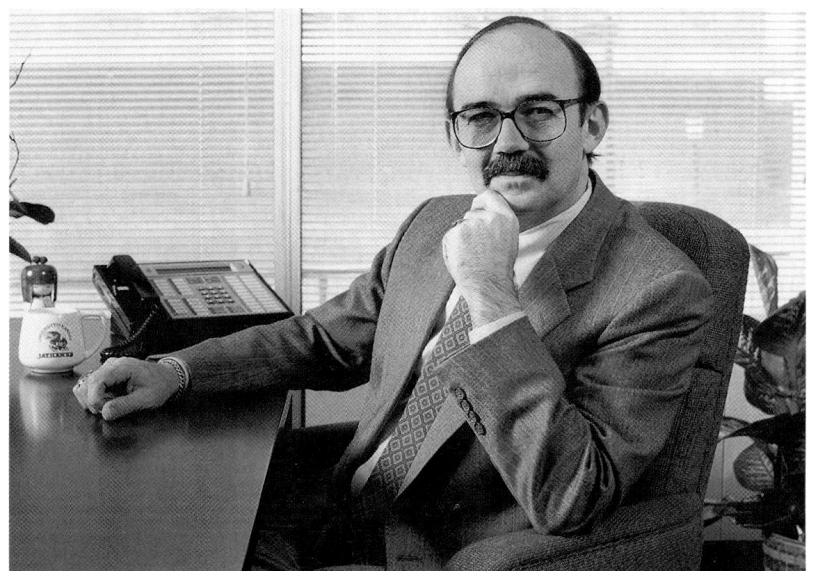

Glenn Potter, vice chancellor for hospital administration.

I was very impressed with the university and with the outstanding medical center. I sensed a commitment to excellence that makes the med center a plum in the nation.
—Glenn E. Potter, vice chancellor for hospital administration, *Lawrence Journal-World,* March 24, 1990.

Many feel, as I do, that as we prepare to enter the Twenty-First Century, we find ourselves in a crisis. As a nation, we are spending over $650 billion on health (a sum in excess of eleven percent of the gross national product), and yet we are not able to provide adequate health care for 25 to 35 million Americans, particularly those in rural America and our inner cities. Our medical schools and academic health centers are faced with a series of problems that challenge their very existence as we have known them. We are forced to practice in a cost-conscious environment with intense competition, all of which we have produced. By virtue of our locations and our heritage, we are caring for a disproportionate share of the underprivileged. At the same time, we are expected to educate future physicians as well as advance our disciplines through research.

—D. Kay Clawson, M.D., executive vice chancellor, Kennedy Lecture, May 25, 1989.

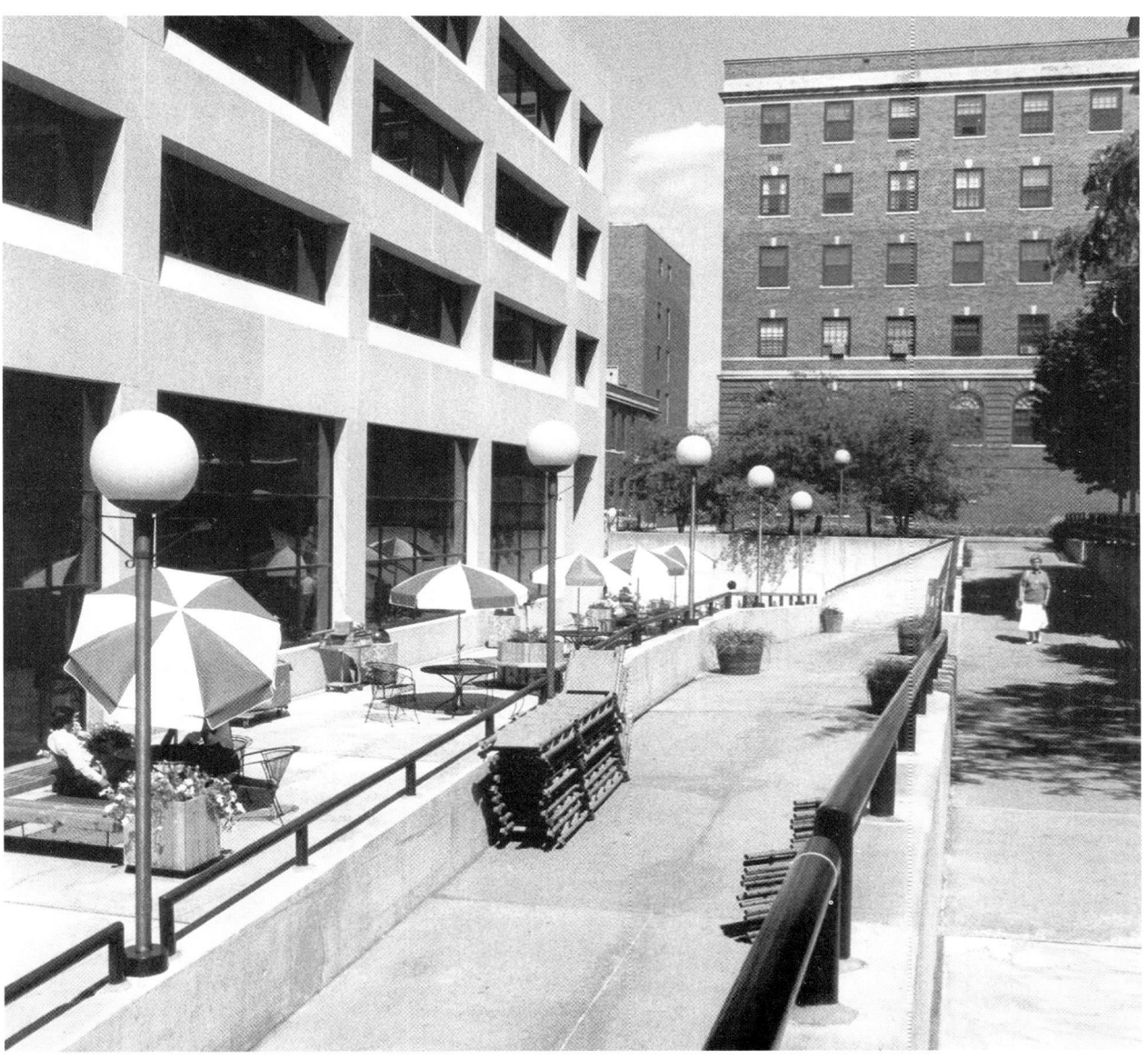

Orr-Major and Sudler Hall.

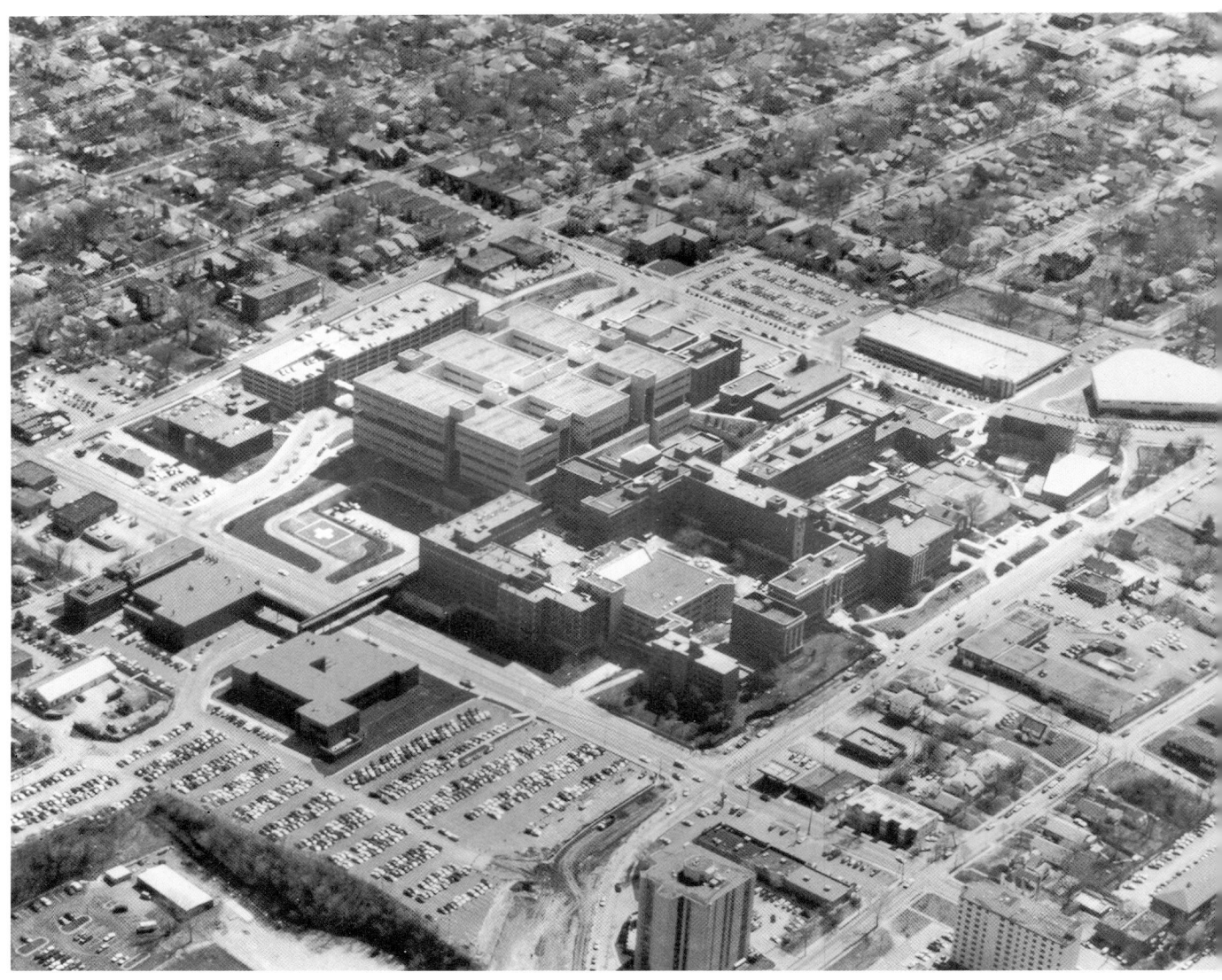

Aerial view, 1990.

Additional Reading

The starting point for more information on the University of Kansas Medical Center is an intimate and informal study, *An Account of the University of Kansas School of Medicine* by Ralph H. Major (Kansas City: University of Kansas Medical Alumni Association, 1968). Two monographs by Helen M. Sims, *Simeon Bishop Bell, M.D.* (Kansas City: University of Kansas Medical Center, 1979) and *The Wahl Years at the University of Kansas Medical Center, 1919–1948* (Kansas City: University of Kansas Medical Center, 1983), contain valuable material on institutional development. For the history of the 77th Evacuation Hospital Unit, see *Medicine under Canvas,* edited by Max S. Allen, M.D. (Kansas City, Mo.: Sosland Press, 1949). Important data pertaining to the rise of the Medical Center can be found in *The Kansas Doctor: A Century of Pioneering* by Thomas Neville Bonner (Lawrence: University of Kansas Press, 1959); *A Pictorial History of Kansas Medicine* by John B. Runnels and George F. Sheldon (Topeka: Kansas State Historical Society, 1961); and *The University of Kansas: A History* by Clifford S. Griffin (Lawrence: University Press of Kansas, 1974). Crucial to understanding the genesis of modern American medical education is Abraham Flexner's report, *Medical Education in the United States and Canada* (New York: Carnegie Foundation for the Advancement of Teaching, 1910). Additional information on the Medical Center can be found in Margaret Landis's *The Winding Valley and the Craggy Hillside: A History of the City of Rosedale, Kansas* (Kansas City, Kansas: n.p., 1976). The pictorial history of the Lawrence campus is covered in Virginia Adams et al., comp., *On the Hill: A Photographic History of the University of Kansas* (Lawrence: University Press of Kansas, 1983). An interesting history of health care in the Kansas City area can be found in *From Shamans to Specialists: A History of Medicine and Health Care in Jackson County, Missouri,* by Barbara M. Gorman, Richard D. McKenzie, and Theodore A. Wilson (Kansas City, Missouri: Jackson County Medical Society, 1981). For a sociological perspective on medical students, see Howard S. Becker et al., *Boys in White: Student Culture in Medical School* (Chicago: University of Chicago Press, 1961).

Many of the letters, speeches, manuscripts, correspondence, and printed items quoted throughout this book can be found in the University of Kansas Medical Center Archives or the Clendening History of Medicine Library. The University of Kansas Archives in Lawrence, Kansas, and the Kansas State Historical Society in Topeka also contain materials relevant to the Medical Center's history. Additional information on key figures in the Medical Center's history and administration is available through the oral history collection housed in the Medical Center's archives.

Photographic Credits

All photographs are from the University of Kansas Medical Center Archives except those listed below, which are used courtesy of the following individuals and organizations.

AV Services, KUMC: bottom left p. 211, bottom right p. 211, top p. 213

Clendening History of Medicine Library: top p. 9, middle p. 9, top p. 10, top p. 11, bottom p. 11, p. 16, p. 29, top p. 43, bottom p. 43, bottom p. 100

Facilities Operations, KUMC: bottom left p. 166

Shari Hartbauer, University Relations, KUMC: p. 196, bottom p. 199, top p. 201, bottom p. 201, top p. 204

Larry Howell, Design and Illustration, KUMC: p. 44

Jackson County Historical Society: p. 13, all of top row and left and middle of middle row p. 69, bottom left and right p. 70

Kansas Collection, University of

Kansas Libraries: bottom left p. 148

KUMC Archives, Dorothy Early Collection: top p. 79, middle p. 79

KUMC Archives, Hostetter Collection: top p. 61, p. 62, right p. 67, p. 80, p. 81, top p. 82, middle p. 82, bottom p. 82, top p. 83, bottom left p. 83, top p. 86, bottom p. 89, left p. 90, right p. 90, top p. 93

Noel Klein, AV Services, KUMC: bottom p. 197

Channon H. Krupsky: top p. 192

Lightfoot Photography: p. 216

Dale Monaghen, AV Services, KUMC: top left p. 209

Elissa Monroe, AV Services, KUMC: p. viii, middle p. 210

John Tyler Motsinger, KUMC Archives: p. 191, p. 215

Rick Robinson: bottom p. 192

Stephan L. Spector, AV Services,

KUMC: top p. 109, p. 170, p. 179, top p. 189, bottom p. 189, p. 190, top p. 193, top p. 195, top p. 197, bottom p. 198, p. 200, p. 202, p. 203, bottom p. 204, p. 205, top p. 206, bottom p. 206, left p. 207, right p. 207, top p. 208, bottom p. 208, top right p. 209, bottom p. 209, top p. 210, bottom p. 210, top p. 211, p. 212, bottom p. 213, top p. 214, bottom p. 214

University Archives, Spencer Research Library: p. 6, p. 7, top p. 8, bottom p. 33, bottom p. 34, bottom p. 37, top p. 41, bottom p. 55, bottom p. 61, p. 84, bottom p. 86, top p. 92, top p. 98, bottom p. 124, top p. 125, top p. 166, bottom p. 174, bottom p. 176, top p. 177, bottom p. 180, p. 181, top p. 182, top p. 183, bottom p. 183, top p. 184, bottom p. 184, p. 185, top p. 186, bottom p. 186, top p. 187, bottom p. 187, p. 188, top p. 194

University of Kansas School of Medicine–Wichita: top p. 163, bottom p. 163, bottom p. 194

Wyandotte County Historical Society and Museum: bottom p. 10, p. 15, top p. 68

Index